Dear Betsy -

I can't believe it's been four years since you and I taped "Y"s on your backs when you ran out to the lagoon - and four years since our novice boat won nationals (twice!). Although you're too modest to agree, I think you've been a huge factor in keeping us 5 seniors together and "on an even keel," to use crew terminology. Your quiet determination, fun-loving spirit, and unending patience have made you a role model for us all. A natural leader and sympathetic listener, you've helped us weather Nat attacks, injuries, and seat racing traumas. I know that you've inspired me and taught me a lot.

All these qualities make you a great friend outside of crew as well - I'll be sad to graduate and say goodbye. I've had so much fun rowing with you and hanging out with you, Jube. We have to stay in touch so we can reminisce and make fun of one another's laughs. You're great, Bets.

Thanks for four terrific years.

Love,
Stephanie
May, 1991

THE
ATHLETE WITHIN

A Personal Guide to Total Fitness

THE
ATHLETE WITHIN

A Personal Guide to Total Fitness

Harvey B. Simon, M.D.
Steven R. Levisohn, M.D.

Illustrations by Sheila Boss-Concannon

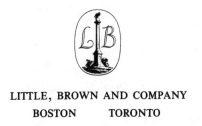

LITTLE, BROWN AND COMPANY
BOSTON   TORONTO

Before embarking on any strenuous exercise program, including the activities described in this book, everyone, particularly anyone with a heart, blood pressure, or back problem, should be evaluated by a physician.

FIRST EDITION

Library of Congress Cataloging-in-Publication Data
Simon, Harvey B. (Harvey Bruce), 1942–
    The athlete within.

    Bibliography: p.
    Includes index.
    1. Physical fitness. I. Levisohn, Steven R.
II. Title.
GV481.S55   1987   613.7′1   86-33766
ISBN 0-316-52250-3

BP

Designed by Jeanne Abboud

*Published simultaneously in Canada
by Little, Brown & Company (Canada) Limited*

PRINTED IN THE UNITED STATES OF AMERICA

For our families

*Those who think they have not
time for bodily exercise
will sooner or later have
to find time for illness.*

— EDWARD STANLEY, EARL OF DERBY, 1873

*I have two fine doctors —
my right leg, and my left.*

— RUNNER'S ADAGE

Contents

Introduction

Why *another* fitness book?

Fred Epstein may be able to tell you the answer. Mr. Epstein is not a household name; he has never appeared on TV, endorsed a running shoe, or signed a multiyear sports contract. Yet he is an athlete just the same. Unfortunately, Fred did not discover the athlete within until *after* his heart attack.

In 1979, Fred was a forty-eight-year-old, highly successful advertising executive who smoked two packs a day, weighed 268 pounds, had a 48-inch waistline, and exercised only by going to the refrigerator for food or drink. His success was built on stress, but he didn't know it until January 1980, when he developed severe chest pain. He was admitted to the Massachusetts General Hospital, where a heart attack was diagnosed. Despite the best medical treatment available, Fred continued to have chest pain, so he underwent urgent heart surgery to bypass a blocked artery. His recovery was excellent, and he left the hospital ten days later, entirely free of pain.

Fred Epstein's story is a common one, and his progress up to this point followed the path of traditional American medicine — excellent treatment of a life-threatening disease. What happened next is not so conventional: Fred Epstein became an athlete. He did not do it on his own — anyone with heart disease needs careful evaluation and supervision in order to learn how to exercise safely. Fred was referred to Harvard's Cardiovascular Health Center, where he underwent a comprehensive evaluation. A careful, graded exercise program helped Fred greatly — at first, he could barely walk one-half mile without fatigue, but he gradually built up to eight miles of steady jogging with ease. But exercise was not the whole story: Fred underwent detailed nutritional counseling, which enabled him to assume a healthful diet, lose 116 pounds and 16 inches from his waistline, and lower his blood cholesterol level. He also learned to recognize and control stress in his life, and got the help he needed to stop smoking. Fred's running has made him an athlete — but the comprehensive program of nutrition and stress control in addition to exercise is what has made him fit. And, we trust, healthy and happy.

Mr. Epstein does not need this book — he has had the benefit of an intensive cardiac rehabilitation program. But if his story represents a triumph of medical care in America, it also represents a tragic failure: in large part, his heart attack signifies a failure of preventive medicine. Our profession has made enormous strides in *treating* disease but has a long way to go in devising strategies to *prevent* illness. Nor is medicine alone in this failure — our society as a whole has repeatedly overlooked some surprisingly simple aspects of disease prevention.

Good health and longevity involve many factors. Some of these factors are beyond our control; heredity is the most prominent example of an uncontrollable factor, since each of us has a genetic destiny that may predispose us to certain diseases or toward longevity. Many other important influences on our health require societal action if they are to be controlled. Pollution and other environmental hazards, sanitation, access to medical care, availability of adequate nutrition, and the risk of war can all be crucially important to health, but require collective rather than individual action in order for improvements to occur. However, in addition to these genetic and societal considerations, there are many important health factors that *are* under individual control. Collectively, these factors can be grouped together as health habits or, more appropriately, as life-style. The way in which you choose to live can, in fact, directly influence your health and your longevity.

Life-style modification is very important for your health. Nine of the ten leading causes of premature death in the United States can be significantly affected by behavior and life-style. In fact, if we include high blood pressure as a risk factor that can be modified by behavioral changes (diet, exercise, stress control, and compliance with medication), *all* of the leading causes of death can be related to life-style. The figures are awesome. In 1982, over 985,000 Americans died of heart attacks or strokes — accounting for nearly half of all the deaths in the country, at a cost of ninety billion dollars in medical care and lost productivity. By age sixty, one of five American men and one of seventeen American women have had a heart attack. Three hundred fifty thousand people die in the United States each year from disease directly related to smoking. Another two hundred thousand will die needlessly of problems related to alcohol abuse, and one hundred thousand die in accidents, of which 50 percent occur on our roads and highways (including many which are alcohol-related).

Modern medicine has made enormous progress in treating disease, yet the overall impact on longevity is a bit disappointing. For example, the life expectancy of an American man who was forty-five years old in 1977 was only five years greater than the life expectancy of a man who was forty-five in 1900. So although we spend enormous sums of money on medical care, amounting to at least one thousand dollars per person per year, our overall impact on longevity has been surprisingly slight. In contrast, government studies show that life-style modification could increase the life expectancy of an average forty-five-year-old male by over eleven years. The message is obvious: The *way* you live accounts in large part for how *long* you live and how *well* you live.

We have written this book to help you achieve a healthful life-style. At the Massachusetts General Hos-pital, we have a comprehensive program to treat patients like Fred Epstein who have heart disease. But we can reach only a few people in this way. For every Fred Epstein who has heart disease, there are hundreds of people who are starting out healthy, and this book is for them.

The time to begin your fitness program is *now*. These facts and figures about heart attacks and early death can be depressing, but you can fight back. In this book we'll show you how to determine your starting point, plan an individualized fitness program, and implement that program safely, effectively, and enjoyably. We cannot promise you an Olympic medal — our goal is not to train competitive athletes, but to help ordinary people achieve optimal health through fitness. And in this we can promise success. If you follow our plan for building your own fitness program, you will achieve your goals and enjoy yourself in the process.

Our goal is fitness in its broadest sense. We define fitness as the ability of the organism to withstand stress. Many kinds of stress can affect you: the stress of athletic competition, the stress of social and career pressures, the stress of illness, and even the stress of the aging process itself.

Fitness can help you withstand all of those stresses. But fitness does not come easily. The first challenge is to understand yourself: where you are starting from, your strengths and weaknesses, and your personal goals. Part I of this book defines the four facets of fitness and explains the scientific basis of each. You will also find a series of self-assessment tests, which will enable you to determine your own fitness level.

Unfortunately, understanding fitness will not itself make you fit. Part II will help you translate theory into practice. Because each of us has a unique set of potentials and problems, the key to our plan is individualization — each of you will be able to construct your own personal program based on your starting point, your interests and abilities, and your goals. Not all of us can run a 6-minute mile or press 200 pounds — any plan that tried to force each of us into an arbitrary mold would be doomed to failure, but this program, which allows you to tailor a plan to fit your own needs, is bound to succeed.

Nutrition and stress control are essential to total fitness, which is why we've devoted a full chapter to each. But exercise is the key to our program; we believe that the human body has a minimum daily requirement (MDR) for exercise just as it has an MDR for nutrients and a need for mental relaxation. In Part II, you'll learn how to exercise correctly. The core of this program is a progressive exercise training regimen we call FAS(S): Flexibility, Aerobics, Strength, and Speed (which is optional). You'll construct a balanced program for musculoskeletal fitness, which includes exercises for flexibility, strength, and endurance. You'll also learn how to use aerobic exercise as the central component of your program. Aerobic exercise is the unifying element, giving you the stamina to enjoy an active lifestyle and the cardiovascular conditioning to improve your health. You'll learn how to coordinate all this with a healthful life-style including preventive medicine, but we'll build your total package around exercise. Exercise is what makes fitness fun.

You could stop reading this book at the end of Part II and still have a program that will keep you fit. But exercise for fitness quickly leads to exercise for sports. Part III will show you how to apply the principals of fitness to a wide variety of sports. Our stress will be on *lifesports* — sports that you can do at your own pace on your own terms, both today and tomorrow, for a lifetime of fitness. We'll also give you an overview of competitive and team sports; you'll learn how to get into shape for each, and how each sport can in turn help keep you in shape.

We hope to show you that you can all become athletes. Each of you has surprising potentials; most of you will never be sports stars, but all of you can greatly extend your horizons through careful planning and diligent training. If you exercise regularly and develop your potentials to their fullest, you will be a true athlete, even if you never win a race or compete on center court. We have made the transition to fitness ourselves and we have helped many friends, colleagues, and patients to do the same. But we are doctors, not coaches, and we are not trying to recruit you for our favorite sport. Instead, we will present a comprehensive, balanced program. We will explain the pros *and* cons of *many* forms of exercise and sports, so that you can find the program that's best for you. Exercise can also have excesses and even perils; we'll explain these too, so that you can maximize your benefits and minimize your risks.

Part IV of this book looks further into exercise-related health problems. Here, too, our goal is balance and objectivity: we are not trying to gloss over the potential complications of an active life-style but to explain them in detail so that you can learn how to recognize, manage, and above all prevent these potential difficulties. But we can't turn you into doctors any more than we can turn you into professional athletes — in Part IV we'll also tell you when and how to get professional help for your sports medicine needs.

This book is for healthy adults who are out of shape but want to reform. It is also for weekend athletes who want to know if they are doing enough for their health. This book should help the amateur athlete who wants to learn about nutrition and balanced training for improved performance and health. And although we don't presume to help advanced athletes with their training, we may be able to help competitive performers avoid injuries and build their sport into a comprehensive fitness program.

Clearly we are not the first people to recognize the central role of fitness in health. There are many excellent books by nutritionists, psychologists, and doctors on nutrition and stress management. There are also many fine books by physicians that tell you how to prevent or "live with" heart disease and high blood pressure. And it goes without saying that there are lots of good books by athletes and coaches, which can instruct you about sports and exercise ranging from walking to Nautilus. Perhaps as a result of this enthusiasm, there has also been a proliferation of sports medicine books, which tell you how to treat your athletic injuries. We have an ambitious goal: to unify all of these diverse elements into a single fitness program that will take you all the way from the scientific basis of fitness to the proper use of ice and ace bandages. But our goals go beyond completeness alone — we are striving for balance and for flexibility so that each reader can construct an individually tailored program with success built right in. If you achieve your goals, we'll achieve ours — and this will be the last fitness book you'll ever need to buy.

Harvey B. Simon, M.D.
Steven R. Levisohn, M.D.
Boston, February 1987

Acknowledgments

Many people have been instrumental in making this book possible. We are grateful to numerous colleagues in Boston and around the country for all they have taught us about fitness and sports medicine. Our patients, too, have been invaluable sources of encouragement; whether cardiac patients or athletes, they have convinced us to make the effort required to get our fitness program into print. Even with all this encouragement, our task would have been impossible without the editorial skills of Bill Phillips and Laura Fillmore at Little, Brown, and without the patient efforts of Judy Feiner, who prepared the manuscript.

Above all, we thank our families for their encouragement, help, and forbearance. Medical practice produces great demands on the families of physicians, and our families have been unfailingly supportive in all of our efforts.

THE
ATHLETE WITHIN

A Personal Guide to Total Fitness

I

THE FOUR FACETS OF FITNESS

Understanding the Medical Basis
for Your Fitness Program

1

Cardiovascular and Pulmonary Fitness

When people think of fitness, they think first of strong muscles. Imagine, then, a single muscle strong enough to lift a seventy-pound weight a distance of one foot. Impressive, but hardly of Olympic caliber. But imagine that muscle lifting the seventy-pound weight once a minute, every minute of every day of your life. A world-class muscle indeed: it's your heart.

Your heart is strong enough to perform work equivalent to lifting seventy pounds per minute. And with appropriate training, your heart, like any of your muscles, can be made even stronger. But your heart is also vulnerable to diseases that can sap that strength; heart attacks occur in America at the rate of two per minute. Fortunately, you can help protect yourself from this epidemic of heart disease at the same time that you increase your heart's strength and efficiency.

THE NORMAL HEART AND CIRCULATION

All athletes spend a great deal of time worrying and fussing about their muscles. Few of us, however, give even a moment's thought to the most important muscle of all, the heart. Because your heart's functions are automatic, they really don't require any thought on a day-to-day basis. A little thought about your life-style, however, will help keep your heart healthy over the years. And a little thought will also remind us what an extraordinary muscle the heart is. Although your heart is no bigger than your clenched fist, it is responsible for pumping over two thousand gallons of blood through some sixty thousand miles of blood vessels *each day*. To do this, your heart beats over one hundred thousand times per day each and every day of your life.

The heart is separated into four pumping chambers; two of these chambers (the right atrium and the left atrium) are relatively weak pumps but are very important to collect blood from outside the heart. The other two chambers, the right ventrical and the left ventricle, are the strong pumps that distribute blood to the rest of the body (see Figure 1–1).

Blood from all the body's tissues is collected into veins that finally empty into the heart. The right atrium collects the blood and pumps it into the right ventrical. From there the blood is pumped into the lungs. In the lungs the blood passes through tiny vessels called capillaries. The walls of capillaries are so thin that gases and nutrients can pass back and forth through the capillary walls. Carbon dioxide (CO_2), one of the waste products of tissue metabolism, passes from the blood into the lungs and is then exhaled into the air. At the same time, oxygen (O_2), which is required to nourish all tissues, enters the blood from the lungs and binds to the hemoglobin of the red blood cells so it can be carried to all the body's tissues.

The oxygen-rich blood now enters the second set of veins — called pulmonary veins — which empty into the heart. What happens next on the left side of the heart parallels exactly the events on the right side of the heart. Blood from the lungs collects in the left atrium

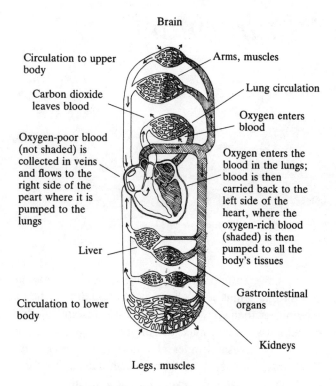

Brain

Circulation to upper body

Arms, muscles

Carbon dioxide leaves blood

Lung circulation

Oxygen enters blood

Oxygen-poor blood (not shaded) is collected in veins and flows to the right side of the peart where it is pumped to the lungs

Oxygen enters the blood in the lungs; blood is then carried back to the left side of the heart, where the oxygen-rich blood (shaded) is then pumped to all the body's tissues

Liver

Circulation to lower body

Gastrointestinal organs

Kidneys

Legs, muscles

FIGURE 1–1: *The Normal Heart and Circulation*

and is pumped into the left ventrical. The left ventrical is the strongest pump of all, sending blood to all of the tissues that are outside of the lungs. En route to the body's tissues, the blood goes from the left ventrical to the body's largest artery, the aorta. The arteries divide into successively smaller vessels, like the branches of a tree. Finally, the blood is once again in thin-walled capillaries so that oxygen and nutrients can enter the tissues and waste products can be carried away to the lungs, the liver, and the kidneys for elimination.

Just about now you are probably telling yourself that you wanted to read a book about sports and fitness, not a biology text. Granted this anatomy and physiology seem a long way from the gym, but just as athletes have to go through training camp before they begin the season, so too should we lay careful foundations for our understanding of fitness. And these considerations can also help you understand the causes and prevention of heart disease.

As a muscle, the heart needs its own arteries and capillaries to provide oxygen and nutrients. The job of

carrying oxygen to the heart falls to the right and left coronary arteries, which branch off from the aorta just beyond the left ventrical of the heart itself. The coronary arteries are small vessels with very big jobs. If the flow of blood to the heart is interrupted, illness or death will result. It's easy to see why a small blockage in the coronary arteries can have such disastrous consequences. Indeed, coronary artery disease is the number-one killer in the United States, being responsible for angina, heart attacks, congestive heart failure, and sudden death due to disorders of the heart's pumping rhythm.

Obviously, in pumping blood to the whole body the heart generates substantial pressure. The exact magnitude of this pressure is measured quite accurately each time your blood pressure is checked. The first or higher number you are given is the "systolic" blood pressure and the second, lower, number is the "diastolic" blood pressure. The systolic blood pressure measures the pressure in your arteries while the heart is pumping blood into the aorta, while the diastolic pressure reflects the lower pressure present when the heart is refilling with blood between beats. In healthy people, there is no single value of blood pressure that is considered normal, but a broad range of readings that are within normal limits; pressures that are consistently above 150 systolic and 90 diastolic (written as 150/90) are considered abnormally high. High blood pressure (hypertension) means extra work for your heart and arteries; hypertension rivals coronary artery disease as a crucial health problem in the United States today.

The heart does not work alone but is intimately linked to the lungs and blood vessels. Your lungs are a bellows, which bring oxygen to the blood and remove carbon dioxide from the blood. Your blood vessels are a vast network of canals, which supply channels for the distribution of oxygen to your tissues and for the removal of waste products from your tissues. Among these tissues, of course, are the skeletal muscles, which work so hard when you exercise. So each sprint down the track or swing of the racket requires enormously complex interaction among your heart, your lungs, your blood vessels, and your muscles.

HOW YOUR HEART RESPONDS TO EXERCISE

Strenuous exercise places tremendous demands on your body. The metabolic demands of your muscles are fifty times greater when they are exercising then when they are at rest, and the oxygen requirements of your entire body increase more than ten times as the result of vigorous exercise. Obviously your heart, lungs, and circulation have to work a lot harder to supply the oxygen needed to power exercise.

The way your heart responds depends on the *intensity* and *duration* of exercise; the faster and longer you run, the harder your heart will have to work. The *type* of exercise is also extremely important in determining the way your circulation responds (see Figure 1–2). Static exercise, such as pushing against a wall or lifting a heavy weight, causes your blood vessels to constrict or narrow. When you perform static exercise, your muscles contract in a way that increases the pressure in the muscle tissues, and this increased tension in turn causes your blood vessels to constrict. As a result, your blood pressure rises substantially, but the volume of blood being pumped by your heart does not increase very much. Dynamic exercise, such as running or swimming, causes your blood vessels to dilate or widen. This is because your muscles do not increase their tension when they are exercising dynamically; instead, blood vessels dilate to bring more blood to the muscles. As a result, your blood pressure will increase only slightly, but the volume of blood pumped by your heart increases dramatically.

Both types of exercise can be very useful to your muscles. True isometrics, such as pushing against a fixed resistance, is the purest form of static exercise. But lifting heavy weights is also a high-resistance form of exercise that resembles static or isometric exercises, in terms of its effect both on your circulation and on your muscles. Chapter 2 explains how high-resistance exercise builds muscular strength and power and how dynamic (or low-resistance) exercise builds muscle endurance. Although athletes need both types of exercise to improve performance, our hearts benefit much more from dynamic or high-volume work. Dynamic exercise has an extraordinary ability to improve the endurance of the heart and the efficiency of the circulation. High-resistance contributes much less to these adap-

FIGURE 1–2: COMPARISON OF TYPES OF EXERCISE

	Dynamic or Isotonic Exercise	Static or Isometric Exercise
Examples	Running, swimming, rowing, biking	Pushing against fixed resistance (pure isometrics) Weight lifting and shoveling snow (relatively isometric)
Effect on muscles	Muscle fibers contract and shorten, but muscle tension remains constant	Muscle fibers contract but instead of shortening, muscle tension increases
Effect on blood vessels	Vessels widen	Vessels narrow
Effect on blood pressure	Slight increase	Marked increase
Effect on heart	Heart rate increases greatly More blood pumped with each beat	Heart rate increases slightly No change in amount pumped with each beat
Effect on circulation	Great increase in volume of blood pumped by heart	Great increase in pressure in blood vessels

tations. In fact, if you have heart disease or hypertension, the high pressures generated during static work tend to be harmful. The heart attack suffered while shoveling snow is the classic example. We don't mean to frighten you away from weight lifting. On the contrary, we've already said that this type of exercise is important for many athletes. But if you are in the older age groups or if you have any circulatory disorders, you should approach high-resistance exercise with special precautions and supervision.

Let's concentrate on how your body responds to dynamic exercise. As you sit in your chair reading these words, your heart is pumping approximately five quarts of blood through your body each minute. Although we're happy that you're reading our book, our ultimate goal is to have you close the book, stand up, and run around. When you do so, your heart will be pumping much harder. Your heart rate will increase by as much as 300 percent, and the volume of blood it pumps will increase from five quarts per minute to twenty quarts per minute or more.

Not only is the amount of blood pumped increased, but the distribution of the blood is altered dramatically. When you exercise, all of this extra blood flow is directed toward the tissues that need it most: your exercising muscles. Because your heart is an exercising muscle, it gets its share of increased blood flow as well, but the circulation to other organs actually decreases. Less blood is pumped to your digestive tract, your skin, your kidneys, and to various other organs that are not involved in the work of exercise. Obviously, this redistribution allows maximum delivery of oxygen to your working muscles, but it also means less oxygen elsewhere. Like other circulatory responses to exercise, this redistribution of blood is automatic and beyond your control. However, you can help things along in at least one important respect. Be sure not to eat heavy meals before you exercise. Since your digestive tract actually gets significantly less blood during exercise, digestion will be impaired and a heavy meal can lead to sluggishness, cramps, and abdominal discomfort.

The acute circulatory responses to exercise are impressive, but the long-term adaptations enjoyed by athletes are even more extraordinary. We'll give you plenty of facts and figures to show how your heart and circulation improve with regular exercise training. For now, an actual case history will show you what we mean.

Our subject grew up in New York City and never played anything more strenuous than the radio during his entire childhood. "Physical Education" in college amounted to nothing more than six horrible months of mandatory remedial posture. Needless to say, subsequent professional training and a high-stress job did not provide any additional impetus to get into shape. By age thirty-five the subject was rotund, inert, and unfortunately endowed with a high blood cholesterol level and a marginally high blood pressure reading.

This story is all too common in twentieth-century industrialized America. Not even the most doting mother could mistake our subject for an athlete. However, on his thirty-fifth birthday the pleadings of his athletic wife finally induced him to engage in voluntary exercise for the first time in years. Not surprisingly, slow jogging for only four-tenths of a mile resulted in total collapse. The subject spent the afternoon in a hammock, but although he was stiff and sore the next day, he went out and did it again. His first days and weeks were much more work than fun, but ever so gradually distances and speed increased and effort was rewarded by enjoyment. Over a year, repeated exercise training resulted in a thirty-pound weight loss, a waistline decrease of four inches, a substantial decrease in blood pressure, and a dramatic lowering of blood cholesterol. But the most striking change of all was the increase in his physical work capacity. Whereas this subject could barely jog for four-tenths of a mile at age thirty-five, at age thirty-nine he was able to complete a fifty-mile race with comfort.

This hundredfold increase in work capacity did not occur instantly and is not the story of Clark Kent. The subject is surely not a superman, and the transition took months and years of patient training rather than a trip to a telephone booth. This is not the story of a famous athlete, for the subject is hardly that. Nor is it the case history of a patient or friend, though we have seen many patients and companions undergo similar transformation. In fact, this little tale is the true story of one of the authors of this book (HBS).

Hopefully this story will help inspire you to attain fitness. But first, let's return to our discussion of the heart, lungs, and circulation so that we can learn how these organs are able to change so dramatically in response to regular exercise training.

We've already told you that the heart of a healthy untrained person beats about seventy times per minute at rest, and pumps about five quarts of blood during each minute. During maximal exercise that same heart may beat up to two hundred times per minute and can pump up to twenty quarts of blood each minute. The endurance athlete is quite different. At rest his heart also pumps five quarts of blood per minute but requires many fewer beats to do so (see Figure 1–3). Many trained athletes have heart rates of fifty beats per minute or even less; champion cross-country skiers and marathon runners often have resting heart rates in the high thirties or low forties. When these extraordinary athletes exercise, their heart rates also rise, but the athlete's heart rate will be much lower than the "normal" heart rate at the same submaximal work load. The athlete's heart rate is slower because his heart is more efficient; hence his heart will save thirty-six thousand beats per day, beating thirteen million times less often each year than the heart of a sedentary person.

The athlete's heart is able to pump much more blood each minute than is the heart of the sedentary individual. Whereas an untrained heart may pump twenty quarts of blood each minute during maximal exercise, an athlete can pump thirty quarts or more per minute. This means that much more work can be done. More oxygen can be delivered to muscles, and these muscles can carry the athlete much faster. In addition, the athlete is capable of sustaining this peak for much longer, so he can run much farther.

What enables the athlete's heart to perform in this extraordinary fashion? Actually there are two factors at work, one in the heart itself and one in the blood vessels and muscles. The cardiac effects of exercise training involve an actual increase in the strength and thickness of the muscular walls of the heart's main pumping chamber, the left ventrical. In experimental animals who have been exercise trained, an increased number of capillaries (small blood vessels) supply oxygen to the heart muscle, and the heart muscle of these animals also has an increased content of enzymes. In man, our measurements are much less direct, but with new techniques we can measure the strength of contraction of the human heart and the volume of blood pumped with each contraction. Exercise training does, in fact, increase the amount of blood pumped with each contraction, and the actual strength and efficiency of each heartbeat are also improved.

Another circulatory benefit of exercise training is on the blood pressure. People who play sports regularly have 35 percent less hypertension than do sedentary people. In fact, endurance exercise can be used along with weight reduction, stress control, and dietary salt restriction as the first line of treatment for hypertension.

While these changes in the cardiovascular system of trained athletes are very important, they do not tell the whole story. Important contributions are also made by the circulation and by the muscles. Training increases the number of capillaries in muscles, allowing the heart to pump more blood to where it's needed during exercise. In addition, training increases the activity of certain enzymes in the muscles themselves, so that they can extract and utilize oxygen more efficiently. All in all, trained muscles get more blood, extract more oxygen from that blood, and use that oxygen more efficiently to burn glycogen (sugar) and generate energy.

Both the cardiac and the muscular adaptations to exercise training are important. For people with normal hearts, they seem to contribute about equally. How-

FIGURE 1–3: THE ATHLETE'S HEART

		Sedentary person	Well-conditioned athlete
At rest	Heart rate	70	50
	Amount of blood pumped by heart	5 quarts	5 quarts
During moderate dynamic exercise	Heart rate	150	100
	Amount of blood pumped by heart	15 quarts	15 quarts
All-out effort	Heart rate	200	200
	Amount of blood pumped by heart	20 quarts	30 quarts

ever, for people who have heart disease, the muscular effects are more important, because their hearts cannot improve as much as an entirely healthy heart can.

Muscle improvement as a result of exercise is highly specific for the muscles that are trained, but the heart's improvement will occur with any type of effective dynamic or aerobic training. If you have a healthy heart, its function will improve whether you swim, run, play tennis, or row — as long as you exercise often enough, long enough, and hard enough. However, if your training is confined exclusively to running, your leg muscles will improve but your arm muscles will not. When a long-distance runner switches to swimming, he has to go through a period of retraining to get a new set of muscles into shape. Chapter 2 explains that when you train for sports and competition you have to train specifically all the muscles you will be using in that sport. But if you are training for your heart and your health, any combination of activities will do as long as they are done right.

EXERCISE AND YOUR LUNGS

When our patient Nancy G. decided to get into shape, her first goal was to improve her "wind." As she trained over the weeks and months, her exercise capacity increased dramatically. She now jogs at least twenty miles a week, and she's happy with her svelte figure and her ten-kilometer (6.2 miles) racing time. Yet every time she starts to run she still gets "winded" for the first two or three minutes — even though she is breathing easily at the end of an eight- or nine-mile run. And although she is in very good shape, she is always forced to gasp for air if she sprints all out.

Nancy's experience is very typical; it is common knowledge that training improves your "wind" and that many athletes feel short of breath early in a race until they get their "second wind." It may surprise you to learn that neither the improvement in your "wind" with training nor the breathlessness a competitor feels during a sprint has anything to do with the lungs themselves.

The job of your lungs is to exchange gases. When you breathe in, oxygen-rich air enters the trachea or windpipe and then travels through successively smaller branches of the breathing tubes until it reaches millions of tiny air sacs, or aveoli. Oxygen travels from the inspired air across the filmy membranes of the air sacs into the very fine blood vessels or capillaries that sur-round the air sacs. The oxygen is then carried in your blood to the organs and tissues of your body. But at the same time your tissues are producing waste products, including carbon dioxide. Carbon dioxide travels from the capillaries into the air sacs and is expelled from your body every time you exhale. The lungs themselves are actually quite passive during this process. The energy for pumping blood is, of course, provided by the heart, and the bellow apparatus that exchanges the air is powered by the muscles of your chest cage and your diaphragm.

If you have healthy lungs you have a tremendous capacity to diffuse oxygen into your body and carbon dioxide out of your system. This capacity, in fact, greatly exceeds the pumping capacity of your heart, the delivery capacity of your blood vessels, and the oxygen uptake capacity of your muscles. So when you get into shape you improve your heart, the delivery capacity of your blood vessels, and the oxygen uptake capacity of your muscles to the point where they can make fuller use of the extra capabilities of your lungs. Your lungs themselves don't actually improve with exercise training — they don't have to because they already have such great capacities. Your "wind" and maximum oxygen uptake do improve, but this improvement is caused by beneficial changes in the pumping of the heart and the ability of your muscles to use oxygen rather than any changes in your lungs. Kelly Evernden is a good example of the tremendous capacity of healthy lungs. This twenty-four-year-old All-American tennis star reached the round of 16 in the 1985 U.S. Open tennis championship — playing with only one lung. Kelly lost one lung in a childhood accident, but his remaining lung has more than enough capacity for him to be a top athlete.

Before we go any further, one qualification is in order. If you smoke, your lung capacity is diminished. So smokers do, in fact, have to get their lungs into shape in order to exercise to full capacity; you must stop smoking to really get fit (and stay healthy). A variety of other lung diseases can also impair lung capacity, either temporarily or permanently. People with chronic lung disease such as emphysema may have diminished breathing capacities, which limit their exercise tolerance. Exercise training may have some benefit for these people by strengthening respiratory muscles. But the lungs do not undergo adaptive changes with exercise *per se*, so exercise training has a much smaller role in rehabilitation of patients with lung disease than it does in heart disease.

Even nonsmoking superstars such as Joan Benoit or Carl Lewis experience a feeling of breathlessness at some time during exercise, but this is very different from the smoker or emphysema patient who gets "winded." One type of shortness of breath is always present at the start of exercise. This is the normal breathlessness associated with warming up. As soon as you start exercising, your muscles demand increased oxygen, but it takes a while for your heart to gear up to pump that oxygen. Your lungs are ready to go, but your heart takes several minutes to rev up; even though your lungs aren't to blame, the oxygen debt is interpreted by your body as breathlessness.

This warm-up phenomenon lasts only a few minutes. At the end of three to five minutes you should be over this early phase of breathlessness. There are several important lessons here. The first is to warm up before you start strenuous exercise (see Chapter 7). It is very important to give your heart a chance to get started gradually. It can be every bit as damaging to start running at full speed a it is to try to start your car in fourth gear: needless to say, the consequences of stalling are much greater when it comes to your heart! And when you start exercising, build up the intensity gradually to minimize the breathlessness of the warm-up period. Even with these precautions, you'll still experience some shortness of breath when you begin exercising. Many people make the error of throwing in the towel at this point. Don't give up too soon. Remember that this early breathlessness is perfectly normal, and that if you keep going at a modest level you will soon become comfortable once again. You'll get your "second wind."

Once you pass through this warm-up period, you should be able to exercise at moderately high intensity without feeling winded. During this phase of exercise your breathing rate remains constant, as does your heart rate. Your lungs are able to take up enough oxygen and your heart is able to pump it to your exercising muscles.

If you increase the intensity of your effort by sprinting, running up a hill, or charging the net, you will once again feel short of breath. This is a very different type of breathlessness, but here, too, your lungs are really not at fault. When you exercise at moderate intensity, your lungs and circulation are able to provide your muscles all the oxygen they need. Muscles that get enough oxygen are able to use oxygen to burn fuel efficiently in what is called aerobic metabolism. But when you exercise at maximum intensity, your muscles need a lot more oxygen. As the intensity of your exercise in-

creases, you will eventually come to a point at which your heart simply cannot deliver enough oxygen to your muscles. This is the infamous "anaerobic threshold." When you cross that threshold, your muscles will have to burn fuel to generate energy without the benefit of oxygen. This so-called anaerobic metabolism is much less efficient, so that your muscles burn up their glycogen stores faster and run out of energy quicker. They also generate more waste products, including lactic acid. Lactic acid produces muscle fatigue and cramps. To get rid of it, the body neutralizes it and generates large amounts of carbon dioxide in the process. It is this extra carbon dioxide that makes you breathe faster to expel the waste gases.

When you cross the anaerobic threshold, your breathing rate increases very steeply and you feel short of breath. You don't have to know anything about metabolism to know when your muscles are anaerobic — you'll be huffing and puffing and your lungs will feel a characteristic discomfort called "air hunger." There are two morals to this story. First, train properly to raise your anaerobic threshold (see Chapter 6). And second, when you are in an event that places a premium on endurance, keep the intensity of your effort just below the anaerobic threshold so that you won't run out of oxygen.

In addition to these normal types of shortness of breath there is a third type of breathlessness. This is the *abnormal* breathlessness associated with various diseases of the heart or lungs. Exercise itself does not produce lung damage, but heavy air pollution or exercise-induced asthma can sometimes limit athletic performance. And exercise can unmask symptoms of underlying illness. If you feel unduly short of breath for the amount of exercise you are doing, listen to your body and back off. If the breathlessness is associated with a pale or gray complexion, coughing up phlegm or blood, fever or chest pain, be sure to consult a physician as soon as possible. Above all, get a checkup before you start exercise training so that you can identify potential problems before they cause breathlessness.

For healthy people, however, lung capacity *per se* does not limit the intensity or duration of exercise. As we have seen, breathlessness during exercise is produced when your muscles demand more oxygen than your heart and circulation can deliver. Oxygen is the driving force that provides the power for aerobic exercise. The best overall determination of fitness is the measurement of oxygen uptake and delivery.

Let's look in a little more detail at oxygen uptake

tests. In the exercise laboratory, physiologists are able to measure the volume (V) of oxygen (O_2) which can be utilized during maximum exercise — the "VO_2 max." VO_2 max is an excellent overall measurement of fitness because it measures simultaneously all the links in the oxygen delivery chain: the ability of the lungs to take up oxygen, the ability of the heart to pump the oxygen-rich blood, the capacity of the circulation to deliver oxygen to exercising muscles, and the ability of the muscles to extract and utilize oxygen. In short, this single measurement, VO_2 max, reflects the integrity of the entire "supply side" of oxygen delivery and utilization.

Enough theory! Why not get on the bike ergometer and taken an exercise test to find our your own VO_2 max? You arrive in the lab, and are ushered into a small room filled with computer equipment, panels, gauges, and the poorest excuse for a bicycle you have ever seen. Hanging on a boom over the bike is complex headgear with a mouthpiece connected to air-collecting bags. Nose clips are used to prevent you from breathing through your nose. Cardiac monitoring leads are attached. You are finally hooked up — only to discover that you can-

not swallow, so your saliva becomes a major preoccupation until the test begins. Then the challenge of the machine takes over. Doubt about your ability to put out a decent effort under these conditions begins to build up along with the sweat and heat from the poorly ventilated surroundings. Nevertheless, after you have warmed up and accommodated to the conditions, you begin to rise to the challenge. The resistance is raised only twenty-five watts every minute, and for the first five or six minutes it's child's play. By six minutes and 150 watts the going is getting tough and your breathing rate begins to pick up. The computer is spitting out numbers and the technician is looking pleased. But the resistance rises again and again — pretty soon you are breathing rapidly as you cross your anaerobic threshold. The pain starts, but the technician is encouraging you to continue. The last twenty seconds seem longer than the first five minutes. Then it's over. You can breathe the real air again as you spit the mouthpiece out and wait for your numbers.

What can you learn from this torment? Let's look at the data generated by Dr. Bengt Saltin in his important 1968 study of five healthy people (see Figure 1–4). As

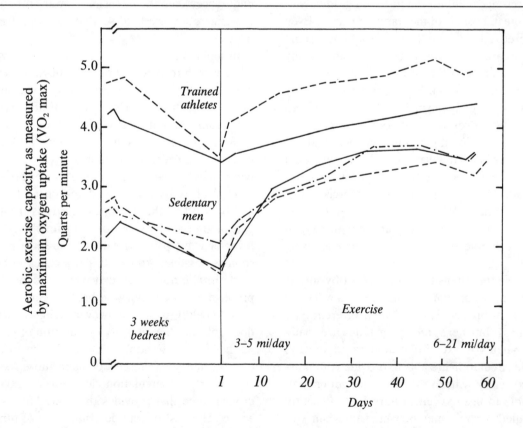

FIGURE 1–4: DR. BENGT SALTIN'S STUDY OF THE EFFECTS OF BEDREST AND ENDURANCE TRAINING ON EXERCISE CAPACITY

you can see, he tested two world-class athletes and three sedentary men at the beginning of a three-month experiment. Not surprisingly, the athletes had much higher values for VO$_2$ max. Next, all five men were put to bed for three weeks. All five volunteers had a substantial decline in VO$_2$ max as a result of inactivity. Finally, the subjects were all placed on an exercise training program — and VO$_2$ max rose steadily before plateauing during the second month of training.

Many factors influence fitness as measured by oxygen uptake. First off, *genetics* is an important factor. Note that in Saltin's experiment the sedentary men never managed to catch up with the world-class athletes. Hereditary factors limit how good you can get, even with diligent training.

Exercise is the second major variable in oxygen uptake, and is the most important because it is under your own control. Regular endurance training will increase your VO$_2$ max, just as it did in Saltin's subjects. In fact, you can expect to increase your VO$_2$ max by 50 to 100 percent with three or four months of training. How much you improve depends on your starting point; if you are really out of shape, you have the greatest potential for improvement. But continued exercise is necessary to maintain fitness. You are dealt a certain hand at birth — but the way you live determines how well you play your cards, how fully you realize your potential in terms of fitness, health, and longevity.

VO$_2$ max also depends on *body weight* and especially lean body mass. Obviously, it takes more energy and more oxygen to move a heavy body than a light one. Therefore, when comparing studies on different people, it's important to correct for body weight. To do this, divide VO$_2$ max by weight — you'll come out with the amount of oxygen in milliliters per kilogram per minute (ml/kg/min). This correction also serves to equalize men and women; because women are generally smaller, they would have artificially lower VO$_2$ max readings without this correction.

The final important variable is *age*. VO$_2$ max rises during childhood but peaks at about age twenty before beginning a gradual but progressive decline. By age sixty the average person will have only two-thirds the VO$_2$ max he or she did at age twenty. But here's the good news — regular endurance exercise greatly attenuates the effects of age. Fit people have much higher VO$_2$ max levels at all ages than do their sedentary peers.

What can VO$_2$ max tests tell us about athletes? If you are really out of shape, you could have values as low as 25 or 30; an average person will have VO$_2$ max read-

ings in the 35 to 40 ml/kg/min range at age thirty. Further training might increase this to 50 or so. But world-class endurance athletes are a breed apart. The numbers generated by champion marathoners are an awesome illustration: Bill Rodgers: 78.5, Alberto Salazar: 76.8, Grete Waitz: 73.5, and Frank Shorter: 71.5. Remember that because these runners were tested in different labs at different times, the absolute numbers are not strictly comparable — but they all bespeak an incomparable level of talent and training. Figure 1–5 shows you representative VO$_2$ max levels of champion athletes from a variety of sports.

But important as it is, VO$_2$ max does not tell the whole story. Two athletes tested at our hospital are a case in point. Greg Meyer is a Boston Marathon winner who has held American roadrunning records at distances ranging from ten to fifteen miles. His VO$_2$ max was an impressive 68. But Dave Hemery, tested when he was the Boston University track coach, scored "only" a 50. Well, you may say, he's just a coach. But he also holds an Olympic gold medal in the 400-meter hurdle. The difference is that Hemery is a sprinter, a "jet fuel burner" who has an extraordinary capacity to generate lots of power and work *an*aerobically — for short

FIGURE 1–5: REPRESENTATIVE MAXIMUM OXYGEN UPTAKE (VO$_2$ MAX) FOR ATHLETES FROM VARIOUS SPORTS

	Women
Sedentary	38
Basketball	45
Speed skating	52
Sprinting	52
Rowing	58
Long-distance swimming	60
Long-distance running	72
Cross-country skiing	74

	Men
Sedentary	43
Baseball	54
Tennis	58
Hockey	60
Long-distance swimming	68
Bicycling	70
Rowing	75
Long-distance running	85
Cross-country skiing	90

periods of time. In contrast, Meyer is typical of endurance athletes. He's a "coal burner" whose VO_2 max is so high that he can generate energy aerobically for incredibly long periods of time.

But even these precise measurements will never predict the outcome of athletic competition. Sports are won on the playing field, not in the exercise laboratory. The VO_2 max is an excellent measure of the "supply side" of exercise. In other words, it measures the ability of the lungs, heart, and circulation to provide energy to working muscles. But VO_2 max does not predict the *output* of work. Energy is obviously critical — but so is the *efficiency* with which that energy is transformed into work. Musculoskeletal structure, style, and technique are major variables in work output (see Chapter 2). And no one has yet figured out a way to measure the other major competitive variables: experience, strategy, self-confidence, and above all the determination to persevere and the will to win (see Chapter 3).

Heredity determines your athletic potential, and training allows you to express that potential by achieving your VO_2 max. But once you are at VO_2 max, is there any point in training harder? For health and fitness, perhaps not. But for competitive sports, yes!

This is the bottom line for you. Once you are trained, stop paying attention to your heart and lungs. They achieved their maximum contribution to your performance long ago. The improvement you will see from now on will come from increases in endurance, strength, quickness, style, efficiency, form, mental attitude, and experience.

EXERCISE, YOUR BLOOD COMPOSITION, AND BODY FATS

Your blood is a combination of plasma and blood cells. The plasma or fluid component contains many complex types of chemicals. In terms of exercise and fitness, however, there are only a few important components. Two of these are so-called electrolytes (body chemicals), namely sodium and potassium. Most of the sodium or salt in your body is stored in the circulating plasma and in the tissue fluids of your body. When you exercise strenuously, you lose salt and water in your sweat. You lose relatively more water than salt, and it is very important to restore that water by drinking before, during, and after exercise. However, the normal American diet contains plenty of salt, so you should *not* have to replace lost sodium. Nor should you have to replace potassium. Only a small amount of this second blood chemical is lost in sweat, because the majority is stored not in the plasma but within the cells. In fact, your muscle cells may actually deliver some of their potassium stores to your blood and circulation when you exercise, so your blood potassium levels may rise for a brief time during and just after exercise (see Chapter 4).

Exercise training changes the volume of plasma itself. If you exercise regularly, you will tend to have an increase in the absolute volume of plasma in your circulation. This produces a slight dilution of your red blood cells, which can be thought of as a mild "thinning" of your blood. Although we don't know for sure, this may be beneficial for your circulation because your blood will be a bit less viscous or sticky and will therefore flow to the tissues more easily.

Does this mild diluting effect impair the ability of your blood to deliver oxygen to your tissues? Not at all. Oxygen is carried from the lungs to your tissues by your red blood cells. Regular exercise training will actually produce a slight increase in the number of red blood cells in your body and in their ability to carry and deliver oxygen.

The red blood cells are one of the three types of cell in your bloodstream. A second type, the white blood cells, are important to fight infection. Exercise can very briefly produce a slight increase in the white blood cell count, but this minor effect is not sustained. In fact, there are no long-term effects of exercise on the white blood cells, and exercise does not really affect your body's capacity to fight infection. As enthusiastic as we are about exercise, we cannot find any scientific evidence to support the claim that active people get fewer colds or other infections.

Exercise may beneficially affect the third type of blood cell in your circulation, your platelets. Platelets are very important in forming the blood clots that stop you from bleeding if you are injured. Exercising does not influence this aspect of platelet function. But like so many other good things, platelets may possibly produce some harm as well as good. Some theories suggest that platelets may have a role in initiating atherosclerosis, or "hardening" of the arteries, and in causing spasm of blood vessels, which may contribute to heart attacks and strokes. Regular exercise seems to modify platelet function in ways that may help fight atherosclerosis. Exercise also increases the body's ability to dissolve small blood clots, which may clog the vessels. This clot-dissolving activity is called "fibrinolysis." We don't know if this increased clot-dissolving ability helps protect fit people from heart disease, but it is another intriguing piece of the puzzle.

The puzzle is much more complete when it comes to the effects of exercise on a critically important component of your blood, your blood fats. This is one of the most highly publicized areas of exercise research, and justly so. It's also a very complex area, involving subtle interactions between diet and heredity as well as exercise. Although blood fats have gotten a bad reputation when it comes to heart disease, the situation is actually quite complex. Fats are obviously essential to life: they provide the building blocks for the membranes that surround all the cells in the body, and they are essential to retain and store vitamins and other important chemicals. But excessive amounts of fats can indeed lead to atherosclerosis, the leading cause of death in the United States today.

Not all fats are equally guilty, however. At the risk of oversimplifying, we will discuss three different types of fats in your blood (Figure 1–6). All of these fats are carried in your circulation as lipoproteins, so called because they bind lipid (fat) with protein. One important group of blood fats are the triglycerides. These are carried in your circulation on very light lipoproteins, the so-called very low density lipoproteins, or VLDL. Although it was once thought that elevated blood triglyceride levels were linked to heart disease, the evidence at present suggests that triglyceride levels are rather weak risk factors. The other two major types of blood fats are the blood cholesterols. For many years it has been known that elevated cholesterol levels are directly linked to increased risk of heart disease and stroke. While this relationship remains unchallenged, it turns out that things are more complex, because there are two major types of cholesterol in your blood. Most of your blood cholesterol is carried on low-density lipoproteins. The "LDL cholesterol" is, in fact, the "bad" cholesterol, which is linked to atherosclerosis: the higher your LDL cholesterol levels, the greater your risk for atherosclerosis.

But in the past few years we have learned that there is a second form of cholesterol in your blood. This type of cholesterol is carried on high-density lipoproteins and is therefore called "HDL cholesterol." In layman's terms it is also known as the "good" cholesterol. And indeed, this nickname is well earned. Many studies ranging from Framingham, Massachusetts, to Norway, Japan, and Honolulu have shown an inverse relationship between HDL levels and heart disease. In other words, *higher* HDL cholesterol levels are linked to *lower* risks or heart disease. For example, people with HDL cholesterol levels *below* 35 have *eight times* more heart disease than people with HDL cholesterol levels above 65. Women and children tend to have relatively high HDL cholesterol levels — and they have less heart disease. Lower HDL levels are found in people who are overweight, smokers, or diabetics — and all have a higher risk of heart disease. It may surprise you to learn that alcohol raises blood HDL cholesterol levels. In fact, *small* amounts of alcohol (about two ounces per day) may help to protect against heart disease.

Doctors are just now beginning to learn how these various blood fats affect blood vessels. Atherosclerosis is a disease in which fatty deposits build up in plaques on blood vessel walls (see Figure 1–7). Many factors can accelerate the buildup of these fatty plaques, including high blood pressure, smoking, and diabetes. An elevated blood level of LDL cholesterol also accelerates the formation of fatty plaques, because much of the

FIGURE 1–6: YOUR BLOOD FATS

	Triglycerides	Low-Density Cholesterol	High-Density Cholesterol
Carrier proteins	Very low-density lipoproteins (VLDL)	Low-density lipoproteins (LDL)	High-density lipoproteins (HDL)
Effect of high blood levels on heart-attack rate	Possible increased risk	Increased risk	Decreased risk

cholesterol in these plaques comes from the blood LDL cholesterol. If these plaques build up to the point where blood flow is impaired (either by the plaques themselves or by clots forming in the greatly narrowed vessels), serious damage can result. If this happens in coronary arteries, the result is a heart attack; if this happens in the blood vessels of the brain, a stroke results. Fortunately, the body has a way of removing cholesterol from the blood vessel walls. That's where high-density lipoprotein comes in. It now appears that the HDL cholesterol represents cholesterol that is being carried *away* from blood vessel walls into the circulation. We have no direct evidence that this mechanism will open up blood vessels once they are already clogged, but it does appear that increased HDL levels will prevent plaques from forming in the first place by carrying cholesterol away from the blood vessel walls before the damage is done.

While our understanding of the exact mechanisms involved remains a bit speculative, the protective effects of HDL cholesterol are well established. What is the effect of exercise on HDL cholesterol? In a word, the

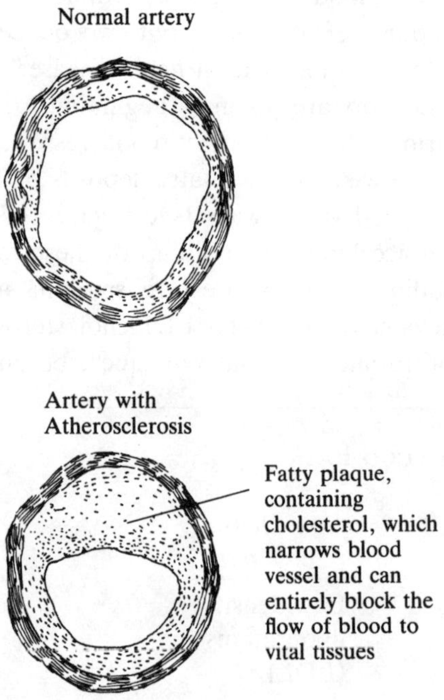

effect is good. Many different population groups have been studied in many parts of the world. In all cases, active people have higher levels than do sedentary people, no matter if the activity comes in the form of chopping trees for a living or playing soccer or tennis for fun. But if the type of exercise doesn't seem to matter, the *amount* of exercise surely does. For example, scientists in Houston found that joggers have much higher HDL levels (58) than do sedentary people (43) — but marathon runners are much higher still (65).

The beneficial effects of exercise on your body fats may be hard to appreciate when couched in these rather complicated terms. But you don't have to be a doctor to see these effects for yourself — just look at your waistline. The percentage of body weight that is fat decreases with exercise. For many people, weight reduction is a major reason to begin an exercise program. We're all for it. But fitness is more than skin deep. The unseen fats in your circulation are more important for your health than for your vanity — but as you adopt a program of regular exercise and sound nutrition to attain fitness, your blood fat profile will improve as surely as your visible profile.

Does exercise protect against heart disease and prolong life expectancy? The answer is yes. You may be surprised to hear doctors take such a definitive stand on this important question. We think our emphatic answer is well justified by the facts, even though other doctors may be a bit more equivocal on this point, perhaps because exercise "treatment" is in the hands (and legs) of you, the public, instead of us, the doctors. On purely scientific grounds, it is true that not all the facts are in, but even the most conservative elements of the medical establishment are now beginning to recognize the benefits of exercise. Hopefully, your own doctors will no longer repeat the traditional advice of our mothers and grandmothers: "Take it easy — you'll live longer." Instead, you should be hearing what we tell our patients, our friends, and even our children: "Get off your duff — you'll live longer."

Two important bodies of evidence support the beneficial effects of exercise: intensive study of experimental animals, and epidemiological investigations of human population groups.

Dr. Dieter Kramsch and colleagues at Boston University studied three groups of monkeys. The first group was fed a normal diet and maintained in sedentary living conditions. They did not develop heart disease and had a normal life span. The second group of monkeys, however, was fed a high-fat diet while maintaining an in-

Normal artery

Artery with Atherosclerosis

Fatty plaque, containing cholesterol, which narrows blood vessel and can entirely block the flow of blood to vital tissues

FIGURE 1–7: *The Normal Artery and One with Atherosclerosis*

active life-style. These animals had a terrible problem with heart disease. Their cardiograms reflected severe heart damage and there was a high incidence of sudden death caused by heart attacks. Autopsies disclosed severe atherosclerosis and coronary artery disease as well as damage to the heart muscle itself. The third group of animals was fed exactly the same harmful high-fat diet, but these monkeys were placed in a daily program of strenuous exercise. Sure enough, the exercise was highly protective. These monkeys had a normal life expectancy and had no evidence of heart disease on their electrocardiograms or heart X rays. When their tissues were examined microscopically, their coronary arteries were actually wider than normal and their heart muscles were stronger and heavier than normal. As you might have guessed, these exercising monkeys had elevated HDL or "good" cholesterol levels and lower LDL or "bad" cholesterol and triglyceride levels.

Needless to say, human studies rely on much less direct techniques. The basic approach to finding out how exercise affects human life span is to study large population groups. These groups are surveyed with regard to their exercise habits as well as to other cardiac risk factors, such as smoking, weight, diabetes, family history, and so forth. The incidence of heart disease is then tabulated and examined as a function of each of these risk factors. It sounds complex, and indeed it is. Because of these complexities, many of these studies are subject to some technical criticisms, and there are some discrepancies in the fine details of the results that have been reported. But by now a great number of these studies have been performed, and they overwhelmingly agree on the essential point: sedentary living is an independent risk factor for heart disease, and, conversely, regular exercise exerts a protective effect.

The first important study of exercise and longevity was performed by Dr. J. N. Morris and his colleagues in 1953. These doctors found that conductors on double-deck buses in London had only half the incidence of heart disease as bus drivers who sat behind the wheel all day instead of walking up and down the stairs. A few years later Morris did a similar study of postmen; mail carriers had significantly less heart disease than did sedentary post office clerks. And nearly twenty years after their first study, Dr. Morris and his colleagues have investigated the effects of leisure-time exercise on nearly eighteen thousand English white-collar workers. During a nine-year period of observation, the men who played vigorous sports during their leisure time had less than half the incidence of heart attacks that their sed-

entary peers had. None of these beneficial effects could be explained by differences in smoking, blood pressure, family history, diabetes, or obesity.

During the past two decades, similar investigations have been performed in diverse population groups ranging from Finnish lumberjacks to Israeli kibbutz workers, Masai tribesmen, and the townspeople of Framingham, Massachusetts. It's a long way from the forest of Scandinavia or the plains of Africa to your swimming pool or tennis court, so let's concentrate on two American studies that may be easier to relate to your own daily life-style.

The leading American investigator of exercise and longevity is Dr. Ralph Paffenbarger of Stanford University. Dr. Paffenbarger and his colleagues studied the effects of activity during work on 3,686 San Francisco longshoremen. These men were extensively evaluated and then were closely followed medically over a twenty-two-year period. The results were striking. A high-energy output at work significantly reduced the risk of fatal heart attacks, especially in younger men. In this population group, vigorous physical activity could reduce the incidence of fatal heart attacks by 49 percent. Paffenbarger did not stop with an evaluation of the effects of exercise. In this same population group, non-smokers had 30 percent fewer incidences of heart disease than did smokers, and men with normal blood pressure readings had a similar 30 percent reduction in risk. Dr. Paffenbarger estimated that a combination of all three — exercise, smoking cessation, and control of blood pressure — might reduce the incidence of coronary heart disease by up to 88 percent, an impressive figure.

If 3,686 San Francisco longshoremen don't convince you, perhaps seventeen thousand Harvard graduates will. The Paffenbarger group has recently presented a very interesting study of 16,936 Harvard alumni who entered college between 1916 and 1950. These subjects were evaluated by means of questionnaires and alumni records; the validity of these techniques was confirmed by close study of a smaller subset of the men. All subjects were followed until age seventy-five or until heart attack, death, or the conclusion of the study. All in all, there were 117,680 person-years of observation.

The findings of this study are impressive. High activity levels reduced the risk of heart attack by a dramatic 26 percent, and this protection was valid for all age groups between thirty-five and seventy-four. Importantly, the benefits of exercise apply only if you keep on exercising. Even those who were varsity-level competitors during their undergraduate years were no better off than their sedentary classmates unless they continued to exercise. The converse is also true: men who took up active life-styles later in life still got the benefits of exercise.

What do these results mean for you? Even if you don't start until midlife you can benefit greatly from exercise. For example, if you spend three hours each week doing aerobic exercises, starting at age forty, by age seventy you will have earned an extra *thirteen months* of life expectancy. In other words, for each hour you exercise, you can expect to live *two* hours longer. And you'll live better, also.

In order for you to plan your exercise schedule, you have to know how much exercise is required to produce this protective effect. The Stanford investigators have provided an excellent guide for you: they found that a total energy expenditure of 2,000 calories per week provides optimal benefit.

Obviously there are many ways to get your weekly 2,000 exercise calories. Paffenbarger found that active sports were somewhat more beneficial than less strenuous activities such as walking and stair-climbing. There is nothing to suggest that one sport is better for you than another. The bottom line is the intensity, duration, and frequency of exercise; Figure 1–8 shows the efficiency of various sports by comparing the amount of time it takes to get your 2,000 calories through each activity.

FIGURE 1–8: HOW LONG IT TAKES TO USE 2,000 CALORIES AT VARIOUS ACTIVITIES

Strolling	10 hours	
Housework	10 hours	
Bowling	8 hours	30 minutes
Golf	8 hours	
Raking leaves	7 hours	
Doubles tennis	6 hours	
Brisk walking	5 hours	30 minutes
Biking (leisurely)	5 hours	30 minutes
Ballet	4 hours	30 minutes
Singles tennis	4 hours	30 minutes
Racquetball, squash	4 hours	
Biking (hard)	4 hours	
Jogging	4 hours	
Downhill skiing	4 hours	
Calisthenics, brisk aerobics	3 hours	30 minutes
Running	3 hours	
Cross-country skiing	3 hours	

In addition to sedentary living, there are a number of other things that increase the chance of getting heart disease. Some of these risk factors are beyond your control, while others may be subject to modification by you and your doctor. There are three risk factors that are beyond your control. The first is *heredity;* if your family history includes an excess of heart disease, particularly early deaths from heart attack, you are at greater risk than you would be if your family tree were notable for longevity instead. Similarly, in our society men are at a higher risk for heart disease than women, so *male sex* is the second uncontrollable risk factor. Third, *age* itself is a risk factor insofar as the incidence of coronary heart disease increases with age.

Another major risk factor is *diabetes*. In most cases, diabetes is an inherited problem. Along with their abnormal sugar metabolism, diabetics inherit an increased risk for disease of the heart and vessels. Diabetes can be controlled with diet, weight reduction, and medication, but even with the best of control there is an increased risk of heart disease. One of the oldest treatments for diabetes is actually exercise itself, and in the past few years doctors have confirmed the ancient observations that regular endurance exercise improves sugar metabolism in diabetics.

Even if you have uncontrollable risk factors, you should not give up on your health. On the contrary, it is even more important for you to work on those risk factors that can be modified or controlled. You can't trade in your grandparents, but you can do quite a lot to help yourself in other areas. For example, *cigarette smoking* lowers HDL cholesterol levels and damages blood vessels, including the coronary arteries. There can no longer be any doubt that cigarette smoking is a major hazard to health, causing disease, disability, and death from both heart and lung disease.

Another major risk factor that you can control is *hypertension* (high blood pressure). In some cases excess salt intake can contribute to high blood pressure (see Chapter 4). Anxiety and tension can also elevate your blood pressure (see Chapter 3). Hypertension places an excessive stress on your heart and blood vessels. Over the years this stress can produce vascular damage, resulting in heart attacks, heart failure, stroke, or kidney disease. But almost all of these important complications of hypertension can be prevented if treatment is started early enough. The trick is to detect high blood pressure before damage has occurred. Unfortunately, you cannot count on nosebleeds, headaches, flushing, or tension as warning signs. In fact, in most cases high blood pressure is present for years before these symptoms are evident. Clearly the name "silent killer" is well earned. Even world-class athletes have high blood pressure without knowing it, and without having it interfere with record-setting performances. The message is clear. You have to have your blood pressure checked at reasonable intervals in order to detect hypertension at its earliest, treatable stages.

Even if your doctor does discover hypertension, you do not have to give up sports. In fact, exercise, salt restriction, weight reduction, and mental relaxation can control hypertension in a surprising number of patients, without medication. If these techniques don't do the job entirely, many drugs are available so that in almost all cases excellent control can be achieved.

Another factor that can increase your risk for coronary heart disease is *stress* or tension. Certain personality types — especially the "Type A" peronality — seem to have a greater incidence of heart disease (see Chapter 3). Exercise can help you relax and may modify this risk factor.

Obesity is another potential cardiac risk factor. Note that we have qualified obesity as a potential risk factor only. Although fat people do have more heart attacks than thin people, this difference may not be accounted for by obesity *per se*, but by other adverse factors associated with obesity, such as high blood pressure, diabetes, and high cholesterol.

Exercise can have a beneficial effect on all of the above risk factors, as well as on the final independent risk factor of sedentary living. Dr. Kenneth Cooper, one of the earliest and most forceful proponents of aerobic exercise in America, has demonstrated that exercise increases aerobic power or fitness and also decreases body weight, body fat, blood pressure, cholesterol, and blood sugar. Dr. Cooper did not measure the effects of exercise on Type A behavior — but how often have you seen anyone reading the stock pages while jogging? Exercise alone is not enough, but it is an important unifying link, which can help protect you against heart disease.

With all the publicity given to these risk factors, we have already started to see some benefits in our population. Between 1963 and 1983, cardiovascular death rates in the United States fell by 36 percent. Even so, cardiovascular disease remains by far our leading cause of death, taking 550,000 lives in 1984. We are headed in the right direction, but there is still plenty of room for improvement.

Appropriate exercise, sound nutrition, stress control, smoking cessation, and the detection and treatment of hypertension will help our society control its epidemic of heart disease. Each of these elements can help you as an individual. But you need not be preoccupied by risk factors. Fitness has its own immediate, tangible rewards: you will look better, feel better, and be more energetic and upbeat. As you exercise your way to fitness, you'll be thinking about how good you feel, not about how your cholesterol is improving. When all is said and done, fitness is fun.

EXERCISE AND AGING

Many people regard aging as a somber issue. In truth, there is nothing grim about growing older — especially when you consider the alternative. We haven't discovered the fountain of youth and we certainly don't pretend that we will show you how to turn back the clock. Yet there are ways to grow older without getting old, to stay vigorous in mind and body as the years and decades go along. Part of the secret is mental. To quote the noted contemporary American philosopher Muhammad Ali, "Age is a question of mind over matter. If you don't mind, it don't matter." In addition to a youthful mental attitude, regular physical activity is also important to keep you young.

The aging process is gradual, continuous, and inevitable. All of the organs of your body are involved. Muscular strength declines, and flexibility of ligaments and joints decreases. Bones may lose calcium and have less strength and resistance to stress. Whereas muscle mass diminishes, the percentage of your body composition that is fat increases over the years.

Your metabolism also changes. Older people tend to burn fewer calories each day. Blood sugar levels increase, and many older people develop a mild form of diabetes as a result. Your blood cholesterol levels also increase, and in some cases fatty deposits in blood vessels produce narrowing or even occlusion of arteries (atherosclerosis). Blood composition also changes, so that you tend to have fewer red blood cells and also less plasma as you grow older. This may partially explain another phenomenon seen in advanced years, which is greater tendency toward the formation of blood clots.

The nervous system is also affected by age. Changes in the speed and clarity of thought and memory are extremely variable. In some people, mental quickness and concentration diminish, but in others creative and retentive thinking remain unimpaired. However, other changes in the nervous system are more uniform. For example, hearing and vision tend to become less acute over the years. In addition, reaction time increases, so your "reflexes" slow.

Your heart and lungs are not immune to the effects of age. Blood pressure tends to increase, largely as a result of narrowing and thickening of the blood vessels themselves. Your maximum heart rate declines very predictably to the tune of about one beat per minute per year. Moreover, the amount of blood that your heart can pump with each heartbeat also tends to decline. The combined effect of a slower maximum heart rate and a smaller pumping volume is a decline in the total amount of blood that your heart can pump. Similar changes occur in the lungs as your chest wall becomes stiffer and your maximum breathing capacity is decreased, so that oxygen delivery declines. The net effect of these changes is that your body's capacity to perform work diminishes over the years. In fact, work capacity declines by about one percent per year beyond age twenty-five — at age seventy-five it would be only half of what it was at age twenty-five.

These changes collectively produce a profile of increasing cardiac risk factors over the years. Between ages thirty and fifty, the average American man gains thirty pounds, loses 30 percent of his aerobic capacity, and has a 30-point rise in his serum cholesterol. It's not surprising, then, that heart disease tends to be more common in the elderly.

You may be surprised to learn that it does not take forty years to produce these changes. In fact, very similar alterations can be produced in healthy young people in just forty *days*. Simple inactivity, such as bed rest, will do the trick. The effects of disuse on your muscles and bones, metabolism and body composition, nervous system, and circulation are in many ways identical to the effects of age.

You can modify almost all of these changes in a favorable direction. The old adage "Use it or lose it" holds up scientifically; in the fourth century B.C., Hippocrates observed: "That which is used, develops, that which is not used wastes away." The answer is physical activity, particularly in the form of endurance training. This will tend to increase heart and lung capacities, lower blood pressure, and decrease body fat. Blood cholesterol and blood sugar levels tend to decline. Muscles become stronger. In fact, endurance training will even improve reaction time so that you have faster "reflexes." All in all, endurance training can maintain an excellent total work capacity even in the face of advancing years.

There are many examples of outstanding athletic achievement beyond age seventy. Clarence Chaffee was the tennis and squash coach at Williams College for forty years but did not begin competing nationally until age seventy. Since then he has collected forty-one national Super Seniors' tennis titles. Exercise will not make you immune to heart disease, and even the remarkable Mr. Chaffee demonstrates this point, for he had a heart attack at age eighty-two. But five months (and one pacemaker) later he was back on the courts, and so far he's won seven more national titles for his age group. Another inspirational case in point is Albert Gordon, a well-known businessman and philanthropist. Mr. Gordon has been a competitive runner throughout his life but did not enter his first marathon until age eighty, at which time he completed the difficult London Marathon in an excellent six hours and thirty minutes.

Both of these men, of course, are extraordinary athletes whose achievements as octogenarians were built upon a lifetime of regular exercise. Most of us cannot attain these achievements at eighty or, or that matter, at forty. But if we set realistic goals — not too high and not too *low* — we can achieve an amazing amount at any age.

Clearly, the best time to start is when you're young. In fact, the youth of America need a fitness program just as badly as the rest of us. Only 36 percent of school-age children passed a physical fitness test administered by the American Athletic Union in 1984. Even more shocking are the results of a Michigan survey, which showed that 98 percent of elementary school students have one or more major risk factors for developing coronary heart disease, including body fat levels averaging 5 percent above ideal, elevated cholesterol in 41 percent, and high blood pressure in 28 percent. Is it a wonder that when the Cincinnati Reds baseball team began their "youth movement" in spring training in 1985, they turned the conditioning program over to Walter (Doc) Eberhardt — age eighty?

Fitness and exercise are not the fountain of youth, but they can favorably moderate the physiologic changes of aging. The surest way to get old is to "act your age," to think and act old. Don't celebrate your birthday by hanging up your running shoes! Age will, of course, alter your exercise capacity and style. But with appropriate precautions and medical clearance, you can begin an exercise program at any age. It's never too late to get fit.

Are there limits? Of course. Few of us can get to center court at any age, and none of us can win the U.S. Open at age fifty. Don't be discouraged if you're not a brilliant senior athlete like Clarence Chaffee or Albert Gordon. After all, younger athletes are not deterred from tennis or running because they are not a Jimmy Connors or Alberto Salazar. With appropriate precautions and medical backup, you can exercise and play sports at any age, with great dividends in terms of pleasure and health. Helen Hayes says it best: "Resting is rusting."

THE OTHER SIDE OF THE COIN: PERILS, PITFALLS, AND PRECAUTIONS OF EXERCISE

Jogging did not kill Jim Fixx. The noted writer and running enthusiast died while jogging in Vermont in July 1984. An autopsy showed that Fixx had advanced arteriosclerosis of his coronary arteries. Coronary artery disease, not running, killed Jim Fixx. But his death at age fifty-two raises important questions and reminds us all that exercise is a serious business that requires certain precautions in order to be safe.

Fixx was a former two-pack-a-day cigarette smoker; his father suffered a heart attack at age thirty-five and died of the disease at forty-three. Fixx himself avoided medical checkups, so we do not know his cholesterol levels. And it appears that before his fatal attack he had symptoms of angina, which he ignored.

We can explain the tragedy of Jim Fixx as a combination of risk factors, self-neglect, and denial of symptoms. But how about Miami Dolphin linebacker Larry Gordon, who died while jogging at age twenty-eight? Or J. V. Cain, a tight end for the St. Louis Cardinals, who died during a football game? And Arturo Brown, the captain of the Boston University basketball team, was only twenty-one when he died during a practice session.

The sudden death of an apparently healthy young athlete during competition is a rare but well-documented phenomenon. These tragic events can occur even in high school as well as in college or pro sports. In addition, we can all think of examples of highly trained, apparently healthy athletes who have suffered nonfatal heart attacks. John Hiller of the Detroit Tigers, Dave Stallworth of the New York Knicks, and tennis star Arthur Ashe are three illustrations of young athletes

who survived heart attacks and were able to return to active life-styles, including sports. Nor are examples confined to skilled competitors. From time to time you will read about others who die during jogging or racing, as in the case of U.S. Congressman Goodloe E. Byron of Maryland.

All of these examples are, of course, tragedies for the individuals and families involved, and they make us wonder about the safety of running and other sports. What causes sudden death in athletes? Can these tragedies be predicted and prevented? Can exercise be harmful to your heart?

These are difficult questions, but the last one is the easiest to answer. Exercise will *not* cause heart disease if your heart is healthy to begin with. Most highly trained athletes do have distinctive changes in their hearts. Whereas these changes do, indeed, result from regular vigorous exercise, we now know that they are signs of a strong healthy heart, not a diseased heart. Athletes tend to have lower blood pressures, and as a group they have strikingly slower heart rates. Careful cardiac examinations may reveal enlargement of the heart and heart murmurs. Chest X rays may also disclose enlargement of the heart's main pumping chamber, the left ventricle, and electrocardiograms may show similar changes. These changes are easy to understand when you remember that the heart is a muscle; like other muscles, the heart muscle becomes larger and stronger with regular exercise. And like other muscles, the heart will lose its extra strength unless you maintain exercise training.

In the past, this cardiac enlargement was labeled with a diagnosis of "athlete's heart," which was considered to be a disease. We now know, however, that the athlete's heart is a healthy heart with a strong, efficient pumping mechanism. Although most doctors are aware of this nowadays, you may still want to remind your physician of this entity if you are endurance trained. Insurance companies are even more likely to need reminders. My own experience is fairly typical. I (HBS) was required to submit a routine electrocardiogram in order to purchase a new life insurance policy, but the policy was delayed because of supposed "abnormalities." The issue was not clarified until I underwent an exercise stress test, which I am happy to say produced more pain to the treadmill than it did to my chest.

Although exercise does not produce disease in healthy hearts, deaths do occur during sports. Why is this?

First of all, not all sudden deaths in athletes are due to heart problems. Sad to say, a surprising number of athletes, both in the professional and amateur ranks, use illicit drugs in an attempt to improve athletic performance. Occasionally these drugs, such as amphetamines (or "speed") and cocaine, can produce critical elevations in the blood pressure or disorders in the heart rhythm, which can lead to death. In other cases, inborn abnormalities of the blood vessels in the brain can lead to sudden death if one of these so-called aneurysms ruptures. Cerebral aneurysms can rupture anytime. Whereas death during sleep gets little publicity, this kind of sudden death during exercise gets a lot of attention and is often erroneously attributed to exercise in general and the heart in particular. Additional noncardiac causes of death in athletes are heat stroke and allergic reactions to insect stings. The leading cause of death during contact sports is direct trauma causing brain damage.

Athletes who die of heart trouble during training or competition fall into two distinct groups. In the older age groups, beyond age forty or forty-five, the cause is generally preexisting coronary artery disease. Most often these individuals have had known heart disease, major risk factors, or warning symptoms, but have persisted in unsupervised exercise despite these warnings. However, in other cases the first manifestation of coronary artery disease can occur as collapse or even death during exercise. This latter group is uncommon but is particularly worrisome for doctors and for patients.

In people with coronary heart disease, exercise can produce problems in several ways. Exercise produces an increase in heart rate, in the strength of the heart's contractions, and in the blood pressure. All of these factors mean that the heart is working harder. Just like all exercising muscles, the heart muscle will need more oxygen to do its work efficiently and safely. If the coronary arteries have blockages, however, not enough blood and oxygen can get to the hardworking heart muscle. In most cases this will produce chest pain and pressure called angina, which is a signal to stop exercising at once and get appropriate medical attention. But sometimes exercise can precipitate an actual heart attack, if the oxygen demands of the working heart muscle exceed the oxygen supply enough to damage or kill heart muscle fibers. In other cases, the lack of oxygen may cause a disorder of the heart's pumping rhythm, which can cause an abrupt fall in blood pressure, collapse, or even sudden death.

The other category of sudden death occurs in younger competitors. Ordinary coronary heart disease is very unusual in young people, and the major causes of these rare events are congenital or inborn abnormalities of the heart muscle or circulation. For example, some people are born with "anomalous coronary arteries," in which the coronary arteries themseves are either abnormally small or abnormally positioned so that the heart muscle does not get enough blood. Unfortunately, this condition is almost never suspected until a heart attack occurs.

An entirely different but equally important cause of sudden death in young athletes is an abnormality of the heart muscle called "idiopathic hypertrophic subaortic stenosis," or IHSS. In this problem, the walls of the main pumping chamber or left ventricle become excessively thick so that the flow of blood from the heart into the circulation can be impaired. This can lead to a drop in blood pressure or to abnormalities of the heart rhythm. Sudden death can be the result. In fact, IHSS was responsible for the deaths of Larry Gordon and Arturo Brown. Can IHSS be detected before it kills? Brown is a case in point. Just a week before he died he had a fainting episode while jogging. Fainting during exercise, chest pain during exercise, or undue breathlessness during exercise should always raise this possibility in young people. A family history of sudden death at an early age may provide an additional clue in some cases. Unfortunately, most doctors don't think of this entity because it's quite rare, and because the victims typically appear healthy. Routine physical examinations, X rays, and electrocardiograms can provide important clues in some people, but in others the abnormalities are very subtle or even absent. If this condition is suspected, however, a relatively simple test called an echocardiogram can lead to a diagnosis. Needless to say, people with IHSS should exercise only with extremely careful precautions as outlined by their cardiologists.

All of these potential heart problems are intimidating and even scary. Do they mean that we shouldn't exercise? Of course not. First, all of the risk factor and epidemiological studies we discussed earlier in this chapter demonstrate that exercise is beneficial for longevity. Second, although cardiac complications do occur, they are really quite rare. Dr. Cooper and his colleagues in Texas have kept careful records of exercise-related complications at the Aerobics Center. They found less than three heart problems for every *ten thousand hours* of exercise in healthy men of all ages. None of these complications was fatal; in fact, there were no deaths in 374,789 person-hours of exercise, which included over *1.2 million miles* of jogging and walking. Dr. Roy Sheppard, a preventive medicine authority at the University of Toronto, is equally reassuring; he estimates the odds of dying during a heavy workout as one in five million for middle-aged men and one in seventeen million for women.

Perhaps the best perspective on the risk of sudden death during sports comes from the 1984 study of Dr. Siscovick and his colleagues in Seattle, Washington. They found that the risk of sudden death is increased during strenuous exercise, but that the risk is much smaller in people who exercise regularly than in people who are out of shape. Moreover, people who are physically fit have a marked decrease in their overall risk of sudden death, which more than compensates for the risk incurred during exercise itself. All in all, this study agrees with one of our major themes: exercise is good for your health and your heart, but for safety's sake you should get into shape gradually, warm up and cool down before each workout (see Chapter 7), and discuss things with your doctor to see if you need special supervision or precautions.

This is the third reason not to avoid exercise, and it is of the greatest practical significance to you. Although some of these complications are totally unpredictable, many of them *can* be prevented by appropriate precautions and screening procedures. Your job is to report risk factors and early symptoms. Your doctor's job is to perform appropriate medical examinations. Chapter 5 details the medical screening we recommend to help make exercise safe. But the warning symptoms of heart disease are important enough to merit mention here as well. Chest pain is the most obvious distress signal. Cardiac pain typically causes a dull, heavy pressure in the midchest. The pain may radiate to the neck, arms, or jaw. It is usually brought on by exertion or emotion, but it can come on after a large meal or even without apparent precipitating causes. In general, this type of cardiac pain, which is called angina, is relieved by rest or by certain medications such as nitroglycerin. In some people, however, the pain of angina can be quite atypical and can be confused with indigestion, gall-bladder attacks, or asthma. The converse is also true, in that noncardiac problems can cause suspicious chest pain. Other symptoms that require prompt medical evaluation include undue shortness of breath, disproportionate fatigue, unexpected nausea, sweating, or light-headedness, and a sensation of skipped beats or erratic heart rhythm. Obviously, any of these symptoms should lead you to get a prompt and competent evaluation.

Don't let these gloomy considerations keep you from exercising. From time to time you will read somber warnings about exercise and the heart in newspapers and magazines. You should be very suspicious of any oversimplified, exaggerated claims about exercise — either pro or con. Exercise is safe and beneficial for your heart if you follow a few simple commonsense guidelines. Although it is no panacea, a balanced exercise program can, in fact, go a long way toward preventing heart disease, as well as prolonging and enriching your life.

SELF-ASSESSMENT

One of the questions we are asked most often is "How can I get into shape?" Before answering this key question in Parts II and III, we must ask you an equally crucial question: What shape are you in right now? You have to know your starting point in order to plan a safe and effective fitness program.

Cardiovascular fitness can be measured in the laboratory with great precision. An exercise tolerance test, popularly called a stress test, will measure your total work capacity, maximum heart rate, and blood pressure response to exercise as you jog on a treadmill or pedal a bike. And because your electrocardiogram is monitored continuously during the test, these studies can be used to screen for coronary artery diseases. With some additional equipment to monitor your breathing, exercise testing can also give you a precise measurement of your work capacity, or maximum oxygen uptake, as well as your anaerobic threshold.

Exercise tolerance tests, however, are not for everyone. They are expensive, time consuming, and can even be misleading — particularly in younger people with a low risk of coronary heart disease. In Chapter 5, we'll set down some guidelines for who should be stress-tested. If you are younger than fifty and free of known cardiovascular disease, worrisome symptoms, and major risk factors, you can safely estimate your own level of fitness with some simple self-tests.

You can assess your level of fitness in three different ways: a risk-factor profile, an analysis of your current exercise level, and a test of your present endurance capacities. We suggest that you take all three tests. Keep a record of the results in your fitness log (Chapter 7) and retest yourself every eight to twelve weeks. You'll have a clear record of where you are starting from and will be able to chart your progress toward your fitness goals.

You can tabulate your risk-factor profile by filling out

a simple questionnaire, totaling your point score, and tallying up the results (see Figure 1–9). Note that some of the information will have to come from your doctor, but you can also take this test without this medical information; you can retest yourself simply by retabulating Part B.

FIGURE 1–9: RISK-FACTOR PROFILE

A. *Uncontrollable Factors*

1. Age	Under 30	0	Score _____
	30–44	1	
	45–54	2	
	55–64	4	
	Over 65	6	
2. Sex	Female	0	Score _____
	Male	5	
3. Family history of heart disease (parents, siblings, uncles and aunts)			
	None	0	Score _____
	1 or 2	1	
	2 or more	3	
	(Younger than 50, add 4 points)		
4. Diabetes	Absent	0	Score _____
	Present	3	
		Part A	Subtotal Score _____

B. *Controllable Risk Factors*

5. Stress	Low	0	Score _____
	Moderate	2	
	High	4	
6. Regular exercise			Score _____
	Very active	0	
	Moderate	1	
	Little	2	
	Sedentary	4	
7. Smoking	Never	0	Score _____
	Cigar or pipe	1	
	Cigarettes		
	None for at least 8 yrs. or more	0	
	None for 3–8 yrs.	1	
	In past 3 yrs:		
	Less than ½ pack/day	4	
	Up to 1 pack/day	6	
	1–2 packs/day	8	
8. Weight	Less than 15 lbs. over	0	Score _____
	15–30 lbs. over	1	
	More than 30 lbs. over	2	
		Part B	Subtotal Score _____

C. *Medical Data*

9. Total cholesterol			Score _____
	Under 190	0	
	190–209	1	
	210–219	2	
	220–239	4	
	240–259	6	
	Over 260	8	
10. HDL cholesterol			Score _____
	Over 50	0	
	45–49	2	
	35–44	8	
	25–34	6	
	Below 25	8	
11. Triglycerides (fasting)			Score _____
	Below 150	0	
	151–200	1	
	Over 200	2	
12. Blood pressure			Score _____
	Below 140/85	0	
	Below 150/90	1	
	Below 160/95	2	
	Below 170/100	4	
	Below 175/105	6	
	Higher readings	8	

Part C   Subtotal Score _____

Grand Total Score _____

Risk score interpretation:

Below 12	Low risk
13–26	Modest risk
27–37	Moderate risk
Above 38	High risk

If medical date (Part C) is not available, use the following interpretation scale:

Below 10	Low risk
11–15	Modest risk
16–21	Moderate risk
Above 22	High risk

Remember that "risk" is a relative term. A low-risk profile does not mean that you are immune from heart disease. Conversely, a high-risk profile does not mean that a heart attack is inevitable. But since many of these risk factors *can* be improved, you should modify your life-style to lower your score.

A second way to assess your fitness is to evaluate your current level of physical activity. The method is simple: just keep a log of your exercise for a week. Using Figure 1–10, calculate the total caloric cost of your activities, and total them up. To score your activity level use Figure 1-11.

FIGURE 1–10: CALORIC COST OF VARIOUS ACTIVITIES

Daily living:		
	Rest	60 cal./hr.
	Desk work	90 cal./hr.
	Standing	120 cal./hr.
	Light housework (dusting, etc.)	150 cal./hr.
	Heavy housework (vacuuming, etc.)	250 cal./hr.
	Scrubbing floors	300 cal./hr.
	Raking leaves	300 cal./hr.
	Average sexual activity	300 cal./hr.
	Snow shoveling	420 cal./hr.
	Heavy digging	480 cal./hr.

Walking/running:		
	Strolling, 1 mile/hr.	120 cal./hr.
	Level walking, 2 miles/hr.	150 cal./hr.
	Level walking, 3 miles/hr.	240 cal./hr.
	Brisk walking, 4 miles/hr.	360 cal./hr.
	Jogging, 5 miles/hr.	480 cal./hr.
	Jogging, 6 miles/hr.	660 cal./hr.
	Running, 7 miles/hr.	760 cal./hr.

Biking:		
	6 miles/hr.	240 cal./hr.
	10 miles/hr.	360 cal./hr.
	12 miles/hr.	480 cal./hr.

Racquet sports:		
	Table tennis	300 cal./hr.
	Badminton	300 cal./hr.
	Doubles tennis	300 cal./hr.
	Singles tennis	420 cal./hr.
	Squash, paddleball	480 cal./hr.

Dance:		
	Ballroom	340 cal./hr.
	Ballet, disco	460 cal./hr.
	Aerobic (vigorous)	600 cal./hr.

Skiing:		
	Downhill	480 cal./hr.
	Cross-country	660 cal./hr.
	Water	500 cal./hr.

Others:		
	Bowling	240 cal./hr.
	Golf (pulling cart)	240 cal./hr.
	Golf (carrying clubs)	300 cal./hr.
	Canoeing	480 cal./hr.
	Volleyball	580 cal./hr.
	Rope jumping	660 cal./hr.
	Soccer (brisk)	660 cal./hr.
	Basketball (full-court)	660 cal./hr.
	Rowing (vigorous)	660 cal./hr.
	Swimming (hard)	660 cal./hr.
	(butterfly)	740 cal./hr.

NOTE: These are typical values for people of average size exercising at moderate intensity. Highly trained athletes can utilize substantially more calories per hour at competitive sports.

FIGURE 1–11: MEASURING YOUR LEVEL OF PHYSICAL ACTIVITY

Weekly exercise	Fitness level
Less than 500 calories	Poor
501–1,000	Fair
1001–1,499	Good
1500–1,999	Very good
2000–2,999	Excellent
Above 3,000	Superior

Remember to include your physical activity at work and around the house as well as your workouts and sports. And be sure to pick a typical week; if you have any doubts, just repeat the tally for another week, and average the results.

To give you a feel for this method of evaluating your fitness, let's look at the log of one of our friends, Anne S., a healthy thirty-eight-year-old physician.

	Activity	*Calories*
Monday	Calisthenics, 15 min.	75
	Walking, 1.5 miles	150
Tuesday	Calisthenics, 15 min.	75
Wednesday	Calisthenics, 20 min.	100
	Jog, 3 miles	300
Thursday	Walk, 1 mile	100
Friday	Calisthenics, 20 min.	100
	Jog, 3 miles	300
	Walk, 1 mile	100
Saturday	Calisthenics, 15 min.	75
	Tennis (doubles), 1 hr.	300
Sunday	Calisthenics, 20 min.	100
	Jog, 5 miles	500
	Gardening, 45 min.	275
	Total	2,550

Anne's score clearly puts her in the excellent category. She didn't get there all at once, but built up to this level little by little. If she can fit all these activities into her busy schedule, you probably can, too. Most importantly, Anne feels great and enjoys her exercise. Try it; you'll like it too.

The third way to estimate your fitness level is with Dr. Kenneth Cooper's famous 12-minute test. The idea is simple: See how far you can get by walking, jogging or running during a 12-minute period. For precision, it's best to do this on a track so that you can count laps and measure distance accurately. If you are out of shape, you should not push yourself too hard for your first test; instead, take a 6- to 8-minute pretest to get an idea of your capacity. Wait a few days, and then pace yourself appropriately during your self-test. Be sure to dress appropriately, warm up gradually, and avoid eating for at least two hours prior to your test.

Cooper's scoring system can be simplified for adults between twenty and fifty to give you an approximate fitness level:

Distance covered	*Fitness level*
Less than 3/4 mile	Poor
3/4–1 mile	Fair
1–1¼ miles	Good
1¼–1½ miles	Very good
1½–1¾ miles	Excellent
More than 1¾ miles	Superior

Anne covered slightly more than 1½ miles in her 12 minutes, putting her in the excellent category.

Each of these three self-assessment tests will provide an estimate of your fitness level, but no self-test is as precise as an evaluation in an exercise lab. The important thing is not what you score now, but how much you improve. So keep a record of your scores and retest yourself every eight to twelve weeks until you are convinced that fitness is part of your life-style.

2

Musculoskeletal Fitness

Asound heart is the key to fitness for health as well as for sports. But aerobic fitness is only one of the major components of a true, balanced fitness program. Having a good cardiovascular system doesn't necessarily mean you are in shape for playing on your local touch football team or even for an hour of vigorous, winning tennis. A healthy heart doesn't mean you can carry out the garbage or even carry your heavy briefcase.

For these types of activities and stresses, you need to develop the musculoskeletal component of fitness. It is not strictly musculoskeletal since it also involves all of your connective tissues — your muscles, bones, cartilage, tendons, and joints — and how they function coordinated by complex neurological and psychological systems. This aspect of fitness enables you to maintain your posture or to throw a football.

Until recently, fitness has been defined subjectively and has followed certain fads. Fifty years ago, fitness was defined as the ability of a muscle-bound bully to kick sand in the face of some ninety-seven-pound weakling. Charles Atlas promised that if you followed his regimen, you would put on one hundred pounds of muscle and give that bully his just desserts. On the other hand, in 1972, when Frank Shorter won the Olympic marathon and long-distance running broke into the American consciousness, fitness meant weighing ninety-seven pounds and running like the wind, and all thoughts of the muscular component were lost. These days, the pendulum has swung back again. With the growth of fitness clubs, pumping iron has moved from the neighborhood gym to the high-tech salon and the corporate culture. Being fit has come to mean developing a body by Nautilus.

These extremes lack the balance we are trying to help you achieve. Good muscle tone is only part of the picture. Looking good is fine, but doing well is better; how your body works is more important than appearance as far as fitness and health are concerned. Thus, we will stress functional characteristics such as strength, endurance, flexibility, and other neuromuscular aspects such as reaction time and coordination.

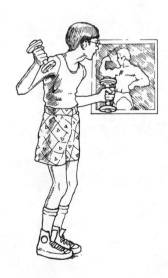

On the other hand, there is nothing wrong with good appearance, and one aspect of muscular fitness that Charles Atlas's promotion accurately portrayed is the self-confidence and self-reliance that derive from being in good muscular shape. The result doesn't follow from a macho build, but rather from knowing what your body can do and how elegantly function and appearance are linked.

Consider the factors involved in a good backhand stroke in tennis (see Figure 2–1). You need arm, shoulder, and upper-back strength, but also good flexibility in these joints, your back, and legs, quick reaction time, good coordination and balance, speed to reach the ball, and the endurance to continue this for a full match. A good training program should enhance all of these aspects as well as your appearance.

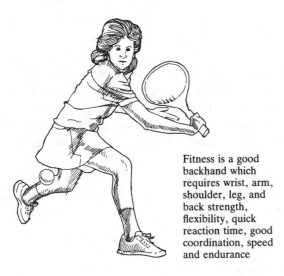

Fitness is a good backhand which requires wrist, arm, shoulder, leg, and back strength, flexibility, quick reaction time, good coordination, speed and endurance

FIGURE 2–1: *A Good Backhand Stroke*

A tennis swing is one thing. But the same principles affect your health. Just as cardiovascular fitness helps protect you against the nation's major killer, heart disease, musculoskeletal fitness protects you against the major causes of injuries and disabilities: musculoskeletal pains, strains, and sprains. Musculoskeletal fitness means you have to know your body, even more than for aerobics. And by knowing about your joints and muscle groups, you can assess your level of fitness, train for specific goals, and avoid injuries. Nowhere is this clearer than in protecting your back, the most vulnerable part of the entire musculoskeletal system.

Obviously, understanding the principles of fitness isn't enough. We encourage you to develop fitness for health through sports for fitness. First of all, building endurance, strength, and flexibility will help to do away with

everyday bad back, stiff neck, or sore knees — that's health fitness. But hitting a forehand like Borg, jumping like Doctor J, or skating like Eric Heiden (relatively speaking) — that's the joy of sports fitness. It has to do with your muscles and your joints, your strength and your power, your flexibility and quickness. Sports fitness means playing touch football with your kids even if *they* are pushing forty; it means being ready to play year-round and build, as the proverb says, "from strength to strength." By outlining the functional anatomy and physiology of your body and helping you assess your own level of fitness, this chapter will allow you to train intelligently and efficiently.

YOUR BODY: THE ANATOMIC BASIS FOR ACTIVITY

Sigmund Freud wrote, "Anatomy is destiny," and while his viewpoint was different from ours, his words are correct. None of us is going to run as fast as a greyhound, but then no dog will hit a forehand smash. That much is obvious. So is the fact that a 5'6" man is going to have problems slam-dunking a basketball, although he may be able to sink twenty-foot jump shots with ease if he is willing to practice.

Human beings tend to have certain basic body types — so-called ectomorph, endomorph, and mesomorph (see Figure 2–2). The ectomorph is your conventional skinny kid. Eat as much as she can, she never seems to put on weight. As an athlete, she tends to be wiry and fast. If tall enough, she'll be on the basketball court; if not, she'll lead the pack in a road race. The mesomorph tends to be at the other extreme: compact and muscular if he's in shape, obese if he's not, he's the classic "big-boned" individual. A mesomorph may be on the wrestling team or play football (as a lineman) in college, and later have problems with his waistline. Between the two is the endomorph: broad shoulders, narrow waist. At 5'8" he plays soccer, and at 6'2" he swims or plays tennis.

Of course, these body types are only the ends of the spectrum; most of us have body types between these extremes. Likewise, all types of individuals can play at any given sport, sometimes with success that defies all categorization. You don't have to give up roadracing if you weigh twice Bill Rodgers's 128 pounds — but don't expect to beat him very often, either. The ideal body type for volleyball may be over six feet tall; but regardless of your body type, if you enjoy the quickness, competition, and strategic aspects of the sport and are willing to practice and to develop your timing and your jumping muscles, you will be able to play an enjoyable game even if you may not compete in the Olympics. Fundamentally, your competition is with yourself — to what extent can you improve and enhance the tools you were born with? The rewards will be the health you gain through being fit.

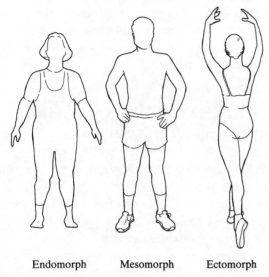

Endomorph   Mesomorph   Ectomorph

FIGURE 2–2: *Basic Body Types*

Another anatomic factor is body composition, in particular, the difference in the physical makeup of men and women. On the average, women tend to be shorter, carry more body fat at similar levels of fitness, and pound for pound are not as muscular or strong. For example, women roadracers tend to average 6 to 10 percent body fat compared to 4 to 8 percent for men. Even that 10 percent level, however, is far below the body fat level of men and women who are out of shape. In addition, women's muscles cannot get as big and bulky as men's, no matter how much they exercise, because they lack the male hormone testosterone. But women can achieve remarkable muscle definition, strength, and endurance by conditioning. On the other hand, women are favored by having joints that are more flexible than men's. This gives them advantages in such activities as figure skating, dance, and gymnastics, while reducing their chances of getting muscle pulls from routine daily activities or sports.

Besides body type and body composition, your physiologic characteristics and capabilities include strength, flexibility, speed, and coordination. You were born with certain anatomic and physical characteristics, but many

other factors determine your success and your enjoyment as well: your level of conditioning, mental attitude, and the amount of hard work you are willing to do to sharpen your skills and get into shape.

Your body's characteristics will establish certain priorities when it comes to getting into shape. This is particularly true of the effects of age. You can modify many of the effects of advancing years by conditioning. But being fit does not mean turning yourself into somebody else, somebody younger, or taller, or more broadshouldered — rather, it involves becoming what you were meant to be.

THE BASIC MACHINERY — FITNESS AT THE TISSUE LEVEL

Whether you are a 4'8" gymnast, a 5'8" accountant, or a 6'8" power forward, your body is constructed of the same components and tissues. For our purposes, the important ones are bones, muscles, tendons, ligaments, cartilage, and the nervous system. The human body is composed of individual bones linked together in a series of complex substructures called joints. The movement of joints depends on muscles and ligaments and is controlled by highly complex sets of nerves. However, we will have to understand more about the individual components — and their functional anatomy — before we can understand how these body parts work together and how conditioning helps.

BONE

Bone is a living tissue composed of a matrix of protein, collagen, to which calcium adheres. The ends of bones are covered with a soft slippery material called cartilage (see page 31). Bone constantly remodels itself in response to stress and use. If your bones are not used, they lose calcium and strength. This is seen most dramatically in astronauts during periods of weightlessness in space. It also occurs in sedentary people, leading to osteoporosis and increased susceptibility to fractures. It is proven, though, that activity enhances the mineral content and strength of bone. For example, tennis Super Seniors (in their seventies and eighties) have increased amounts of calcium and increased density of their bones compared with their less active contemporaries. While many factors influence the composition of bone — dietary calcium, vitamin D, and, in women, estrogen hormones — exercise is one of the most important.

Bone is a very dynamic tissue, and its continued strength and good function is a major determinant not only of your ability to play sports, but of your health. Bone weakness is especially dangerous for older individuals. Hip fractures, degenerative arthritis, and compression fractures of the vertebral bodies of your back are major causes of pain and disability as you age. Some of the worst degenerative arthritis we have seen has occurred in individuals whose most vigorous activity was brushing their teeth. Exercise may not give the resiliency of youth back to your bones, but for most people, fitness produces obvious and impressive improvements.

The way your bones are put together and their relative proportions determine your body type (see Figure 2-2). And what you see is what you get, since bones can remodel at the tissue level but cannot change much in terms of their length, bulk, and shape. Bones can become stronger, but not longer.

Thus, bones primarily play a limiting role. For example, the size of your rib cage is one of the major determinants of your maximal lung capacity. Another example is the female pelvis, which is larger than the male's. In turn, this larger pelvis necessitates a greater angle between the bone of the upper leg (the femur) and the major bone of the lower leg (the tibia). The greater this angle (called the Q-angle), the shallower the groove in which the kneecap (the patella) rides, and the more susceptible to injury it is. This, in part, explains the greater propensity for women to develop knee pain from certain sports, such as running. But whereas you can't affect the size and shape of your bones, you *can* affect the strength of the knee muscle, the quadriceps, and protect the knee against injury by maintaining good muscular fitness.

CARTILAGE

Adults have various forms of cartilage, the most important of which is found on the ends of bones where it provides a slippery surface and shock absorption. When cartilage is damaged, arthritis can result. Cartilage is a living tissue, also comprised of a matrix of the protein collagen. This matrix absorbs a great deal of water, so much, in fact, that water is the chief constituent of cartilage. When joints are used, cartilage is compressed, forcing some of this water out; during relaxation of the joint, the water returns again. This "sponge effect" accounts for the resiliency of cartilage and how it works during exercise.

Unlike most other tissues, cartilage does not have a blood supply to bring in nutrients or allow repair processes to occur following damage; for example, a torn knee cartilage will not heal itself, so it may ultimately have to be removed by surgery. Cartilage gets its nutrients from the joint fluid that flows in and out during compression and relaxation of the cartilage. Inactivity leads to thinning of joint cartilage and to damage, a sequence seen often in older people. This in turn leads to osteoarthritis — so-called wear-and-tear arthritis, which seems paradoxically to affect so many less-active people. On the other hand, regular exercise increases nutrient flow and helps maintain the health and integrity of joint cartilage.

CONNECTIVE TISSUES

A number of specialized tissues connect muscles and bones. These connective tissues include tendons, ligaments, fascia, and other elastic tissues found throughout the body, including those enveloping and holding muscle fibers together. Connective tissue also forms the joint capsules, which are important components in maintaining joint integrity. Connective tissues are passive, since they don't participate in muscle contraction, but they are still very important in exercise and in injury prevention.

Tendons

Tendons are formed when the sheaths that envelop muscles and converge into the strong fibrous bands that attach the muscles to bone (see Figure 2–3). These bands are characterized by tensile strength, but they also have some degree of elasticity. Most tendons are surrounded by their own sheaths, which provide lubrication. The best-known tendon is the Achilles, which you can feel just above your heel, where it attaches the large calf muscle to the ankle.

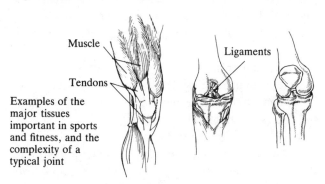

Examples of the major tissues important in sports and fitness, and the complexity of a typical joint

FIGURE 2–3: *The Knee*

Tendons are living tissues, and their intrinsic strength is increased by exercise. Because they function as anchors transmitting enormous forces, they are especially susceptible to injuries, particularly those arising from overuse. This produces inflammation in and around the tendon — "tendinitis" — often limiting motion and causing pain.

In the last few years, the sports world has discovered what dancers and martial arts devotees have known for millennia — that tendons are important determinants of flexibility, and that flexibility enhances athletic performance and reduces injury.

Flexibility is simply the range of motion at a given joint. The greater the range of motion, the greater the flexibility. Flexibility, for most of us, is limited by the tightness or degree of elasticity of our tendons, although it is influenced to some extent by muscular tightness and by joint structures themselves.

Paradoxically, flexibility may be decreased by exercise, if training is not balanced by a conditioning program that includes stretching exercises. As muscles become stronger, they may become shorter, stiffer, and tighter. Tendons, because they are specialized for strength, not for elasticity, may also become less flexible as you get stronger. Examples of this tendency toward musculotendonous tightness are found in the hamstring muscles of runners and the shoulders of swimmers. Each is associated with reduced flexibility around the relevant joints, and each is associated with an increased risk of injury as well.

But you can prevent this side effect of fitness by carrying out a balanced fitness program (see Chapter 7), including flexibility training as well as strength and endurance work.

Ligaments

Ligaments are fibrous bands that connect bones across joints (see Figure 2–3). Because they are crucial for joint stability, ligaments sacrifice elasticity for strength; they are generally very strong but inflexible. For example, the knee's integrity depends on its four sets of ligaments even more than on its muscles and tendons. Ligaments tend to be injured only when too much force is applied, when subjected to overstress rather than overuse (see Chapter 11). Contact sports are the best example. The most common ligament injuries are sprains, partial to complete tears. But if you build up your muscles and tendons properly and if you warm up before you exercise, you can help prevent ligament damage.

JOINTS

That brings us to joints, the very complex structures that determine the nature of all athletic motion. Joints perform a seemingly impossible task. On the one hand, they need to allow flexibility and motion, while on the other hand, they must still provide support and stability. To achieve both these goals, nature has worked out a series of wonderful compromises, unique for each of the joints. The joint can be relatively simple, like the ball-and-socket joint of the hip, or very complex, like the knee (see Figure 2–4).

While each of our joints is different, each one contains the same basic elements. Fundamentally, joints are the juxtapositions of two or more bones, held together by a variety of structures, including muscles and tendons, ligaments, and the joint capsule. These structures allow a defined, controlled motion of one bone relative to the other, propelled by muscles. The two basic types of joint are the ball-and-socket joint and the hinge joint, but there are varieties within each type. The crucial joints for most of us, athletes or not, are the back (in truth, a complex series of joints linked together), the knee, the ankle, the hips, and the shoulders. Each joint uses a different cast of supporting characters to allow its specialized function. Let's discuss these major joints in detail.

The Back

Your back is a series of vertebrae, twenty-five in all, resting on one another. But functionally it is like one large joint with the mobility of a slinky toy. Each vertebra is attached to its neighbors by a series of very strong ligaments, and separated from them by a small gelatinous pad, the infamous disc, which functions as an organic shock absorber. Furthermore, it is important to note that your back is not straight. Rather it is a series of gentle curves beginning with the neck, reversing at the chest, again at the lower back, and reversing a final time in the tailbone area (see Figure 2–5).

As we indicated before, each position of your back depends on the integrity and strength of adjacent structures to carry out its function. When, for example, your neck muscles are weak, injured, tight, or under stress and go into spasm, the actual curve of the neck is lost and all the weight of the head is then lined up over the back's cervical vertebrae — a prescription for trouble.

The thoracic portion of the spine is actually the most protected since its curvature is linked to the bony struc-

FIGURE 2–4: MAJOR JOINTS AND ADJACENT STRUCTURES

Joint	Bones	Type	Motions	Supporting Structures	Injury Risk in Athletes
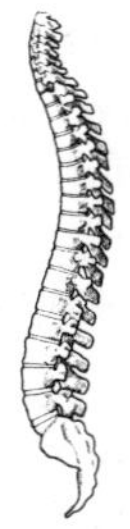 Back	Vertebrae	Simple hinge	Small amounts of flexion, extension, rotation	Paravertebral muscles Ligaments Adjacent structures (abdomen, pelvis)	Moderate
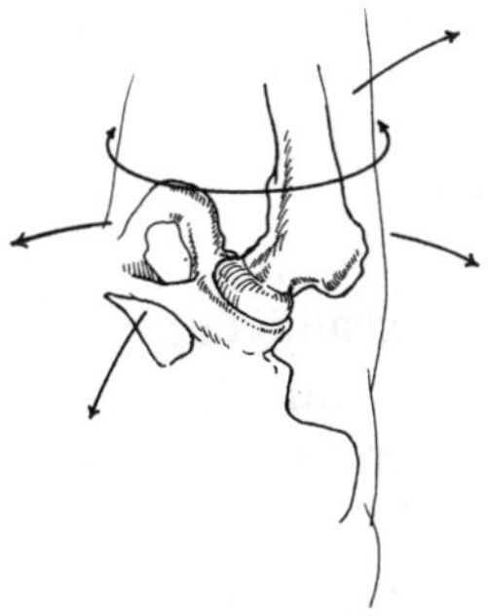 Hip	Pelvis, femur	Ball and socket, simple	Rotation, flexion, extension	Bones, muscles, ligaments	Low
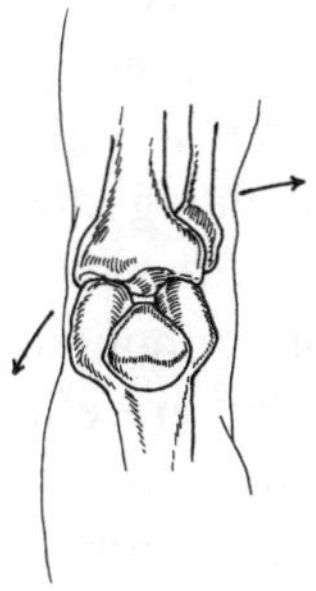 Knee	Femur, tibia, fibula, and patella	Complex hinge	Full flexion, extension, and rotation in certain positions	Ligaments, cartilage, quadriceps muscle, and patella tendon	High
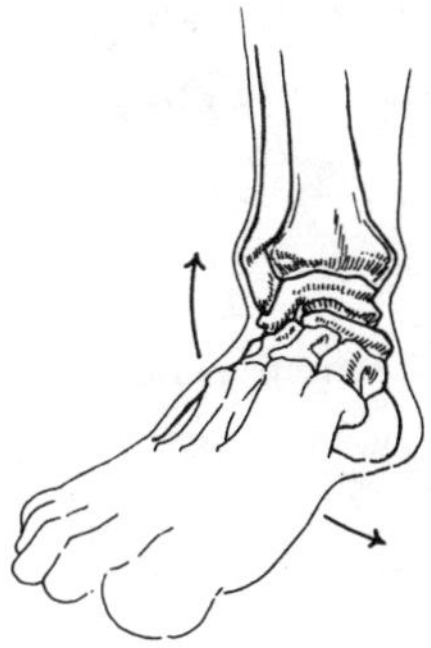 Ankle	Fibula, tibia, and heel bone	Simple hinge	Flexion, extension	Ligaments	Moderate
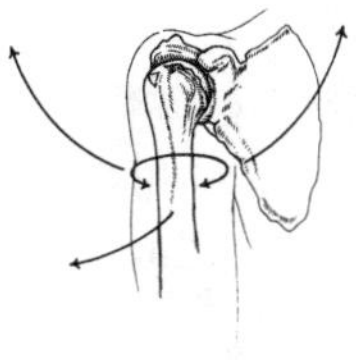 Shoulder	Scapula, clavicle, and humerus	Ball and socket, complex	Rotation, flexion, extension	Ligaments, tendons, muscles, joint capsule	High

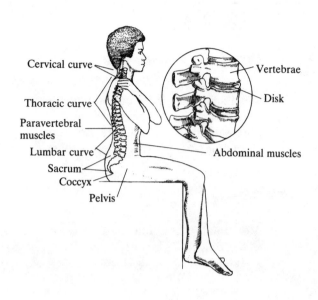

FIGURE 2–5: *The Back and Adjacent Structures*

ture of the ribs and chest. It has limited flexibility and is rarely injured. Its primary motion is only rotation.

However, the lower back is the most beautifully engineered and potentially the most vulnerable portion. On it and its adjacent structures rest the entire upper body. To deal with this, the lower back forms a column with the abdominal muscles, rather than carrying the weight by itself. Bear down as if you are going to lift something and you can feel how your abdominal muscles tighten up to form a rigid cylinder. Of course, if your abdominal muscles are weak or your gut hangs out and cannot carry its weight, you can't depend on your abdomen and you've set the scene for back trouble.

Just as your lower back depends on your abdomen for strength, it depends on your pelvis for flexibility. While the vertebrae can bend forward and backward somewhat, most of the forward flexion of your trunk occurs by rotation of your pelvis, and thus depends on good flexibility of the hamstrings and iliopsoas muscles. If they are too tight, the natural curve will be distorted and lead to chronic aches. At the end of this chapter we will have a special section to help you assess your back's level of fitness.

The Hip

Your hip is probably your strongest joint, a ball and socket formed by the femur and the pelvic bones, which

also allows moderately good mobility. It is surrounded by strong muscles and ligaments. It is rarely injured itself, but the surrounding structures include thirteen bursae and muscles that are subject to overuse and injury. The hip moves forward and backward and rotates. Because of its strong surroundings, it is particularly prone to inflexibility. We have already discussed the importance of hip flexibility in the pelvic component of back flexion, and the same need for hip flexibility is true in all running sports where tightness leads to hamstring, groin, and thigh injuries, usually muscle pulls or strains. Flexibility, more than strength, is the key conditioning mode for your hips.

The Knee

There are at least three hundred thousand athletic knee injuries in the United States each year. Although the knee can be injured during any form of exercise, some sports are more hazardous than others. Skiing leads the list, with football, basketball, skating, track and field, soccer, and baseball rounding out the top seven.

Why are knee injuries so prevalent in sports? The joint's anatomy accounts for its vulnerability. Although the knee is fundamentally a hinge joint, it is actually much more complex than its simple bending and straightening motions would suggest. In fact, the knee also allows sliding and rotary motion. These motions permit the knee the mobility that is essential for graceful athletic movements. But to permit these motions, the knee is a fundamentally unstable joint prone to injury.

The integrity of the knee does not depend on the alignment of the bones themselves, but on surrounding structures (see Figure 2–6). On the outside of the knee,

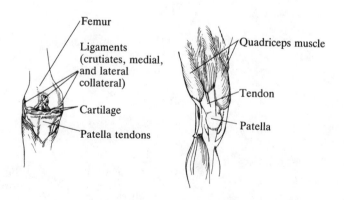

FIGURE 2–6: *The Knee and Its Critical Structures*

ligaments at the sides and rear provide stability. At the front is the kneecap, or patella, which gives protection. The inside of the knee joint is also stabilized by ligaments and by the two knee cartilages, which also act to absorb shock and to provide a smooth surface for the bones to glide on. Additionally, the thigh bone (the femur) and shinbone (the tibia) are themselves covered by shiny cartilage, which allows gliding with low friction. The knee joint is lined by a fine joint membrane, which produces fluid that lubricates and cushions the entire apparatus. Finally, additional cushioning and lubrication are provided by the ten fluid-filled sacs, or bursae, in and around the knee.

Movement of the joint is controlled by the large thigh muscles that also support and stabilize the knee. The fibrous tendons of these muscles pass across the knee, so that inflammation or tendinitis of these structures can also produce knee pain.

The Ankle

Your ankle is among the simplest of joints. It is fundamentally a hinge that allows only restricted motion, merely up and down. The twisting motions all occur in your foot. The ankle is formed by the two lower leg bones, the fibula (on the outside) and the tibia (on the inside, making up the shin), which create a socket that fits over the heel bone. It is entirely supported by ligaments that hold the three bones together, and there are no muscle attachments. The ligaments at the front and back of the ankle are relatively weak, but the ones on the sides are strong and thick and provide good lateral support. The ankle is probably the most commonly injured joint, generally because of sprains and tears of the ligaments holding the fibula to the heel. As with the back and knee, strength and flexibility of adjacent tendons and muscles, as well as strength of the ankle ligaments themselves, are essential to the continued integrity of the joint.

The Shoulder

Finally, among the key joints, your shoulder allows the most complex motions. In order for you to understand both the strengths and weaknesses of the shoulder, just imagine yourself passing a football, hitting the backhand in tennis, or swimming the butterfly. Each of these motions requires an extraordinary degree of mobility at the shoulder, and each of them puts great stress on that joint. Although the shoulder is engineered for maximum mobility, this very freedom of motion means that

it also is susceptible to injuries. Starting out as a ball-and-socket joint like the hip, the shoulder evolved until it now sits in a very shallow groove and so has a remarkable freedom from constraints and a remarkable range of motion. The head of the humerus (arm bone) is the ball, and the socket is composed of a smooth, depressed surface at the outer margin of the shoulder blade (scapula). Part of the scapula also comes around the top rear of the shoulder joint where it joins with the collarbone (see Figure 2–7). The bony structures

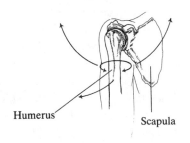

Humerus   Scapula

FIGURE 2–7: *The Shoulder*

of the shoulder girdle are surrounded by numerous muscles, both big and small, which move the shoulder through its extraordinary range. In addition, the shoulder is stabilized by a number of ligaments, and also by the capsule that surrounds the joint. Finally, the normal anatomy of the shoulder includes the bursae sacs, which provide the cushioning and lubrication for the shoulder as it moves through its range. This reliance on muscles and connective tissues makes the shoulder the joint most commonly dislocated, which means that you have to develop good strength and maintain good flexibility to keep it functioning well.

Thus you can see that most joint injuries are, in fact, injuries to one or more of the supporting structures of joints — specifically ligaments, tendons, and muscles. By strengthening these, you can reduce the chance of injury to the joint itself. This is an important goal of conditioning for sports as well as for health. Joint and musculoskeletal injuries, especially back, shoulder, knee, and ankle strains and sprains are a major cause of disability in everyday life. Most are preventable by good conditioning. It is merely a question of developing the joints to the point where they can handle the stresses that will be applied in sports and in everyday life. Your joints are the crucial elements in all your life's physical activity.

MUSCLES

Well-developed muscles are the most visible testament to physical fitness. However, you have to look beyond the bulk, the most obvious aspect of muscles, to understand muscular fitness. Physical size is not the most important functional characteristic of muscle.

We each have more than four hundred muscles, some small, some large, and these muscles perform many functions essential to life, whether we are athletes or not. At birth, the number of muscle cells in your body is fixed. Their bulk and function, however, can improve or deteriorate, depending on their use.

Muscles move. They are highly specialized tissues that can shorten and generate tension. *Smooth muscle*, so named because of its appearance under the microscope, controls *involuntary* functions, such as the narrowing and widening of the blood vessels, or the contracting of the intestines. *Skeletal muscle*, which appears striped or "striated" under the microscope, is responsible for *voluntary* function, ranging from a flick of a finger to a leap over a hurdle. The heart muscle, discussed in Chapter 1, is unique, containing some of the properties of both smooth and striated muscle.

Smooth muscle and cardiac muscle depend on the autonomic nervous system for control, but each can function even if the nerves are damaged. Striated muscle depends on the voluntary nervous system but cannot function alone; if the nerve is cut, the muscle is paralyzed, which emphasizes the interdependence of the muscular and nervous systems. Our discussion here will focus primarily on voluntary, striated, muscle.

Voluntary muscles are organized functionally into opposing pairs — the agonist and the antagonist. The agonist is the muscle that contracts to produce a given motion, while its antagonist relaxes. For example, when you bend your elbow, the biceps muscle contracts and is the agonist, while the triceps muscle relaxes and is the antagonist (see Figure 2–9).

Muscles are composed of bundles of muscle fibers held together in an elastic connective tissue sheath, which plays an important role in muscle flexibility, elasticity, and resistance to stress. The muscle fibers themselves are made up of individual muscle cells, lined up end-to-end and firmly bound together. Inside the cells are highly organized rows of specialized proteins called actin and myosin. When the nerve attached to the muscle fiber gives the signal to contract, the actin is pulled over the myosin, thus shortening the muscle and causing a muscle contraction.

The nervous system is responsible for coordinating muscular activity, sending the signals that cause the agonist muscle to contract and the antagonist to relax. Each muscle fiber has its own small nerve, which causes it to contract. Together the nerve and muscle fiber are called "a motor unit." In addition, there are specialized cell units called "spindle fibers," which detect stretching

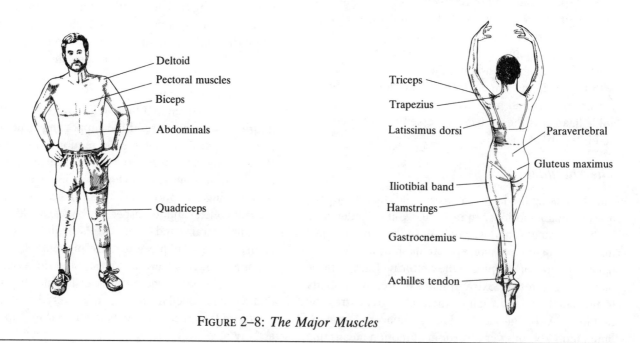

FIGURE 2–8: *The Major Muscles*

Deltoid
Pectoral muscles
Biceps
Abdominals
Quadriceps

Triceps
Trapezius
Latissimus dorsi
Paravertebral
Gluteus maximus
Iliotibial band
Hamstrings
Gastrocnemius
Achilles tendon

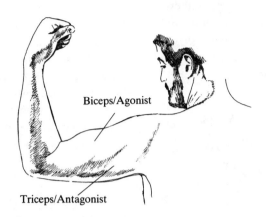

FIGURE 2–9: *The Relationship between Muscle Groups*

or lengthening of the muscle they are part of. These stretch detectors in turn cause a reflex contraction of this muscle when they are stimulated. At the same time, the stretch receptors cause the antagonist muscle to relax.

As esoteric as this may sound, it is readily demonstrable. Just think about the familiar knee-jerk reflex. In that maneuver, the quadriceps muscle is stretched briefly by a tap of the hammer below the kneecap. This brief stretch activates the spindle fiber and causes a reflex contraction of the quadriceps muscle and simultaneously a relaxation of the hamstring muscle, allowing the leg to kick.

Within the muscle cells are subcellular organelles called mitochondria — small, saclike structures packed with enzymes. Mitochondria convert glycogen to glucose, and then break it down further by combining it with oxygen to produce water, carbon dioxide — and the energy muscles need to contract (see Chapter 4). A final essential component of muscles is the network of capillaries surrounding all muscle cells, bringing in oxygen and nutrients and carrying away waste products such as carbon dioxide and lactic acid.

Although all muscles share these same properties, skeletal muscle tissue is not homogeneous. In fact, there are two major types of muscle fibers, which have different structural and functional properties. Certain fibers contract rapidly and are called (naturally) "fast-twitch" fibers; others twitch more slowly, and are called "slow-twitch" fibers.

Fast-twitch fibers contract rapidly, fatigue quickly, and function better anaerobically, that is, without a steady input of oxygen. Not surprisingly, athletes who excel in short, high-output sports like sprinting seem to be richly endowed with fast-twitch fibers. Those athletes who excel at endurance sports seem to have a high proportion of slow-twitch fibers, which function more slowly but for longer periods of time before fatiguing. Basically, these slow-twitch fibers metabolize their energy aerobically. They have large numbers of mitochondria and large numbers of capillaries to bring in oxygen and nutrients and to carry off carbon dioxide. As a result, they look different: slow-twitch fibers are red because of their rich blood supply, whereas fast-twitch fibers are white. White muscle tissue is primarily responsible for strength and speed, and red muscle tissue functions primarily to provide endurance.

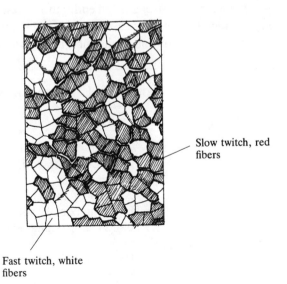

Slow twitch, red fibers

Fast twitch, white fibers

FIGURE 2–10: *A Cross-section of Muscle Demonstrating the Network of Slow- and Fast-Twitch Fibers*

Here again, we see the role of genetics in sports, for the relative proportion of fast- and slow-twitch fiber is fixed at birth and differs from individual to individual. There seems to be relatively little conversion of one fiber type into another, regardless of conditioning. You have to work with what you are born with.

THE PHYSIOLOGICAL BASIS OF EXERCISE AND CONDITIONING: ENDURANCE, STRENGTH, SKILL, AND STYLE

To understand the way to train your muscles, the principle of "specificity" is prominent. Unlike the heart, which is strengthened whether you run or swim, the conditioning of voluntary muscles is highly specific. The muscles you use while running will not help your swimming. Having a good backhand will not help your forehand, at least from the muscular point of view.

The primary hallmarks of good muscular function are strength and endurance. Muscular bulk is not synonymous with strength. Many athletes, both men and women, have lean muscles that are enormously strong. Soccer players, middle-distance runners, and hurdlers, for example, are invariably lean but require considerable degrees of both upper- and lower-body strength. They also have a high degree of muscular endurance — that is, the ability to function for prolonged periods of time without fatigue. Superior muscle function combines these two characteristics, strength and endurance; these functional principles are the true test of muscular fitness.

Muscular strength and endurance are important in sports and in daily life. In particular, your back, shoulders, and knees are stressed repeatedly, and if they are in good shape, they will function well. When you need to carry your suitcase in the airport, walk a few flights of stairs, or pick up some firewood, you depend on muscles to function properly. Most people who are not fit will do even these modest activities reluctantly, not trusting their strength. But if you are in shape, you'll know you can depend on your body, and you will enjoy every opportunity for exercise.

ENDURANCE AND THE ENERGETICS OF MUSCULAR ACTION

It is the cramps that finally do it. Watching the last five miles of a marathon is a primer on endurance, without which runners "hit the wall." This is the point on the course where those runners who are less well prepared run out of gas; where their muscles finally are depleted of stores of energy; where, as George Sheehan says, the hopeful seven-minute-per-mile pace of the first part of the marathon becomes the laboring ten-minute-per-mile slog at the end. But the final blows come as the muscles turn from utilizing sugars to utilizing less-well-metabolized fats for energy, and waste products begin to accumulate, causing spasms, cramps, and pain. Running is not the problem at this point; even walking becomes difficult.

We are not likely to find a more dramatic example of the importance of endurance in athletic activity. But you don't have to be a marathon runner to appreciate the benefits of endurance — or to build up your endurance capabilities, for that matter. Any activity in

FIGURE 2–11: CHARACTERISTICS OF MUSCLE FUNCTION BY FIBER TYPE

Characteristic	*Fast-twitch*	*Slow-twitch*
Aerobic metabolism	+	+ + + +
Anaerobic metabolism	+ + + +	+
Mitochondria	+ +	+ + +
Number of capillaries	+ +	+ + + +
Use in maximal exercise	+ + + +	+ +
Use in submaximal exercise	+ +	+ + + +
Strength	+ + + +	+ +
Endurance	+	+ + + +
Speed	+ + + +	+

+ to + + + + indicate slightly to highly characteristic

which muscles work repeatedly against low levels of resistance increases the endurance of the particular muscle(s) in question.

To understand endurance, we have to look into physiology. We now know, after twenty years of experimental studies, that training muscles for endurance enhances the synthesis and deposition of glycogen, the storage form of glucose, in actively trained muscles. The more you train, the more glycogen your muscles store. Not surprisingly, slow-twitch muscle fibers, responsible for aerobic, low-resistance, high-repetition muscular work, store glycogen preferentially over fast-twitch fibers. They also have the highest concentration of the enzymes ready to convert that glycogen into sugar and then into high-energy compounds to fuel the muscle fibers.

The amount of glycogen a muscle contains directly affects the duration of the exercise it can perform. When glycogen is depleted, fatigue sets in. This is probably what happens when runners "hit the wall." Since the amount of glycogen (and, thus, muscular endurance) depends on conditioning, the work in marathoning is not the race but the months of training that occur before the start. If you put in the work, a marathon can be free of problems and a great deal of fun. Of course, the marathon is an extreme example, but the principle is the same, whether you run two to three miles, bike, walk, or rake the leaves.

The muscle cells, particularly the slow-twitch fibers, utilize both sugars and fats as sources of energy under optimal (aerobic) conditions. But where the muscles rely on a glycogen supply already stored in the muscle cells themselves, fats are actively transported to the muscle cells by blood-borne triglycerides. Scientists still do not understand why the body needs both sources of energy, but it's clear that in most cases the proportion of fat to sugar utilized in the muscle cell at any given time reveals the intensity of the exercise experience. As a rule, the more intense the exercise, the less fat can be used as a source of energy.

But during prolonged endurance activities, fat becomes a very important factor indeed. Take a marathon cross-country ski race, for example. The last stretch may be carried out with only fat fueling the skier's muscles. And as the skiers cross the finish line, breathing hard, observers might sense a sickly, sweet odor — ketones, a waste product from fat breakdown.

Aerobic conditions are the norm in most endurance exercise. On the other hand, when there is insufficient oxygen, whether because of the nature or the intensity of the exercise, the body must generate its energy anaerobically (without oxygen), which results in the inefficient, incomplete metabolism of glucose, releasing smaller amounts of energy and triggering the production of lactic acid. Lactic acid has the undesirable characteristic of lowering the pH (increasing the acid content) of the blood, leading to decreased efficiency of muscular work, cramps, and fatigue.

To better understand the differences between anaerobic activity and endurance activity, let's take another look at running, this time in a few different competitive situations. In the 100-yard dash, you don't really have to generate new energy for your muscles by breathing hard and taking on a lot of oxygen. Your body will call on its fast-twitch muscle cells and use only their preformed energy. By panting afterward, you replenish muscle oxygen stores and get rid of excess carbon dioxide.

At distances of one-quarter to one-half mile, if you're running at full throttle, you will breathe hard, no matter how good your cardiovascular conditioning is. Since your circulation cannot deliver the necessary oxygen, your muscles will rely on anaerobic metabolism of glucose, producing lots of lactic acid and carbon dioxide. Again, your body builds up a large oxygen debt and carbon dioxide excess that need to be dealt with after you run, by panting.

In a ten-kilometer race, however, you'll be running slower, at no more than 85 percent of your maximum. Hence, your body will function aerobically, and you will be much more dependent on slow-twitch fibers and the quality of your circulation, which pumps oxygen-laden blood for efficient use of energy stores. You may breathe hard on a few hills as you temporarily become anaerobic from the extra work, but you should be able to recover afterward without feeling breathless. Finally, when you decide to run a marathon, the limit to your performance might then be the total amount of sugar in your muscles. While a few hills might cause you to breathe heavily, you should be able to talk the whole way, and after the race you should have no oxygen debt or need to catch your breath.

As you will see in Part III, this book emphasizes fitness through "lifesports" — those sports which are more like the 10-kilometer run than the 100-yard dash. They are predominantly aerobic, develop and depend on good cardiovascular conditioning, use slow-twitch muscle fibers, and are associated with high levels of energy stores in the form of glycogen. Lifesports are endurance sports. But to endure you have to be strong.

The relationship between strength and endurance can be illustrated with one simple test: the vertical leap, in which the subject jumps as high as he can from a stationary start. You can use the vertical leap to test yourself for strength or explosive power (see Self-Assessment, pages 45 and 48), and you can learn a lot from top athletes who have been tested. Intuitively, you'd think that a slender distance runner could outjump a much heavier sprinter, to say nothing of a bulky weight lifter. Yet distance runners average only fourteen inches while sprinters average twice that. And Olympic weight-lifting champion Paul Anderson was able to propel his 300-pound body thirty-one inches in the vertical leap.

To be sure, the tremendous explosive power generated by sprinters, swimmers (Mark Spitz's vertical leap was twenty-six inches), and weight lifters is in part due to their inborn ability. But training also plays a role. Speed training and strength training using the high-resistance, low-repetition technique increase explosive power. But a steady diet of endurance training can do just the reverse. In 1968, the year he won the Boston Marathon, Amby Burfoot had a vertical leap of only nine inches. Two years after his "retirement" from a steady diet of endurance training, he was retested, and was able to jump twenty inches.

High-resistance, low-repetition exercise builds strength and explosive power, whereas high-repetition, low-resistance exercise builds endurance. The differences between these two forms of muscle training are summarized in Figure 2–12. Both forms of training are important for fitness and sports, and both are included in our balanced training program (see Chapter 7). But if your sport requires you to emphasize only one form of training, your muscles may actually develop one set of abilities at the expense of the others.

Both types of exercise can improve performance in sports and can help prevent athletic injuries; neither will improve flexibility. Both types of exercise are specific for the muscles you are using; for example, biceps training will improve your biceps but not your triceps, and abdominal muscle strengthening will help your abdomen but not your legs.

Calisthenics and endurance exercises (such as the lifesports described in Chapters 8 and 9) will affect your muscles in the same ways as low-resistance, high-repetition training.

These training methods also affect your heart and circulation (see Chapter 1, pages 6–8 and Figure 1–6). High-resistance exercises produce large increases in blood pressure; they should be avoided by people with hypertension and heart disease, and should be done with caution following medical clearance by people over the age of fifty. If high-repetition exercises are performed faithfully over several months, they will improve your heart function and blood cholesterol, but high-resistance exercise will not.

MUSCULAR STRENGTH

Strength is the other major characteristic of muscular performance. And once again, heredity plays a part by determining to some degree an individual's level of strength. Some people are born with the potential to develop stronger muscles than others, and men are generally stronger than women. But far more important is the degree to which any individual develops and increases muscular strength through exercise and conditioning.

There are two basic types of strength exercises: low resistance and high resistance. Low-resistance exercise calls for stressing a muscle against relatively light resistance — say, a light dumbbell — for a high number

---

FIGURE 2–12: HOW WEIGHT TRAINING BUILDS YOUR MUSCLES

Effects on muscles	Low resistance, high repetition	High resistance, low repetition
Fiber types	Slow twitch	Fast twitch
Muscle metabolism	Aerobic	Anaerobic
Muscle size (mass)	Slight increase	Large increase
Endurance	Large increase	Slight increase
Strength	Slight increase	Large increase

of repetitions over a prolonged period of time and tends to be aerobic. It utilizes more slow-twitch muscle fibers and builds endurance and cardiovascular fitness more than strength.

High-resistance exercise allows you to exert a maximum voluntary force, by lifting a heavy barbell, for example, only a few times before fatigue sets in; it tends to be anaerobic, uses fast-twitch fibers, and builds power more than endurance. High-resistance exercise should be done through a full range of motion, from the most stretched or extended to the most contracted or flexed to avoid muscle tightness.

Full-range, high-resistance, low-repetition exercise can be performed with free weights or with exercise machines, such as the Nautilus apparatus. These exercises provide near-maximum force through the full range of muscle action. If done correctly, they avoid inflexibility while still improving muscle tone and bulk. On the other hand, they contribute little to muscular endurance, since they utilize primarily fast-twitch, easily fatiguing, anaerobic muscle fibers and are performed for a limited number of repetitions. (See Chapter 6 for specific exercise routines.)

One other important aspect of resistance or strength training should be mentioned. Not only do you benefit by lifting a weight up, you benefit by putting it down as well. In both high- and low-resistance dynamic training, conditioning occurs both during the concentric phase (the phase in which a muscle is contracted, while lifting a weight) and the eccentric phase (the phase in which the muscle is lengthening, while setting the weight down again). In fact, muscles are capable of greater force during eccentric motion, and all training programs should provide for both concentric and eccentric training. This is true for sports conditioning as well as weight training. For example, running up hills uses the quadriceps muscle in a concentric fashion, helping the runner bound up the hill; while running down hills uses the quadriceps in an eccentric manner, helping to slow the runner after landing.

Finally, remember the principle of specificity: only those muscles you train will grow stronger. The corollary is that to be generally in shape, your program has to work all the major muscle groups.

Strength: Muscle Mass

Working your muscles against high resistance causes an increase in muscle mass. This increase occurs primarily in the fast-twitch fibers. Each muscle cell increases in size (hypertrophy) and this can produce a striking increase in muscle bulk; however, this phenomenon occurs primarily in men, since it depends on testosterone, the male hormone. For a long time, the fear of bulky muscles prevented women from using resistance exercise to increase their strength, lest they end up looking like Arnold Schwarzenegger. That myth has been largely dispelled in recent years, and most top-flight female athletes now use weights and resistance-based exercises.

Because testosterone enhances muscle bulk, illicit use of male hormones in an attempt to help increase muscle strength began in the 1940s. Synthetic male (androgenic) hormones have replaced testosterone for therapeutic purposes, but their use by athletes has caused continued controversy and the evidence of their effectiveness is mixed. Steroids do increase muscle bulk in bodybuilders, but the benefit in other athletes is uncertain. In women, the muscle-building effect of such steroids is pronounced, but the masculinizing effects of even synthetic steroids are very significant. Furthermore, these steroids may have potential adverse reactions, including alteration of the body's own production of hormones, testicular atrophy in men, skin changes, liver injury, and potentially even liver cancer. We are not alone in believing that steroids should not be used in an attempt to enhance performance or strength. There is no "quick fix" — the only safe and effective way to build your muscles and strength is with training (see Chapter 6).

Strength: Muscle Fiber Recruitment

Strength depends on more than just muscle mass and bulk; another important determinant of strength is the recruitment effect. To illustrate this mechanism, think of the anecdotes about people lifting enormous loads under emergency situations, or athletes producing one performance far in excess of their usual. For example, Bob Beamon's Olympic and world record broad jump in 1968 in Mexico City far eclipsed anything he or his competitors had previously been able to do and stands to this day. These extraordinary feats are as much a physiological accomplishment as they are a mental one. To understand this let's look at the muscles themselves.

These occasional bursts of exceptional strength are related to the way muscle fibers contract and fire — the way muscle fibers are "recruited." Not all the fibers in a given muscle contract at once during a specific motion or action. Rather, different motor units (the nerve attached to its muscle cells) are recruited for different levels of force. Thus, slow-twitch fibers may be recruited for a 20 percent effort, and their nerve cells may be firing at ten times per second. As the force is increased, the nerve may increase its firing rate to twenty times per second and, in addition, other nerves begin to fire, adding other muscle fibers to the effort. This process continues, with some of the slower fibers dropping out and others being recruited, until at a maximum contraction, large nerves attached to fast-twitch fibers are firing at rapid rates of eighty to one hundred times per second, and maximum force is achieved.

The process of muscle fiber recruitment and the nerve's firing rate is not under voluntary control. But training can help. As a motion or activity is repeated, it becomes ingrained, recruitment occurs more effectively, and the body performs the activity with increasing coordination and efficiency. Consequently, there is an increased ability to produce a maximal contraction; and strength increases. Certain things can enhance the process; for example, adrenaline. This is why the excitement of competition can spur you to a super effort. In addition, some of the rituals of the athlete may be more than simple habit or superstition. Bouncing the ball before a foul shot, swinging the bat while awaiting the pitch, practicing your return stroke before the serve is under way, may all facilitate fiber recruitment and allow for a quicker, more coordinated or powerful motion. Even a loud shout has been shown to help muscle fiber recruitment (giving validity to the verbal habits of karate experts). In fact, much of the martial arts repertoire seems to be built on the control and development of these neurophysiologic mechanisms.

As paradoxical as it may seem, another aspect of strength has to do with mechanisms that help muscles to relax. Remember that every muscle is opposed by another muscle, forming an agonist-antagonist pair, such as your biceps and triceps. When the agonist is working, it must spend some of its effort to overcome the tone of the antagonist. If the antagonist is more fully relaxed, the agonist can do more external work. For example, your biceps will be able to lift more weight in the curl if your triceps is more relaxed. And training will help — as you do the curl repeatedly, your triceps will be trained to relax more, even as your biceps is trained to recruit more muscle fibers. For some activities, such as running the 100-yard dash, in which rapid, repeated contraction and relaxation of the quads and hamstrings occur, speed is enhanced by efficient relaxation as much as by rapid contraction, and enhanced by training. Training of this type seems to affect neurophysiologic mechanisms that operate at the level of the spinal cord.

Another aspect of strength applies especially to athletic activity. Often, particularly in competitive sports, pure strength is irrelevant. What is necessary is so-called explosive strength — the ability to produce a maximal output, practically instantaneously. The mechanisms responsible for explosive strength are complex, involving all of the factors we have just described, as well as some psychophysiological factors we can only guess at. Training helps build this form of strength for the competitive athlete, but what makes it all come together is not clear.

In summary, all exercise depends on a combination of muscular strength and endurance. Training enhances these attributes by complex biochemical, neurological, and physiologic mechanisms. It's important to remember that while endurance and strength training generally complement each other, the principle of specificity applies, and excessive reliance on either strength or endurance training can limit the other. Athletes who train only for the marathon have demonstrably less strength than those who use a balanced conditioning program. The conclusion is that to be generally fit, you must engage in a training program that benefits your whole body (see Chapters 6 and 7).

SKILL AND STYLE: OTHER ASPECTS OF CONDITIONING

Certain other components of neuromuscular fitness determine the way you perform and play: speed, reaction time, coordination, balance, and kinesthetic sense. Like all aspects of fitness, they can be improved by training, but only to certain individual limits.

Speed

Speed depends on muscle function. Speed requires strength, but it is more than strength. Speed requires enough endurance to train repetitively, but is obviously different from endurance. For the athlete, speed is defined by the stopwatch, but for the physiologist, speed is rapid repetitive development of maximal force, utilizing rapid-twitch fibers. The potential to develop speed is inherited, but can be enhanced by training. Age is also a factor, as maximum speed declines from its peak at age twenty to twenty-four. Speed can be enhanced by training and conditioning at any age; such training is very desirable for the competitive athlete, but is quite optional for general fitness and health. Finally, as in any muscular activity, speed will develop specifically in the muscles that are trained for it; punching a speed bag will produce quick hands but not quick feet.

Reaction Time

Reaction time is the time needed for a muscle group to respond to a stimulus — your "reflexes." Reaction time can be improved by training. Interestingly, this improvement is not specific to the muscles used in training, but is a function of the body as a whole. If you are fit, you will react more quickly — whether you are returning a serve or reaching for a glass before it topples off a shelf. Not all sports demand quick reaction, nor do all sports produce them. However, quick reactions are a general feature of fitness.

Coordination

Coordination depends on strength, endurance, speed, and reaction time, as well as on athletic skill. It is the ability to shift smoothly from one motion or position to another. Some people are naturally more graceful than others, but coordination can be learned and improved considerably. While training for coordination is relatively specific to the muscles being used, it does carry over to related exercises. Thus, rope jumping will help you develop good footwork for dancing, tennis, and soccer.

Balance

At first glance, balance would not seem to be a function of fitness, since the major control of balance is the inner ear, which functions as the body's gyroscope, orienting you in space. But fine balance also depends on the input from stretch reflexes in muscles, on visual cues, and on reaction time. These aspects of balance can be enhanced by training for fitness and sports.

Kinesthetic Sense

This term describes your ability to know where the parts of your body are in relation to each other and to space. The ability to clap your hands with your eyes closed depends on kinesthetic sense. It is a highly sophisticated neurological function, which relies on many components of the central nervous system. Kinesthetic sense is important to all athletic activity. Champion athletes have a more highly developed kinesthetic sense than the rest of us, but all of us can improve with training.

The study of the body in motion is the science of kinesthesiology. Kinesthesiologists are particularly interested in understanding the efficiency of action. Thus, they have learned that champion discus throwers remain tightly compacted in an isometric contraction during their spin before flinging their discus, while less talented throwers tend to spread out more. Kinesthesiology has taken a leap forward with the use of video and computer technologies, which can analyze the forces at each stage of an activity. So far, results have been more descriptive than prescriptive. In other words, knowing what to do and doing it are still two different things.

FATIGUE: WHY YOU GET TIRED

The sensation of fatigue can result either from changes in your muscles or your nervous system. The first, "peripheral fatigue," results from the depletion of carbohydrate energy stores and/or the buildup of waste products in muscle cells. Anaerobic exercise can resullt in early peripheral fatigue, primarily caused by a buildup of carbon dioxide and lactic acid, even before energy stores are depleted. Aerobic exercise can also result in muscle or peripheral fatigue, but this usually happens after the carbohydrate energy stores are used up and the muscles have to rely exclusively on fat as an energy source.

The second phenomenon, called "central fatigue," occurs when muscles themselves have adequate energy stores and circulation, but you still feel tired. Prolonged or intense exertion can use up *circulating* nutrients, primarily glucose from liver glycogen, and produce fatigue of the nervous system. As central nervous system fatigue occurs, your body may interpret this as muscular exhaustion. In addition, you will notice a loss of concentration and a diminished will to push yourself. Peripheral fatigue is specific to the muscles exercised; central fatigue is not.

Thus, fatigue during aerobic exercise, both "central" and "peripheral," is ultimately related to the depletion of energy stores. The primary goal of aerobic conditioning is to prevent fatigue and to develop endurance. Training builds endurance in several ways. First, by improving circulation, muscle fibers are assured of adequate amounts of oxygen for the generation of energy and for the disposal of carbon dioxide and acid by-products. Second, training stimulates the enzymes that manufacture and store glycogen in muscle. The amount of glycogen available is directly proportional to the amount of time a muscle cell can function. Third, training increases the amount of liver glycogen as well, and this is essential for maintaining the circulating blood glucose levels necessary for adequate central nervous system function.

Fatigue is a critical factor in athletic performance and injury. Peripheral fatigue produces decreased function of exercising muscle groups; you may attempt to compensate by altering style and using other muscles that are not adequately trained. Fatigue produces reductions in force, speed, and reaction time — and often "pulled" or strained muscles. Central fatigue leads to impaired judgment. It frequently shows up in sports, where dramatic declines in performance occur during the latter stages of a match or game. Similarly, injuries that tend to occur late in your exercise — such as the skier's infamous "last run" syndrome — are results of central fatigue and bad judgment, as well as poor muscular performance.

But in a sense, fatigue is not an altogether bad thing. Fatigue is an early warning system, telling you that enough is enough. Listen to your body — push to the point of fatigue and then back off so that you'll avoid injuries and be ready to work out again. Controlled workouts to the point of fatigue also provide a major stimulus for your body to improve. Depletion of your muscle's energy stores stimulates the muscle to store more glycogen than before. Tiring your muscles leads to increases in their strength and increased capillary circulation.

Thus fatigue, when achieved in a controlled fashion, is the gateway to further development; there is no gain without some strain. And when you are fit, you will recover quickly from the fatigue of a vigorous workout, so that the exercise — and even the fatigue at the end — is invigorating, relaxing, and enjoyable. This combination of stimulation and relaxation will be all you'll need to motivate you to work out regularly for fitness, health, sports, and fun.

SELF-ASSESSMENT

Before you begin your fitness program, you need to know your starting point. To assess your musculoskel-etal fitness, you'll have to evaluate your flexibility, strength, and your endurance. In each instance, key muscle groups or joints are the focus of the assessment. To determine your present fitness level, you don't have to push yourself to the absolute extremes of your physical capabilities. You don't have to *prove* anything with a self-test. Listen to your body. Before extrapolating from your general "self-test" to an entire fitness program, bear in mind that a visit to your doctor may be in order to insure that your fitness goals don't outstrip the sane and safe limits necessary to any fitness program. Remember, the poorer your rating at the outset, the greater your improvement range. And improve you will.

FLEXIBILITY

To assess your flexibility, you will have to get used to thinking in terms of angles around the important joints (see Figure 2–4). Use the exercises in Chapter 6 as models for the specific assessment and estimate your flexibility according to the guide on pages 46–47.

While flexibility is specific to the muscle and joint tested, your overall flexibility can also be assessed by your performance on these eight exercises in the guide. Using 1 point for poor, 2 for moderate, and 3 for good, add up your total stretching points. If you score 10 or less, make flexibility a major part of your overall program, devoting extra time and effort to it. If you are in the 11 to 15 range, you should concentrate on those specific areas that these tests show as tight. And if you are over 15, congratulations — but don't neglect a good set of stretches as part of your warm-up or cool-down. Remember, as your muscles get stronger, they will get tighter.

STRENGTH

How strong should you be? There is really no simple answer, since it depends a great deal on what you do in daily life and what sports you play. But we can provide some rough guidelines. As a general guide, your legs should be able to lift, at least in one-time maximal effort, at least 30 percent of your body weight. Similarly, you should be able to handle as a one-time effort 30 percent of your body weight in those exercises that use your back or torso. Your arms and shoulders, however, are less strong and may be able to lift only 20 percent of your body weight. In each case, divide the weight estimate in half if you are using only one arm or leg. If you can handle less than this weight, you are relatively weak and should focus on building strength.

Unfortunately, testing your strength using weights or resistance equipment is a haphazard business, in the literal sense; it is dangerous because lifting with a maximal effort can lead to injury even if you are well trained and know what you are doing. Just as no one would recommend you run a top-speed quarter-mile the first time you put on sneakers, you should not try to bench press at your limit your first time in a gym.

For that reason, we feel that calisthenics offer a good way to assess your muscular strength and endurance. Taken overall, you can decide how important strength training is to your total fitness program.

In the assessment of your strength by calisthenics, there is a range of normal, with women usually toward the lower end initially, and men toward the upper end. Calisthenics are a mixture of strength and muscular endurance, and increased numbers of repetitions indicate higher levels of fitness in both areas.

Muscles: Triceps, chest
Calisthenic: Push-ups (see Figure 6–74)
Repetitions: Less than 5 — poor
                   5 to 15 — moderate
                   16+ — good

Support yourself on your toes and hands with your arms about shoulder width and your body rigid. Slowly lower your chest to the floor and then return to the starting position. Women can do a half push up supporting themselves on their knees rather than their toes.

Muscles: Lower back
Calisthenic: Sit-backs (see Figure 6–92)
Repetitions: Less than 10 — poor
                   10 to 25 — moderate
                   26+ — good

Sit comfortably in a chair with your hands clasped behind your head. Lean forward until your chest touches your thighs and then return to starting position.

Muscles: Lower back, hams
Calisthenic: Toe touches (see Figure 6–89)
Repetitions: Less than 10 — poor
                   10 to 25 — moderate
                   26+ — good

Stand with your feet apart, your knees slightly bent, and your arms above your head. Lean forward slowly until your hands touch your toes, but do not strain. Then slowly unwind, straighten up, and return to the starting position.

Muscles: Quads
Calisthenic: Partial knee bends (see Figure 6–94)
Repetitions: Less than 10 — poor
                   10 to 25 — moderate
                   26+ — good

Stand with your hands on your hips. Bend at the knees but do not bend your knees past 90 degrees. Straighten up.

Muscles: Abdominals
Calisthenic: Sit-ups (see Figure 6–80)
Repetitions: Less than 10 — poor
                   10 to 25 — moderate
                   26+ — good

Lie on your back with your arms across your chest, curl up until your chest touches your thighs, and then uncurl down again. Do not strain or bounce.

A useful additional assessment for your lower back is the lying hyperextension. It should not be tried if you have back trouble! You perform this exercise while lying prone (face down) and raise your upper body off the floor. Score yourself on whether you can raise your upper body and where your arms are: extended adjacent to your ears, hands clasped behind your head, or at your sides (see Figure 6–90).

Arms extended, ribs and upper abdomen off floor	Good
Hands behind head, ribs off floor	Moderate
Hands by sides, head and neck off floor	Poor

One other measure of strength is the standing vertical leap. Obviously, you know by now that no single test can really estimate your strength, since it is specific to the muscles tested. But this test gives you an idea of lower body strength. It is also a measure of explosive power, which is related to speed, both important for sports. They will be improved by the speed training programs we provide in Chapter 6. Stand sideways next to a wall, with your dominant arm (the right for right-handed people) next to the wall. Track your hand up

STRUCTURE	EXERCISE	ACTIVITY	FLEXIBILITY		
			Poor	*Moderate*	*Good*
Ankle, Achilles	Achilles stretch (*Figure 6–2*)	Measure forward lean at heel relative to floor	75–90°	60–75°	45–60°
Calf	Calf stretch (*Figure 6–1*)	Same	80–90°	65–80°	45–65°
Hamstring	Straight-leg raising (*Figure 6–16*)	Measure angle between floor and raised leg	Less than 45°	45–80°	80–90°
Groin, hip adductors	Seated groin stretch (*Figure 6–6*)	Measure angle between floor and knee	45–30°	30–15°	15–0°

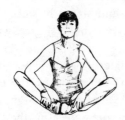

STRUCTURE	EXERCISE	ACTIVITY	FLEXIBILITY		
			Poor	*Moderate*	*Good*
Lower back, hams, pelvis	Toe touch (*Figure 6–11*)	Measure distance between finger-tips and toes. Do not lunge.	Lacks more than 3 inches	Touch top of foot	Touch floor
Hip flexor (iliopsoas)	Anterior thigh stretch (*Figure 6–9*)	Measure angle between knee and floor. Keep back flat.	45–30°	30–15°	15–0°
Knee, quadriceps	Quad stretch (*Figure 6–4*)	Measure angle between heel and buttock	More than 60°	60–30°	30–0°
Deltoid, rotator cuff	Shoulder stretch (*Figure 6–14*)	Measure distance between hands	More than 3 inches	3 to 1 inch	Touch hands

over your head as high as you can, and mark the wall at your maximum reach. Next, jump as high as you can without taking a step; again mark the wall at your highest point (a friend may have to assist you on marking the wall). Jump twice more. Measure the distance between your highest leap and your standing reach — the difference is your vertical leap.

How high should you be able to jump? Your vertical leap does not depend on your height or weight, but on your strength. Anthony "Spud" Webb is a basketball star with the Atlanta Hawks, and won the 1986 "slam dunk" competition. Dunk shots are not remarkable in the NBA, but they are extraordinary if you are no taller than Webb's 5'7". Webb's diminutive stature is offset by an astounding vertical leap of 42 inches. By comparison, David Thompson, one of basketball's great leapers, can jump 44 inches.

We have borrowed from James Counsilman, the legendary swimming coach at Indiana University, who has devised a simple rating system you can use to evaluate your leap. If you jump 10 to 15 inches, you have a relatively poor vertical leap, 16 to 22 inches, a moderate vertical leap, and 23 to 30 or more inches, a good leap.

To rate your overall strength, add up your scores on each of these seven strength tests. Score each poor as one point, each moderate as 2, and each good as 3. If you score 8 or less, make overall strength training a major part of your program. If you are in the 9–17 range, concentrate on the specific areas that are weak.

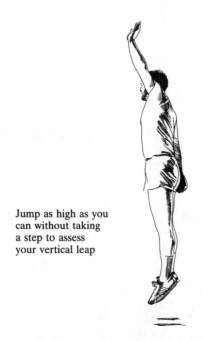

Jump as high as you can without taking a step to assess your vertical leap

FIGURE 2–13: *The Standing Vertical Leap*

And if you score over 17, focus your strength training to complement and support the sports you want to play.

ASSESSMENT OF YOUR BACK

Should you pay extra attention to your back, even if you never had problems there? A good way to know is to go through a careful assessment of your muscles and joints in terms of how they affect your back. Begin by assessing your posture.

As mentioned earlier, the normal configuration of the back is a series of gentle curves (see Figure 2–5) starting at the neck, reversing for the upper back, reversing again at the lower back, and, finally, reversing a last time in the short segment of the sacrum and tailbone. The two areas that most people have trouble with are the cervical spine (do you have the hunched-over look?) and the lumbar curve (is yours absent, indicating a lack of flexibility; or is it exaggerated, because of excessive abdominal weight or iliopsoas muscle tightness?). Compare our figures (2–14) with yours in a mirror, especially at the key areas. If your posture is poor, it is likely that you have poor flexibility and strength in key areas. Systematically check these as follows:

1. Flexibility. The key area of flexibility is the lumbar spine. The gentle lumbar curve, which helps maintain static posture, should be able to reverse completely during forward flexion, or be exaggerated by another 25 to 30 degrees upon backward extension. The simplest test is to bend forward with your knees slightly bent (to avoid any restrictions placed by your hamstring muscles) and ask someone to observe you (see Figure 2–15). Your back should be able to adopt a smooth forward curve. Try bending backward under the same conditions while holding your hips steady to test your extension.

Hamstring flexibility is next on the list. Tight hamstrings are probably the most common factor leading to back problems in younger men. The simplest test is straight-leg raising, already described in the flexibility assessment (page 46). Shoot for 90 degrees or better.

Less well known as a cause of back problems is tightness in the hip flexors and iliopsoas muscles. The test for this group is also covered in our flexibility assessment (page 47). Proper flexibility should allow you to lie with your back flat against the floor and your knee touching the floor. If it lacks 45 degrees of touching the floor, your thigh and iliopsoas muscle are very tight.

2. Strength. Back function depends on the strength of the paravertebral muscles and the abdominal mus-

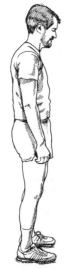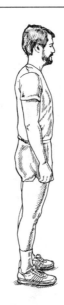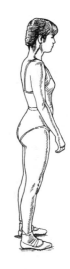

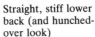

Straight, stiff lower
back (and hunched-
over look)

Normal posture

Exaggerated lumbar
curve

FIGURE 2–14: *Assess the Configuration of Your Back*

cles. Adequate abdominal strength can be assessed by doing conventional bent-knee sit-ups (see the section on strength assessment). Abdominal muscles function well isometrically since they have only a very small amount of shortening available to them. This means that when they are in shape, they have a high degree of tone.

A good assessment of your back muscle strength can be made while sitting in a chair and doing sit-backs (see page 157) or doing the hyperextension test (see page 45).

Set up a check list for your back's flexibility and strength, as discussed above, scoring plus for good and minus for any lower score. Unlike our previous sections, *any* score here less than plus means that you should pay special attention to your back, especially the deficient areas. Your back is truthfully only as good as its weakest or least flexible link. See Chapter 6, pages 158–159 for our back program.

Toe touch — note
the smooth rounded
curve of the lower
back

Back extension —
again note the
smooth curve of the
lower back

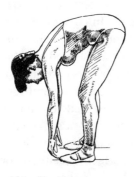

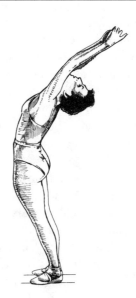

FIGURE 2–15: *Assess the Flexibility of Your Back*

3

Psychological Fitness

Physical exercise is not merely necessary to the health and development of the body, but to balance and correct intellectual pursuits as well. The mere athlete is brutal and philistine, the mere intellectual unstable and spiritless. The right education must tune the strings of the body and mind to perfect spiritual harmony.

— PLATO

Our goal is to show you how sports and exercise can promote your health. You may well wonder where psychological factors fit in. Remember our definition of total fitness: an individual's optimal ability to withstand stress, ranging from strenuous athletic competition, to the demands of everyday life, to illness, and even to the gradual stress of the aging process itself. Now it's time to explore the third fact of fitness: psychological fitness.

It's easy to see how psychological factors affect athletic performance; the will to win often determines the outcome of competition. The media have generated numerous synonyms for the will to win: determination, self-confidence, desire, hunger, drive, guts, toughness, and even the elusive "momentum" factor. And just as some athletes and teams win because they want to win and expect to win, others lose because they expect to lose or are, in fact, afraid to win. These are the competitors who look better in practice than in the game, who crumble under pressure, or who "blow the big one."

Although the psychology of winning — and losing — is a fascinating subject, it's not our subject here. Our goal is not to mold winners in competition but to help you develop yourself into a winner in life and health. We cannot agree with Vince Lombardi that winning is the only thing. In fact, for your health, *playing* is the only thing — winning is a happy plus. Winning can be an important motivator, but it should not dominate your use of exercise and sports for recreation and health.

Let's put aside the psychology of sports for the moment, and discuss how psychological factors affect daily life off the playing field — your happiness, your personal and professional performance, and especially your health. Just as the mind and body are inseparable aspects of every individual, so too are physical and mental fitness inseparably interrelated with exercise and sports.

YOUR MIND AND YOUR HEALTH

It is obvious that emotional factors play a major role in the satisfactions and successes of everyday life. A happy, well-adjusted person can find the silver lining in even the most difficult, stressful situations. He will bounce back from adversity and will have the inner resources to restructure his life so as to minimize future problems. In contrast, a person who brings anxiety or depression to any situation is much less able to surmount obstacles and is liable to crack under stress.

Mental factors determine whether you feel happy and relaxed or unhappy and tense. Your state of mind influences how well you function in your personal life, in your work, and at sports. Psychological factors also are of major importance in determining how you feel *physically*. Perfectly healthy people can feel perfectly miserable because they are anxious or depressed. In fact, many of the patients we see with purely "physical" complaints have no idea that they are depressed — they don't feel overtly sad, but they do lose weight, are sleepless, have abdominal pain or palpitations, and so on. As a result, they see an internist for a medical evaluation rather than a psychiatrist for a mental checkup. We can examine and test these patients in great depth without diagnosing a physical ailment. Nor is symptomatic treatment helpful — until the underlying psychological problems are recognized and dealt with.

We don't mean to imply that anybody with psychosomatic complaints is a hypochondriac or has major emotional problems. Quite the reverse is true: all of us experience functional complaints at one time or another because of transient stress or depression. Similarly, all of us are able to overlook illness or injury at a time of intense competition or excitement or when we are "up" or distracted by other activities.

Mental factors play a major role in modulating messages from your body to determine how you *feel* "physically." More important, mental factors can determine how you *are* physically; your mind can actually produce or exacerbate physical disease. Many of the most common disorders in twentieth-century America can be triggered by stress. Stomach ulcers and gastritis are well-known examples; there are five million cases in the United States, and ulcers are the twelfth leading cause of death. Another illness that is frequently exacerbated by tension is bronchial asthma. Of course not everyone with stress will develop belly pain or wheezing, and not every ulcer patient or asthmatic is under stress. Yet, in many patients a combination of mental stress and a physical predisposition to various ailments acts to produce certain disease states.

The list of diseases that can be caused or exacerbated by stress is quite lengthy. In addition to asthma and ulcers, these problems include hives and other types of skin rashes, high blood pressure, irritable bowel syndrome, ileitis and colitis, various menstrual disorders, tics and tremors, and so forth. As you can see, virtually any organ in your body can be affected. How about your heart — can mental factors contribute to actual heart disease?

John M. is a successful banker, whose rise to the top of his profession was derailed by a heart attack at age fifty-three. There was no heart disease in John's family and he had never smoked. His cholesterol and blood pressure were both normal, and he looked lean and fit. John asked us why he developed heart disease; his wife asked if his twelve-hour workdays and four years without a vacation could have anything to do with it.

The answer is yes — we now know that emotional factors do increase the risk of coronary heart disease. Even more dramatically, stress can precipitate sudden "cardiac" death. How can your mind have such a strong impact on your heart?

We have already hinted at one link between emotions and cardiovascular disease: stress and tension can produce high blood pressure. In turn, high blood pressure puts increased demands on the heart and blood vessels. Over a period of years, atherosclerosis can develop in these damaged blood vessels. All too often the bottom line is a heart attack or stroke.

Even without invoking high blood pressure, there are other links between personality and heart disease. In 1959, Drs. Meyer Friedman and Ray Rosenman found that a specific constellation of personality and behavioral traits greatly increases the risks of developing coronary heart disease.

People manifesting "Type A" personality traits are three times more likely to develop heart attacks than are people without these behavior patterns.

Type A people are easy to recognize in their extreme form. The first clue can come from physical appearance, facial expressions, and speech patterns. Type A people tend to carry themselves very erect and to walk quickly, with short, choppy strides. They are fidgety and rarely sit still for any length of time. Facial expressions are taut. Type A people tend to speak loudly, often in staccato bursts. Even their breathing patterns can reflect a high level of tension: their breathing tends to be irregular and is often punctuated by sighing respirations.

Perhaps the most noticeable behavioral trait of Type A people is the "short fuse" that they have. It doesn't take much to trigger an emotional outburst; even minor frustrations or setbacks can provoke an inappropriate display of temper. You can make a psychological diagnosis of Type A behavior the next time you are in a traffic jam — just listen for the loudest, longest auto horns.

Thus far we have painted a picture of high-voltage tension. Admittedly, our picture is a bit extreme — many Type A people manage to control tension better than this. And all of us will display some of these traits at one time or another in response to external stress. But Type A behavior is more than simple tension. In fact, the single most striking Type A trait is a very strong competitive drive for success.

Again, let's draw the extreme picture: Type A people are workaholics. The Type A person will work twelve hours a day six or seven days a week — and take work home at night. Leisure time is considered a waste, and vacations are eliminated or filled with work. The hard-core workaholic adopts the slogan "TGIM" — Monday replaces Friday as the best day of the week. Type A people are constantly under time pressure and are prompt to a fault. They are typically doing two or three things at once, such as dictating while driving or answering mail while talking on the phone. Moreover, Type A people have extraordinarily high work standards. They are perfectionists who strive constantly for achievement, success, and recognition. Even in recreational sports, Type A people tend to be relentlessly competitive, always striving to reach the top of the tennis ladder or to best their own personal records for roadrunning.

Type A people often are willing to trade other elements of personal happiness for professional success. It's easy to see how this style will affect interpersonal relationships: badly. Yet, how can personality and behavior affect the heart? The answers are not all in, but certain trends are clear. Type A people have higher levels of adrenaline in their circulation. In turn, adrenaline will raise blood pressure and speed the heart. Other hormone levels, including cortisol and testosterone, rise to abnormally high levels when Type A people are subjected to mental stress. Type A behavior may also raise cholesterol levels, increase blood stickiness and clotting, and raise blood sugar levels. As we discussed earlier, all of these changes are risk factors for blood vessel damage and heart disease. Whatever the mechanisms, stress is clearly a "heartfelt" emotion. Even in monkeys, experimental studies have shown that stress accelerates the development of atherosclerosis.

Type A behavior sounds dreadful, and indeed, Type A people do pay the price in terms of an increased risk of heart disease. But remember that the picture we have drawn is the extreme, and that nobody is a pure Type A personality. Our heart patient John M., for example, is a genuinely nice person with many admirable qualities, but he also has hard-driving Type A characteristics that probably contributed to his heart attack. And Type A people do succeed in the workplace. They often are the leaders of business, government, the military, and even the sciences. Type A behavior contributes greatly to social progress, albeit at a high personal cost. Just ask yourself if you would prefer a Type A or a laid-back, easygoing, sometimes even lackadaisical "Type B" person for your accountant, attorney, or physician. For that matter, who would you want to coach your football team? Type A people can have extraordinary

records of success in sports, though they typically earn more respect than friendship along the way.

Not all psychiatrists agree that Type A behavior is the major psychological profile of a person with increased risk of heart attack. Some authorities believe that traits such as hostility or social isolation are more important. To us, these subtle disagreements are less important than the broad consensus of agreement: excessive mental stress can, over time, increase your risk of heart disease.

Granted that stress can gradually lead to heart disease, can a single severe mental stress actually cause sudden death? Although this is not common, it can occur. It is well known that under some circumstances people can literally be "frightened to death." Intense emotions can raise blood pressure, trigger heart attacks, and produce life-threatening irregularity of the hearts rhythm. One patient in Boston even had major heart rhythm irregularities on a recurrent basis just from the excitement of watching the Celtics on television — while they were winning, no less. But remember that most of these people have serious underlying heart disease to begin with.

How does all of this relate to fitness, emotion, and health? First of all, you should be conscious of excessive competitive instincts in sports. If you find yourself *always* going all out to win, you should ask yourself if this reflects other behavioral traits that could increase your risk of heart disease. Not so incidentally, Type A behavior in training and competition often can lead to athletic injuries (to yourself rather than your opponent). If winning is the *only* thing, you may well overlook danger signals from your body so that you push on in the face of pain from minor injuries — only to develop major injuries. Overcompetitiveness can also take some of the fun out of sports. Dave Scott announced his retirement from competition after setting a record in the 1984 Iron Man Triathalon — not because his body couldn't take the incredible demands on it, but because "there is too much anxiety, tension and pressure." Bill Koch, the Olympic medalist cross-country skier, said it better than we can: "I don't like this attitude that winning is everything. The more I win, the more I believe that it is only the icing, not the cake. Doing one's best is most satisfying, not that stupid medal on the shelf."

We are discussing these questions because you can learn to modify Type A behavior and promote your long-term fitness and health. Among Type A people who had heart attacks, patients who received special counseling had a significantly lower rate of second heart attacks and death than did patients whose treatment didn't include counseling.

As impressive as these results are, they amount to secondary prevention after heart disease has already occurred. Clearly, if you have a short fuse, we'd like to get you to lower the flame *before* you get to the point where you need a fire extinguisher! In the next few pages, we'll briefly sketch some of the ways you can recognize and manage stress in your life.

RECOGNIZING AND DEALING WITH STRESS AND DEPRESSION

Even the most health-conscious athlete will have aches, pains, and injuries from time to time. Similarly, even the most psychologically stable of us will have occasional periods of stress or depression. Indeed, in our complex, fast-paced world it is impossible to avoid these ups and downs. Nor should we strive for uniform calm and quiet. The richness of life depends on an admixture of stimulation and excitement; some degree of tension and some episodes of disappointment are the price we will pay, but we'll avoid boredom and mediocrity.

Stress and depression can be acute or chronic, brief and self-limited or long-lasting and recurrent. Transient, relatively mild episodes of stress or depression are universal and require no special treatment if they don't interfere with the quality of life and if they resolve spontaneously. But in many of us, these emotions can gather momentum of their own and gradually begin to encroach on our life-styles and even on our health. In most cases this is not a reflection of emotional instability or "mental illness." Usually you can go a long way to managing these reactions on your own. The trick is to recognize these problems for what they are, so that you can take appropriate corrective action. Finally, you should know what kinds of professional help are available if your problems are not amenable to self-help.

STRESS

In the past few years, stress has become a catchword for many of the shortcomings of our society. We have no quarrel with the concept that excessive, unresolved stress is harmful to health and to function. But stress itself is not always an adverse condition. Rather, stress is a physiological state that can have positive, as well as negative, connotations.

The physiology of stress was classified years ago by the pioneering studies of Dr. Walter B. Cannon of Harvard. The stress reaction is a very primitive human response to threatening stimuli. This response is basically one of arousal, of preparation for "flight or fight." The sympathetic nervous system is activated and the adrenal glands pump large amounts of adrenaline and cortisone into the circulation. As a result, heart rate and blood pressure increase. Blood flow is directed away from the intestinal tract and the skin so that more will be available for the muscles. Muscles are tensed. The pupils are dilated or widened. Blood sugar levels rise. Blood clotting mechanisms are activated. Respiration becomes shallower and more rapid.

You may recognize some of these adaptations from Chapter 1; indeed, in some respects this state of arousal is similar to the physiological response to exercise. Nor should this suprise us: stress is a very basic, primitive physiological response, and as such dates way back to the days when it was just what was needed to evade a saber-toothed tiger. Even today, a hostile chairman will evoke this exact response in a young vice-president making his first presentation to the board of directors.

In these circumstances, the stress reaction is an appropriate, adaptive response to an *external* physical or emotional threat. The arousal reaction may also occur in response to positive or desirable external stimuli ranging from athletic competition to sexual encounters. But sometimes this response can be maladaptive or counterproductive, as in the case of disabling stage fright before a big presentation or performance. Even more strikingly, the stress response can also be triggered by *internal* stimuli. Physical illnesses of many kinds can do this. In addition, internal emotional events can activate the entire gamut of the stress reaction. This is the most troublesome form of stress because it is essentially an *in*appropriate response, which can lead to unhappiness, dysfunction, or even illness. Your goal should be the mastery of "negative" or maladaptive stress so that you can appropriately employ and enjoy "positive" or adaptive arousal states.

How can you tell if you are experiencing stress? You should be aware both of external stress and of internal tension or anxiety. Most of us have no problems in recognizing stressful situations: the demanding boss, the angry coach, impending deadlines, financial pressures, family illness. In fact, stress is everywhere in our cultural milieu of crowded city living, fast food, fast traffic, competitive jobs, and noise and air pollution.

What are the signs of excessive stress within yourself?

In simplest terms, it's a case of the nerves. Agitation, tension, anxiety, nervousness are all synonyms for the stressed state. Whereas some people express stress by overt anxiety, others display stress in more subtle ways. Insomnia, excessive worry, and a mind that is always racing are examples. Stress may also be manifested in physical symptoms including a pounding heart, cold clammy skin, a churning stomach (with or without diarrhea), and excessive perspiration. Muscle tension increases, so that you may get jaw pain from grinding your teeth (even when you are asleep), and you may experience headaches and neck and back stiffness and pain. You will probably be grumpy, restless, or fidgety. Breathing is often rapid, so that you may feel short of breath, light-headed, and tingly — hyperventilation can even lead to fainting. Compulsive eating or smoking can also be manifestations of stress. Finally, and most commonly, stress is expressed by outbursts of anger, hostility, or frustration. Unfortunately, these outbursts rarely serve to dissipate internal stress; instead they put others under stress and hence can lead to a vicious cycle as relationships are strained.

Abuse of alcohol and drugs can also be an indication of stress. Unfortunately, these problems are becoming increasingly common. They can affect people in all walks of life, including professional sports, entertainment, business, and even medicine. Very often, high pressure is responsible. Alcohol or drug use begins modestly for "relaxation," as a refuge from stress. But the stress goes on — and so does the substance abuse, resulting all too often in addiction, illness, or even death.

Another, more subtle, manifestation of stress is the "burnout" phenomenon. If high-stress work goes on without relief for year after year, it may eventually impair production and performance. Burnout can affect all sorts of people, from assembly-line workers to teachers and to football coaches such as Dick Vermeil, who resigned from the Philadelphia Eagles in 1982 because of burnout. Perhaps the best examples are the air-traffic controllers, whose job performance and physical health suffer from constant pressure on the job.

Stress is a part of life; a world without stress would be a dull place indeed. Excitement, challenge, and stimulation are positive forms of stress. But there is a fine line between being "up" and being "up-tight." It's every bit as important to listen to the messages from your psyche during daily life as it is to listen to the messages from your body during sports. If the message you hear is tension and stress, your response should be to eval-

uate the causes of your distress so that you can take corrective action.

DEPRESSION

At first glance, stress and depression seem like different ends of the emotional spectrum. Indeed, stress generally reflects an excess of nervous energy, whereas depression is typically manifested by a lack of mental and physical activity. However, what goes up must come down; anxiety and depression can coexist in the same individual.

Stress or anxiety may be thought of as reactions to a real or imagined threat in the present or future and to a feeling of vulnerability or weakness. In contrast, depression may be thought of as a reaction to past events combined with feelings of hopelessness or helplessness. The prototype of anxiety is fear, of depression, grief.

Most psychologists and psychiatrists agree that the central theme in depression is a sense of loss. All of us feel depressed following the loss of a loved one. In this case, however, the reaction is appropriate and is generally self-limited, though it may take many months to get over. All of us would feel depressed as a consequence of severe illness. All of us feel transiently sad or "blue" after various setbacks or failures. These, too, are realistic and appropriate responses. But when these same feelings occur without an external cause, when they are prolonged, or when they deepen over time, then a true depression exists. Most often, the key element in depression is a loss of self-esteem.

Joseph K. is a fifty-seven-year-old man who came to the office for an evaluation of a seventeen-pound weight loss and fatigue. His appetite was poor, and although he spent most of his time resting, he was more tired than he'd ever been — but at night, his sleep was restless and unsatisfying. He was worried that he had cancer. Fortunately, a variety of tests were negative. When one got to know him, it became clear that his symptoms began shortly after he was passed over for a choice promotion. All of Mr. K.'s physical symptoms were caused by depression; with treatment, he made a full recovery.

Like anxiety, depression can be expressed in mood, in behavior, or in physical bodily function. Dejection and sadness are the major mood alterations, though anger, hostility, and even agitation may occur. Feelings of hopelessness, helplessness, and worthlessness predominate. People who are depressed lose interest in the outside world and become preoccupied with themselves. Despite this preoccupation with self, they often display a marked degree of self-neglect.

In terms of behavior, depression causes a lack of physical and mental energy. Depressed people are typically indecisive and are excessively preoccupied with physical symptoms, many of which are caused by the depression itself. Clearly, even mild depression can lead to failure almost as a self-fulfilling prophecy. Depression is hardly what you would like to see on your side of the playing field — and, in fact, depression may be responsible for various unexpected failures of athletic performance.

Depression also has physical effects. Appetite diminishes, and weight loss is common. Weakness may be pronounced, especially in the early morning hours. Despite all that weakness and fatigue, people who are depressed often sleep poorly, especially in the wee hours before the alarm clock rings.

What we've been describing, of course, is major depression. Symptoms like these cry out for expert medical and psychological attention. But milder depressive states may be so subtle as to go almost unnoticed. If you have an unusual string of "blue" or "down" days or if you find yourself losing interest in your work, your play, or your friends, ask yourself if you might be depressed. If the answer is yes, you too might benefit from a little help.

Exercise itself is a very useful way to dissipate stress and to counter depression. But before exploring this interaction between exercise and mood, let's briefly review more traditional forms of intervention.

COPING WITH STRESS: ALTERNATIVE STRATEGIES

All of us experience periods of stress, and all of us evolve patterns of dealing with stress. Some strategies work better than others. It's important to think about how you deal with stress — and how you might improve your coping mechanisms.

We believe that exercise can be an important aid in stress management. Since this is a fitness book, we will discuss in detail the way exercise affects mood and the way mental attitude in turn can affect athletic performance. But exercise isn't the only road to psychological fitness. Because stress is omnipresent in our society, many diverse approaches to stress management have evolved over the years. At the risk of being arbitrary, it maybe useful to classify these approaches into three groups.

1. The first series of techniques involve *life-style modification*. You change your social environment in order to decrease stress. Improving your interpersonal relationships is vital, enabling conflicts to be resolved at a minimal mental cost to you.

The first task is to identify external causes of stress. You may find that some of the most stressful situations are those you can do without. Eliminate them. However, it is impossible to remove all deadlines and pressures. Establish priorities so that you deal with the most pressing or critical issues first, postponing or omitting low-priority items. If your circuits are just plain overloaded, you can — and should — reduce stress by eliminating nonessential demands on your time and energy.

Learn to pace yourself. Don't try to do everything at once. Alternate stressful and relaxing tasks so that your day has variety. Take breaks — a few minutes of staring into space, stretching and walking, or reading may go a long way toward refreshing you and recharging your batteries. This applies at home as well as at work, and may involve something as simple as taking your phone off the hook, or as structured as booking an appointment with a fictitious visitor so that you have twenty minutes of uninterrupted peace and quiet. Experiment with different variations, but don't overlook the main theme: change gears as frequently as possible so that your mental engine doesn't get overheated with an uninterrupted flow of high-pressure situations.

This approach can be expanded from your daily schedule to your weekly calendar as well. Build in leisure time and vacations. Even a three-day weekend can introduce critical variety and provide an escape valve for pressure. Be careful to avoid overcommitting your leisure — indulge yourself by "wasting" time, and learn to relax by doing nothing at all from time to time.

These tips have proved helpful to many people, but they address only half of the issue. It is important to deal with external stress, but it is equally important to master internal stress. Learn to separate outside events from your own reactions to these events. Analyze your feelings. Learn to temper your reactions to circumstances beyond your control. Try to see the humor in every situation.

Talk to yourself, emphasizing the brighter side of things. Even better: talk to others. It's much better to talk out frustrations and anger than to hold strong feelings in, where they will keep your level of tension high.

You can also accomplish a great deal by learning techniques for coping with stress-producing people. Don't automatically respond to hostility with anger of your own — sometimes just acknowledging anger and trying to understand its causes can defuse an explosive situation ("You sound angry; how can we correct the problem?"). But you can't always fight fire with calming words, nor can you shield yourself from all hostility. Sometimes you'll need a sword of your own to protect yourself from stress. Learn to assert yourself when this is what it takes to solve a problem, but try to assert yourself rationally and effectively instead of emotionally.

All this may sound good on paper but can be hard to put into practice. However, you can learn coping techniques. Many books are devoted entirely to time management and to coping. An ever-increasing number of employers are offering on-the-job stress management workshops and employee assistance programs. Similar programs may be available through your community center, religious organizations, or through the adult education division of your local schools or university. Finally, many organizations offer programs in "sensitivity training" or "assertiveness," which may help you better understand your feelings and those of others. If you can do it yourself — fine. If not, explore one of the many ways to get help with stress.

2. *Self-regulation techniques* focus on the physiological components of stress. Clearly, stress changes your body's functions: your heart rate and blood pressure rise, your skin gets cold and clammy, your muscles tense up, and your stomach may churn or ache. These physiological effects can be reversed by using various relaxation techniques. When your body's stress mechanisms relax, the stress itself diminishes.

Although modern medicine is just now beginning to understand the benefits of the "relaxation response," it is far from new. In fact, Western physicians are in many cases simply rediscovering what has been known to Eastern yoga masters for centuries.

Relaxation exercises come in four basic varieties: breathing exercises, progressive muscular relaxation, biofeedback, and meditation.

Breathing exercises can be performed on their own or can be incorporated into other forms of relaxation (and even into natural childbirth!). Rapid, shallow breathing characterizes most high-tension states; at times, hyperventilation caused by anxiety can be severe enough to cause tingling, muscle spasms, and even fainting. Most of us experience periodic deep, sighing breathing at times of distress. These slow deep breaths are an automatic reaction of the nervous system. People can be taught to voluntarily breathe slowly and deeply, with particular emphasis on exhaling slowly and gently. This breathing pattern helps induce a state of relaxation, and can be helpful in stress management. Breathing exercises are easy to learn. You can do them at any time or place when stress occurs. They are an easy way of slowing down your body's racing machinery and of dissipating stress.

Progressive muscle relaxation is harder to learn, and requires practice to carry out effectively. But once you have the hang of it, it's really quite a simple way to relieve stress. The idea is first to tense a muscle group so that you will develop an awareness of how muscle tension feels. Then you relax the muscles to experience relief from tension. In general, muscle relaxation routines start with one muscle group and then progressively move on to other areas of the body until the whole body is relaxed.

Muscle relaxation exercises should be performed in a quiet room, preferably stretched out on a comfortable mat or firm mattress. Until you master the routine, it is helpful to have a friend read out specific directions. In fact, some people prefer learning muscle relaxation in a group setting, with an instructor providing the directions. You can also tape record the directions if you prefer solitude. Zealots suggest devoting an hour each day to mastering the technique, but many people report benefit from as little as ten or fifteen minutes. You can try this sample relaxation routine for yourself: rest comfortably in a quiet room, preferably lying on a mat or rug. Experiment with quiet background music. Breath in deeply; exhale slowly, feeling the relaxation of tension as you do. Tense each major muscle group, then relax slowly. Inhale as you tense the muscle, exhale as you relax. With practice, you will be able to relax your muscles without tensing them first.

1. Flex your feet up toward your head. Relax.
2. Press your feet downward, tensing your calves. Relax.
3. Tighten your thighs and buttocks, pressing them to the floor. Relax.
4. Arch your back upward. Relax.
5. Tighten your stomach muscles. Relax.
6. Breathe in deeply. Exhale slowly and relax.
7. Shrug your shoulders. Relax.

8. Clench your fists. Relax.
9. Bend your elbows up to tense your biceps. Relax.
10. Press your arms down to tense your triceps and forearms. Relax.
11. Flex your neck. Relax.
12. Clench your jaw and lips. Relax.
13. Close your eyes tightly and frown. Relax.
14. Wrinkle your forehead. Relax.

Biofeedback is the third relaxation technique; it uses medical monitoring devises to record and amplify body functions so that the subject can more readily learn to control them. For example, people who are being taught to lower their blood pressure would watch a graph of their pressure readings while they practice maneuvers to reduce tension. Successful relaxation responses are rewarded by instant evidence of success — the graph displaying blood pressure shows a fall. Positive reinforcement helps facilitate the learning process while these exercises are repeated over and over again. Similar monitoring devices can be used to measure heart rate. Skin temperature can be measured for people learning to control blood vessel spasms that produce finger or toe pain in a condition called "Raynaud's syndrome."

The most common biofeedback devices, however, monitor muscle tension itself. This is usually done by placing two or three small recording electrodes on the skin of the forehead. Muscle contraction requires electrical activity, which can be detected by the electrodes and recorded on a graph or coverted into a series of clicks over an amplifier. The subject practices relaxation techniques, and success is immediately recorded by a slowing of the clicks as muscles relax. Biofeedback clinics are now available at most medical centers, but the machinery is simple enough to be available to individual practitioners as well.

The forth self-regulation technique is also the most popular: *meditation*. Meditation is also one of the oldest techniques, being a central element of yoga for centuries. Although most athletes think of yoga as a muscle-stretching routine, it can be very relaxing in and of itself. Unfortunately, meditation is harder to learn, despite the simplicity of the underlying method: the student is given a special sound, or mantra, and devotes twenty or thirty minutes daily to sitting quietly with his eyes closed while attempting to maintain a constant awareness of his mantra.

Even without meditating, all athletes can benefit from the stretching exercise of yoga to relax stressed muscles. If you experience excessive mental stress, consider a meditation routine to relax your mind. Our colleague Dr. Herbert Benson of Harvard has popularized a simple, effective meditation technique. The technique involves four key elements:

1. Find a quiet environment that is free of distracting sights and sounds. Many people prefer a semidarkened room. Pick a time and place that will minimize interruptions.
2. Assume a comfortable body position. You do not have to cross your legs or to force yourself into an Eastern yoga posture. Instead, find a position that will allow your muscles to relax, so that aches and pains will not intrude. Your goal is not to stretch or relax your muscles but to forget them so that your mind will be free to meditate and relax.
3. Achieve a passive, relaxed mental attitude. Close your eyes and try to block out distracting thoughts and stimuli. Do your best to shift gears so that your mind is in neutral instead of spinning its wheels to cope with pressures and problems.
4. Use a mental device. Most often this is a mantra, which you simply repeat over and over again in a rhythmic, repetitive fashion; you can say your mantra aloud, or just repeat it silently. Pick your own mantra — any word or even syllable will do — or simply repeat the number "one" over and over. Or, if you choose to meditate with your eyes open, you can stare at a fixed object. In either case, the goal is to fix your attention on a neutral object in order to block out distractions, thoughts, and sensations.

These self-regulation techniques may seem mystical, magical, or downright silly. But Dr. Benson and others have done careful studies of Indian yoga masters and of anxious Americans just learning these techniques. There is no doubt that many people can learn to lower their blood pressure, slow their heart rate and breathing, change skin temperature, and decrease muscle tension. Some studies have shown an actual slowing of the body's metabolic processes so that less oxygen is consumed, brain wave activity slows, and decreases in blood lactic acid or adrenaline levels occur during meditation. We don't know *how* muscle relaxation, biofeedback, and meditation work — but there is no doubt that they can produce both mental relaxation and simultaneous changes in the body's neuromuscular activity, circulation, and chemistry.

Much remains to be learned about relaxation techniques, and not everyone can master them. Although many people have reported success in treating headaches, high blood pressure, vascular spasms, and anxiety with these techniques, their long-term efficacy is unproven. Above all, they are not a cure-all. Don't build up unrealistic hopes and expectations — for many people this approach to stress management is worth a try, but you should remember that many other forms of help are available. Finally, beware of unscrupulous individuals who may attempt to take advantage of you by promising great things while extracting exorbitant fees or commitments for teaching these techniques. In general, we'd recommend medical centers or reputable practitioners who combine the best of medical and meditative techniques.

3. *The psychotherapies* are the third group of stress management techniques. Whereas life-style modification and relaxation techniques are basically self-help approaches, formal treatment involves help from a trained therapist. It is very important to emphasize that such treatment does not imply mental illness and should not carry any stigma. Quite the reverse is true: it has been estimated that 15 percent of our population could benefit from some form of mental health care — although only a quarter of this number actually receives it. If those numbers seem high, remember that up to ten million Americans have alcohol-related problems, to say nothing of drug abuse, depression, anxiety, and so forth.

In the past, mental health care was typified by intensive (and expensive) psychoanalysis or depth psychotherapy administered by a psychiatrist or psychologist in an attempt to remove problems by developing insight into their psychological causes. We don't mean to downplay the value of this form of treatment. However, many other forms of therapy are available today, including group sessions, behavior modification, family therapy, and counseling. Similarly, the cast of therapists has expanded to include social workers, psychiatric nurses, counselors, pastoral therapists, and other mental health workers. Each of these individuals has his or her own unique set of skills, but only physicians can prescribe any necessary medications.

If stress or depression interfere with your daily life, you should take action to correct matters. As you can see, many very different approaches are available. It may take some trial and error to find out what is best for you. We'd like to think that your personal physician can still function as a "family doc" and get you started on the right path. You will also find some suggestions for further reading in the Appendix.

So far we've omitted all mention of the role physical exercise plays in mental health; the interaction between exercise and your psyche can also contribute to the control of stress and depression.

PHYSICAL FITNESS AND MENTAL FITNESS: EXERCISE AND YOUR PSYCHE

I (HBS) have just come in from my daily twelve-mile run. It's four below zero here in Boston, with twenty-seven-mile-per-hour winds. Some of you may think I have one of the psychological problems we have just been discussing. Perhaps. But I feel wonderful. I was out on the snow-narrowed streets early enough so that the cars produced no problems for me, nor I for them. The sunrise was spectacular, and the thin air and bright sky outlined the ice-coated trees with unusual clarity. I don't hear celestial music or see shooting stars. I am not high, but I am relaxed, exhilarated, cheerful, and clear-headed. As the day progresses, pressure, stress, and fatigue will return, but for now I am completely happy.

Whereas my feelings are personal, they are not unique. I experience the very same sensations each and every day after I run. True, there is controversy about the "runner's high," but we believe that much of the controversy is caused by inappropriate terminology. In our present culture, "high" implies psychedelic phenomena, which certainly overstates the case. In addition, the mental changes that do occur are clearly not limited to runners, but are shared by all endurance athletes. Perhaps the controversy would dissipate if we could all agree to call it the "exerciser's uplift."

Even the most sedentary of you will remember how good you felt in the shower after you had a vigorous workout. Exercise produces a unique combination of relaxation and exhilaration. But it does not come easily or automatically. First, you have to get into shape physically. Most people report that the mood changes of exercise do not begin until they have been exercising strenuously and continuously for twenty or thirty minutes. As Dr. George Sheehan puts it, the first thirty minutes of a workout are for your body, and the rest, the best part, is for your mind. Obviously your heart, lungs, and muscles have to be in shape for you to do this without pain, exhaustion, or injury. And you have to be in shape mentally as well. If you approach each workout as work, with fierce competitive goals, you may have trouble enjoying yourself. It's fine to extend yourself, and it's important to have goals — but enjoyment should be one of these goals. As in all aspects of life, your training should include variety and balance so that you can improve your performance and still enjoy yourself.

Vigorous exercise does improve mood. We are so used to hearing about "rest and relaxation" that we often overlook the fact that *exercise* is relaxing. Most fit individuals feel mentally better at the end of a workout than they did before. Many adjectives are used to describe those feelings: relaxed, happy, high, exhilarated, calm, peaceful, elated, turned-on, up, floating, and flying. For each of us these feeling differ, but for most of us, the two basic sensations described in these phrases will be present. Exercise is unique in its ability to produce both relaxation and exhilaration simultaneously.

How does exercise produce these changes? Sports psychology is a young field, and there are many unanswered questions about exercise and the mind. But even now, it is clear that many different factors are at work.

Psychological factors are important. Exercise removes you from the mental pressures of everyday life; in addition, team sports or even just working out with a friend can give you the benefits of camaraderie and companionship. Sharing a common sports experience is frequently a rapid path to forming friendships and can give you an opportunity to talk out problems. On the other hand, people who work out alone often value the opportunity for solitude. Even in solitude, you will have time to think out problems and to work out aggression, frustration, and tension.

Physical fitness will improve your self-image and self-esteem. You will experience a sense of accomplishment and mastery when you meet your goals. As you lose weight and develop increased muscle tone, your self-confidence will improve. All the compliments that you get from friends won't hurt your body image either.

Different types of exercise produce different psychological effects. In particular, aerobic or endurance exercise seems to have special benefits. Running, walking, biking, cross-country skiing, swimming, and rowing are examples of these dynamic forms of exercise. In all of these activities, you use large muscle groups in a rhythmic, repetitive fashion for prolonged periods of time. It has been suggested that the rhythmicity and repetitiveness induce a self-hypnotic state similar to that achieved in transcendental meditation by the repetition of a slogan or mantra. Indeed, some endurance athletes do report that they achieve a partial dissociation between sensory stimuli and cognitive processes. Put more simply, they are on "automatic pilot" — time seems to pass very quickly, and the mind is free to wander as the body churns on and on. Perhaps this is why most trained endurance athletes do not use radio or tape headsets. Music may provide a welcome distraction for people just getting into shape, but once you're fit, strenuous aerobic exercise produces its own state of dissociation.

For most of us, this state of dissociation is quite mild. Good thing, too! It's one thing to be oblivious to mild aches and pains, but you would risk serious injury if you were truly detached from your body's warning signals of fatigue and pain (to say nothing of cars and dogs).

What if you were to combine endurance exercise with actual meditation? The results might be awesome. Legend has it that certain Tibetan monks, known as Mahetangs, use meditation to aid their function as couriers between monasteries. Their technique involves staring at a distant mountain peak while repeating their sacred mantra in synchrony with their breathing. Only rough pathways link the monasteries, yet the Mahetangs are said to be able to run up to three hundred miles in thirty hours. This is a spectacular achievement in any climate — but it is superhuman over mountainous terrain at high altitude in cold weather. Unfortunately, scientific studies of these monks are lacking; however, even these legends may tempt me to learn a mantra before my next marathon!

Neurological factors may also contribute to the way exercise affects mood and behavior. Studies here are sparse, but they do suggest that physical fitness improves reaction time, which is a measure of cognitive performance. These changes are particularly notable in older people, which is especially important, since age itself seems to slow reaction time.

Other studies have shown that physical fitness improves the quality of sleep. Sleep is a surprisingly complex phenomenon. It is now clear that only 10 to 15 percent of each night is spent in deep sleep, called "slow-wave" sleep by scientists because of characteristic brain-wave patterns. Physical fitness increases the percentage of sleep that is slow-wave sleep, and it is this deep sleep that is the refreshing and restorative component. Perhaps Americans wouldn't consume thirty million sleeping pills each night if our society weren't so sedentary. Conversely, sleep deprivation impairs athletic performance, so that traditional "good night's sleep" before a big game does make sense. No wonder most teams fare poorly during road trips.

Circulatory factors may play a role in the mental effects of exercise, but this is still speculative. But if physical fitness improves the efficiency of oxygen delivery and utilization — and we know this is good for your heart and your muscles — it is possible that exercise may be good for your nervous system as well.

Chemical factors are of great interest in explaining the influence of exercise on mood. The activity of many hormones and chemicals in your body fluctuates with exercise, and scientists have suggested that various chemicals are responsible for the mood elevation that accompanies exercise. Some of the most exciting research in this area deals with chemicals called *endorphins*. The endorphins are a family of small proteins that are found in the brain and spinal cord and in other tissues such as endocrine glands. Endorphins have some similarity to opium derivatives such as morphine. It appears that these chemicals are important in the body's own defense against pain. In addition, endorphins may directly affect mood, appetite, sexual function, body temperature, and even memory and learning.

Recent investigations have shown that exercise is a potent stimulator of endorphin production and release. Moreover, people who exercise regularly and are physically fit experience an enhanced degree of endorphin production when they exercise. So training seems to improve your endorphin levels as well as your heart and muscles. It may well be that high endorphin levels account for the mood elevation that accompanies exercise, and for the apparent insensitivity to pain demonstrated by some marathoners and other endurance athletes. The possibilities are numerous: endorphins could also account for the changes in appetite and sexual drive noted by many athletes.

Because endorphins are the body's own internal morphine-like substance, they may explain the sense of well-being that accompanies exercise, the elusive "runner's high." Endorphins may also explain the addicting properties of endurance training. The story here is quite familiar — once established, the exercise habit breeds a strong drive for more exercise. Some "exercise addicts" actually experience mild withdrawal symptoms if they cannot exercise, including irritability, insomnia, guilt, restlessness, and lethargy or depression. In general, exercise is a positive, healthful "addiction." However, there is a potential for abuse. Some individuals become so obsessed with exercise and fitness that they allow it to consume all of their time and energy. Professional careers and family life can fall victim to exercise addiction.

Fortunately, exercise addiction and abuse are quite uncommon. For most people, the exercise habit is healthful insofar as it helps dissipate stress and fight depression. Physical fitness will also give you more energy for work (both physical and mental) and more enthusiasm for all aspects of your life. Fitness also promotes other healthful behavior patterns, including good diet and smoking cessation. In fact, a recent study of twenty-five hundred participants in Atlanta's Peachtree Road Race showed that over 75 percent of smokers were able to kick the habit for good after they started running.

If exercise can improve mood and behavior patterns in "normals," what can it do for people with excessive anxiety or depression? Although information is still sketchy at present, a few psychiatrists are starting to study exercise as an adjunct to traditional modes of psychotherapy. Pilot studies suggest that running may be as effective as psychotherapy, and even drugs, in the early management of depression. Long-term results are not yet known, and more studies are needed. Our own experience with cardiac patients has been encouraging in this area. Depression is very common after a heart attack; patients who complete exercise training for rehabilitation experience a clear-cut improvement in mood, sexual performance, and productivity at work.

Exercise is not a wonder drug and it is surely not the answer to all our psychosocial ills; yet every little bit helps, and physical fitness can contribute to mental fitness. This should not be surprising. We all accept the concept of psychosomatic disorders, in which mental factors precipitate physical ailments. The unity of mind and body clearly works both ways. Somatopsychic interactions do occur; physical illness often produces mental depression, and physical fitness can contribute to mental well-being. The Greeks and Romans said it more succinctly than we can: "Mens sana in corpore sano" (a sound mind in a sound body).

In Part II of this book, we will explain exactly how to construct your own physical fitness program. We also believe that a physical fitness program will help your psychological fitness. Physical fitness is one of the few areas of your life that is purely under your own control. When it comes to setting up and sticking to your program, you don't have to answer to your boss, your teacher, or even your mother-in-law — you'll be answering only to yourself. Part II will help you construct a realistic program; if you stick to it you *will* succeed. And this success in achieving physical fitness will have many benefits. You'll feel better, and you'll have more energy and strength for daily life as well as for sports. You'll develop a feeling of self-confidence and well-being. And because you'll look better, all the compliments you'll get will reinforce your newfound mental confidence. Finally, the success you've achieved in attaining physical fitness will give you the confidence you need to succeed in other areas. You will have learned that planning, diligence, and hard work pay off: you have succeeded, you can succeed, and you will succeed.

SPORTS PSYCHOLOGY

The psychology of *exercise* does not account for all of the mental ramifications of *sports*. Competitive sports are more than just exercise. Dr. Michael Sacks, a leading sports psychiatrist, points out that sport can function for adults as an extension of childhood play, as a world apart, with its own time and space, its own rules and regulations. As such, the make-believe world between the white lines can be an ideal way to work off aggression, to take risks and overcome fears, to display exuberance, and to participate in a communal experience. Even physically passive spectators at sporting events can identify with the athletes and experience vicariously some of these benefits. In these respects, sports is play.

"All men," said Aquinas, "need leisure." Recreation allows true re-creation and restoration for mind and body. Exercise and sports are an ideal form of leisure play. Dr. George Sheehan, a cardiologist and running guru, puts it best: "Like most distance runners, I am still a child. And never more so than when I run. I take that play more seriously than anything else I do. And in that play I retire into a fantasy land of my imagination anytime I please. Like most children I think I control my life. I believe myself to be independent. I am certain I have been placed on this earth to enjoy myself. Like most children I live in the best of all possible worlds . . . where nothing but good can happen."*

*G. Sheehan, *Running and Being* (New York: Simon and Schuster, 1978).

But there are also psychological negatives in competitive sports. Professional athletes are not conspicuous for mental health — note the alarming incidence of alcohol and drug abuse, the outbursts of temper, and the examples of violent or irrational behavior. In general, these are not problems generated by sports or intrinsic to the game. Instead, these are widespread problems in our society, which spill over onto the playing field. Sports can become a microcosm for society, encompassing and intensifying financial pressures, aggressiveness and hostility, and excessive competitive pressure to win at all costs. In these negative respects, sports is not play but business.

When sport becomes a business, it loses many of its psychological benefits. Agents, lawyers, arbitration, and strikes have improved players' pay but have taken some of the fun out of sports — for athletes and fans alike. Many players flop after signing lucrative long-term contracts. In part, motivation is lacking because financial rewards are assured. But in addition, performance suffers when the fun is gone. Ask Bjorn Borg — a retiree at age twenty-six because the fun was gone from tennis for him.

In the preceding pages, we have concentrated on the ways in which physical activity affects mental function. What about the other side of the coin: can mental factors affect athletic performance?

The answer is, of course, yes. There is an old joke in which a paunchy ex-athlete says that since exercise is 50 percent mental anyway, he'll skip the physical part. We don't want you to skip the physical part, and we don't want to quibble about percentages. But the message is clear: mental factors can be pivotal in sports.

Athletes themselves know this. Coaches call time out before a crucial foul shot or field goal attempt to let tension build. Mark Spitz defied competitive custom by entering the Olympics with long hair and a mustache instead of a closely shorn head and body. The Cincinnati Bengals' offensive line played the 1982 AFC championship game in short sleeves despite a wind-chill factor of 59 degrees below zero. Mark Fidrich talked to the baseball and Ty Cobb openly sharpened his spikes. True, it's all part of the game — of the mental game of "psyching" opposing players.

"Psyching" works because self-confidence is an important element of success in sports. Many other mental factors also contribute to success. Concentration is crucial, both in practice and in competition. Competition itself requires a state of arousal — which is basically a controlled degree of stress or anxiety. If arousal is insufficient, alertness and intensity will suffer, and play can be sloppy and lackadaisical. If arousal is excessive, anxiety can lead to "choking." Finally, motivation is crucial. Athletes should compete for themselves and for success itself. If they are motivated by other factors, such as fear of the coach, or a desire to please a parent, extraneous psychological conflicts can interfere with performance and success. Moreover, successful team-work requires the motivation for communal success to overcome the drive for individual glory.

Confidence, concentration, intensity, and desire are the psychological ingredients of success in sports. More-over, nothing succeeds like success. A team on a win-ning streak or an individual athlete "in a groove" are good examples. The harmony of mind and body con-tributes to teamwork, to fun — and to winning.

Athletic performance is also improved by subtle neu-ropsychologic factors. The home-court advantage is more than home cooking and self-confidence. The roar of the crowd can actually intensify arousal and improve per-formance. All of us who have run the Boston Marathon have experienced this effect. At mile 13, the course passes through Wellesley College; just when you are starting to tire, there are hundreds of cheering students. The results are predictable: an instant second wind that turns even the tortoises among us into hares (tempo-rarily).

Speaking of hares, the neuropsychology of sports is also illustrated by the "rabbit," a sprinter who enters a distance race to set a fast pace. World records depend on rabbits because pacing allows runners to "lock in"

FIGURE 3–1: *Effects of Relaxation and Arousal on Athletic Performance*

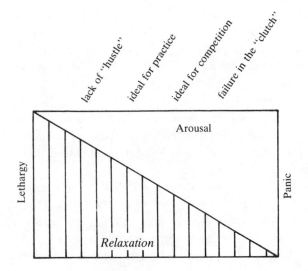

to a smooth, effortless pace and stride. When Eammon Coughlin broke his own world record in running his-tory's first sub 3:50 indoor mile on February 27, 1983, the first person he thanked was Ross Donoghue. Don-oghue, like Coughlin a Villanova product, is a 3:58 miler, and set the torrid pace knowing he would be unable to sustain it. Donoghue dropped out altogether, but Coughlin was launched to a historic record of 3:49:78. Again, this is more than just psychology — it seems likely that performance is actually enhanced by subtle neurological factors as well (see Chapter 2). On a hum-bler level, many of us have set our personal records when running with a speedy friend, and most of us play our best when our opponents are better than we are.

But in other cases psychological factors can lead to failure. Slumps and losing streaks are often caused by a lack of confidence or by excessive anxiety, which causes the athlete to "choke up" or try too hard. Subtle depres-sion can also destroy performance. Recently we eval-uated a national-class runner whose 4:02 best in the mile held great promise. Instead of improving, how-ever, his times began to slip and he was losing to "slower" runners. He had no injuries, but he complained of fa-tigue and he began losing weight. When all of his coach's training tricks failed to help, he was referred for a med-ical evaluation to see if his fatigue was caused by illness. His physical health was perfect, but his fatigue was caused by depression. With appropriate psychological counseling his fatigue is gone, and he's again in the running for a four-minute mile.

Most successful coaches are master psychologists, in-stinctively manipulating arousal, concentration, confi-dence, and motivation. And in this ever more complex and specialized world, a new discipline is emerging, that of sports psychologist.

Coach Mike White hired a psychologist for his 1983 Big Ten champion University of Illinois football team: "The psychologist was able to do things that I couldn't. He was an ear for the players to talk to. He was someone they could trust." The Chicago White Sox felt the same way about hypnotist Harvey Misel, who treated players to achieve "concentration and relaxation for maximum performance and maximal consistency."

Athletes are being taught many of the same relaxa-tion techniques we've discussed. One particularly in-teresting variant is imaging, whereby athletes prepare for competition by mentally rehearsing their perfor-mance in detail, and by mentally reliving previous suc-cessful performances. These techniques can be employed by individuals or by whole teams. For example, the University of Illinois basketball team credits part of its successful 1983 season to relaxation and imaging sessions. The entire team underwent six thirty-minute training sessions in the pre-season. Before each game they spent five minutes in a darkened room, first practicing relaxation techniques and then creating positive mental images of successful shots, passes, and rebounds. Coach Lou Henson feels it helped. And so does assistant coach Dan Smith, who led the sessions — and who just happens to be completing his doctorate in sports psychology.

For those with less imagination (or more affluence), another technique substitutes videotape replays for mental images. Here, too, the player views repeatedly his best and worst efforts. Coaches use these sessions to brush up fine points of technique. Psychologists use similar sessions to improve mental attitude, bringing confidence, arousal, and relaxation to the proper blend.

Many athletes rehearse their performances both mentally and physically before an important effort. Just watch champion high jumpers before they start down the runway: they will stand at the starting line for a minute or more, concentrating intensely and moving their arms and bodies through some of the motions they are anticipating in the big jump. Or listen to Toronto's star pitcher Dave Stieb: "My preparation for the game is simple. I visualize first warming up and getting the right movements on my fast ball, then I think about the first few innings and what I want to do. When I get to the mound, the same thing applies. I see the pitch going and doing whatever I want it to do and accomplishing whatever I want it to accomplish. Then I just wind up and throw it."

You don't have to be a big-league star to use mental preparation to help you in sports. If you are out of shape, you can motivate yourself to get fit by imagining how you'll look and feel twenty pounds lighter. When you're running up a steep hill, don't think about how tired you are — instead, project a mental image of how good you'll feel at the top. Whatever your level, you can help motivate yourself by setting realistic goals and then concentrating your will on achieving them. Above all, think positively; if you approach a tennis match with a fear of double-faulting, you're likely to do so, and if you are confident and self-assured, you'll play aggressive, winning tennis. Yogi Berra said it best: "Ninety percent of the game is mental, and the other half is physical."

PSYCHOLOGICAL FITNESS — SELF-ASSESSMENT

Emotional phenomena are notoriously difficult to quantitate; it's a lot easier to measure your cardiopulmonary fitness on a track or treadmill or your muscular fitness by counting sit-ups and measuring flexibility than it is to assess your mood and temperament. You may be able to evaluate your emotional state simply by reflecting on the discussions of stress and depression in this chapter. But for most of us, it's hard to be objective about our own subtle personality traits. A spouse or a relative or a close friend may be able to inform you about your mental state, and we'd hope that your "family doc" would know you well enough to help out.

Best of all would be an objective test to assess your psychological fitness. In fact, a great variety of personality tests have been developed to fill this need, but most are time-consuming and complex, and many require a skilled psychologist to administer and/or interpret the results. Among the simpler tests, two have been found particularly useful by our psychiatric colleagues; we've modified these tests to make them easier for you to take and score by yourself (see Figures 3–2 and 3–3). Although no test is foolproof, these two should help you evaluate yourself for depression and stress.

For these tests to work, you will have to rate yourself honestly. Read each statement carefully, but don't spend too much time on the answer. There are no right or wrong answers, so just try to pick the statement that describes how you *generally* feel. All of us experience fluctuations in our emotional state, so try to give the most weight to your feelings during the past month.

Take the depression and anxiety tests separately, but complete both tests before you score either of them. To take the tests, simply circle the number under the statement that best applies to you.

To interpret your psychologic self-assessment tests, add up your total points on each test, and compare your scores with this table:

Score	Interpretation
Below 30	No evidence of depression/anxiety
31–45	Mild depression/anxiety
46–60	Moderate depression/anxiety
61 and over	Severe depression/anxiety

Remember that these interpretations are intended only as guidelines, not as medical diagnoses. They are not intended to tell you if you are "normal" or "abnormal" and certainly should not be used to diagnose mental illness. All healthy people have periods of depression and anxiety. But if you find yourself scoring in the moderate to severe depression or anxiety category, you should take measures to improve your psychological fitness.

Just as with the other self-assessment tests in Part I of the book, you can repeat the psychologic self-assessment tests as you carry out your fitness program. The chances are good that as you get your body into shape, your psychological scores will improve as well.

FIGURE 3–2: A SELF-ASSESSMENT TEST FOR DEPRESSION*

	Almost never	Often	Sometimes	Almost always
1. I feel blue or sad.	1	2	3	4
2. I feel confident and hopeful about the future.	4	3	2	1
3. I feel like a failure.	1	2	3	4
4. I don't enjoy things the way I used to.	1	2	3	4
5. I feel guilty.	1	2	3	4
6. I have a feeling that something bad may happen to me.	1	2	3	4
7. I am pleased with myself.	4	3	2	1
8. I blame myself for everything that goes wrong.	1	2	3	4
9. I have crying spells.	1	2	3	4
10. I get irritated or annoyed.	1	2	3	4
11. I am interested in people and enjoy being with them.	4	3	2	1
12. I am unsure of myself and try to avoid decisions.	1	2	3	4
13. I feel that I look attractive and healthy.	4	3	2	1
14. I sleep poorly and am tired in the morning.	1	2	3	4
15. I am energetic and eager to take on new tasks.	4	3	2	1
16. My appetite is not as good as it used to be.	1	2	3	4
17. I am as interested in sex as I used to be.	4	3	2	1
18. I am concerned about my stomach and my bowels.	1	2	3	4
19. I feel healthy.	4	3	2	1
20. I have trouble doing my work.	1	2	3	4

*Modified from the Beck Depression Index.

FIGURE 3–3: A SELF-ASSESSMENT TEST FOR ANXIETY OR STRESS*

	Almost never	Often	Sometimes	Almost always
1. I am "calm, cool, and collected."	4	3	2	1
2. I feel that problems are piling up so that I cannot overcome them.	1	2	3	4
3. I feel my heart racing or pounding without exercising.	1	2	3	4
4. Some unimportant thought runs through my mind and bothers me.	1	2	3	4
5. I feel secure and at ease.	4	3	2	1
6. I feel I am losing out on things because I can't make up my mind soon enough.	1	2	3	4
7. I feel dizzy, light-headed, or faint.	1	2	3	4
8. I wish I could be as happy as others seem to be.	1	2	3	4
9. I feel joyful and confident.	4	3	2	1
10. I feel worried and tense.	1	2	3	4
11. I am afraid of people and things.	1	2	3	4
12. I have stomach pains or indigestion.	1	2	3	4
13. I am inclined to take things hard.	1	2	3	4
14. I sleep poorly or have nightmares.	1	2	3	4
15. I enjoy sitting quietly.	4	3	2	1
16. I feel rushed or hurried.	1	2	3	4
17. I get headaches or neck pains.	1	2	3	4
18. I get flushed or sweaty without exercising or I get hives.	1	2	3	4
19. I am eager for new challenges and tasks.	4	3	2	1

*Modified from the State-Trait Anxiety Inventory.

4

Nutritional Fitness

All people eat to live, but for many, food means much more than sustenance. Epicures eat for pleasure, athletes for energy, and vegetarians for health. No diet can be all things to all people, but your diet can provide you with all three: enjoyment, energy, and healthful nutrients. In order to achieve these goals, you will have to understand the fundamentals of nutrition and your own special needs so that you can plan the meals that will be best for you.

Medical science is just starting to understand all the interactions between diet, athletic performance, and health. The science of nutrition began with the study of deficiency diseases, which led to the establishment of minimal daily requirements for nutrients. But contemporary American society faces a different nutritional problem; instead of diseases of dietary deficiency, we are now confronted with diseases of dietary excess: obesity, high blood pressure, and arteriosclerosis. Within the past few years, doctors have turned to the problems of dietary excess, but even here, the major thrust has been disease prevention. Nutrition means more than fighting off illness — the ideal diet should also be designed to enhance health by promoting optimal function of the body.

Controversies in nutrition also exist because of the very strong influence of cultural, social, and psychological forces on dietary preference. Whereas some cultures equate corpulance with wealth and prestige, America in the 1980s represents the quintessence of the "slim generation." Both extremes are, of course, oversimplifications. But it's hard to buck trends and fads, to say nothing of commercial interests and advertising. Do we buy one-calorie soda because we strive to be slim, or are we obsessed with slimness because of the soda salesman? At the other extreme, will we be healthier if we eat "health foods" and drink bottled water? And will our athletic performance improve if we start each day with the "Breakfast of Champions"?

Unfortunately, the athlete has been the last to benefit from scientific study of nutrition. While medicine has grappled with the more pressing problems of diet and illness, the apparently healthy athlete has been left largely on his own to design a diet for sports. The results have been predictable — no other aspect of fitness has been more affected by both the newest fads and the oldest traditional training regimens, which often amount to little more than "old coaches' tales." Although many athletic skills are learned best by observing and imitating world-class competitors, you must be wary of extending this approach into nutrition. Bill Rodgers is a well-known junk food addict — but don't expect a diet of pizza and potato chips to improve your marathon time. At the other end of the spectrum, while Harold Soloman is an acknowledged vitamin devotee, you cannot expect to improve your serve with megavitamins. To be sure, diet can improve physical fitness in general and athletic performance in particular. The first principle is that good nutrition for the active individual is really very similar to good nutrition for everyone. Athletes require only extra calories, extra carbohydrates, and extra water. So let's look in some detail at the fundamentals of good nutrition so that we can understand what diet is best for fitness and athletics.

Some of this information about nutrition may surprise you, and some of it may even be hard to accept at first. Remember that nutrition, though vital, is just one of the four facets of fitness. This is not a diet book, and we are not trying to convince you to change your diet for nutrition's sake alone. Instead, we encourage you to make these changes gradually as part of a total fitness program. As you feel your body changing and growing stronger, your attitude toward food may begin to change. For many people, dietary patterns are governed by psychological needs; they eat when they are angry, frustrated, or sad rather than when they are truly hungry. Similarly, many of us choose foods on the basis of habit or whim rather than on the basis of what our bodies need for energy and health. Instead of trying to change these deeply ingrained patterns all at once, keep working on dietary improvements as you proceed with your fitness program. The chances are good that as you begin to think of your body as fit, healthy, and strong, you'll begin to choose foods that will enhance your body's total fitness.

The human body is a truly remarkable piece of machinery. Our bodies are composed of thousands of different chemicals — all of which can be synthesized from just thirty-eight essential nutrients plus a source of calories. Of these thirty-eight compounds, fifteen are minerals, eleven are vitamins, ten are amino acids (the building blocks of protein), and one is a fatty acid. The final essential nutrient is often overlooked but is no less important — water.

These thirty-eight nutrients are considered "essential" because omission of any one will result in illness — there are just no substitutes available. But your body requires much more than these thirty-eight chemicals, including balanced amounts of carbohydrates, protein, and fat. These other nutrients are "nonessential" only because within each group, foods can be substituted for each other without causing illness. However, good health and optimal athletic performance require balanced amounts of all of these foodstuffs. Nor does man live for fitness alone — your diet can be enjoyable and tasty as well as being healthful.

The average American adult consumes nearly one ton of food each year. Let's look at what you should include in your ton — and what you should avoid.

CALORIES

In our diet-conscious society, calories have gotten a bad name. In fact, the calorie is neither blameworthy nor praiseworthy — it's just a simple unit of energy. In scientific terms, a calorie is the amount of energy required to raise the temperature of one gram of water by one degree Centigrade. The energy value of all foods can be measured and assigned a calorie count. In addition, the energy required for exercise can be measured and quantified in calories. So this single unit of energy can be used to express the intimate link between the food you take in, the energy you expend, and your body weight.

Your body weight reflects the balance between the number of calories in your food and the calories you burn as a result of all your metabolic processes. After food is digested and absorbed, its energy is used for all your body's functions, including the growth and repair of tissues, the work of your organs, the generation of

FIGURE 4–1: AVERAGE DAILY CALORIC REQUIREMENTS FOR HEALTHY ADULTS

Weight	Sedentary		Moderately Active		Very Active	
	Men	Women	Men	Women	Men	Women
100		1,300		1,800		2,700
120	1,800	1,560	2,520	2,160	3,600	3,240
140	2,100	1,820	2,940	2,520	4,200	3,780
160	2,400	2,080	3,260	2,880	4,800	4,320
180	2,700	2,340	3,780	3,240	5,400	4,860
200	3,000		4,200		6,000	
220	3,300		4,620		6,600	

heat, and the work of your muscles — exercise. If, after all this, calories are left over, their energy will be stored in your body as adipose tissue (fat). Conversely, if you use up more calories than you take in, energy will be mobilized from your body stores, and you will lose weight. It's really just a matter of simple arithmetic — one pound of adipose tissue contains the energy equivalent of 3,500 calories. Popular lore notwithstanding, calories do count.

How many calories do you need each day? Many factors affect the answer to this simple question. First and foremost is your weight — the bigger you are, the more calories you need just to maintain your weight. Another variable is gender; men generally need more calories than women because a larger percentage of their body weight is muscle, so that fewer calories are stored in adipose tissue. Age is another factor. Obviously children and adolescents need more calories to support growth. But even in adulthood, your metabolic rate — and hence your caloric requirements — is age dependent, showing a slight decline for each decade beyond age thirty. A variety of other factors can affect your caloric needs — for example, pregnancy and lacjtation, fever, trauma, surgery, and excessive thyroid activity all increase caloric requirements. But the biggest variable, and the one you can control most readily, is exercise. At rest, a 150-pound man consumes about

70 calories per hour, but intense exercise will increase his caloric consumption up to tenfold. You can easily see the way physical activity influences your caloric needs by taking a moment to calculate your own daily requirements with the use of the simple chart in Figure 4–1.

If your weight is normal, the wisdom of your body can substitute for these calculations — in general your appetite will make automatic adjustments for your level of exercise and your weight will stay fairly constant. Unfortunately, many of us should lose a few pounds to obtain optimal fitness. To do so, you should curb your appetite and increase your expenditures of energy in exercise.

Caloric balance is the bottom line for your weight. If you want to lose weight, keep track of the calories you eat. A detailed listing of caloric values is beyond our present scope, but some useful reference sources are listed in the Appendix.

How about exercise? Obviously, the more you exercise, the more calories you will burn. Athletes in training can require enormous numbers of calories to give them the energy they need. Daily intakes of 5,000 or 6,000 calories (two to three times the "normal" consumption) are not unusual. But world-class athletes don't have to count calories — their appetites will automat-

FIGURE 4–2: "RUNNING IT OFF": HOW MUCH TIME IT WILL TAKE YOU TO WORK OFF THE CALORIES IN SELECTED FOODS

Food	Minutes
Celery	1
Cauliflower	2
Spinach	3
Peas, tomato juice	4
Melon	6
Banana	7
Orange juice, bread	8
Raisins, chicken, soft drink, cookie (1), wine, whiskey (1 oz.), peanut butter	10
Cereal, cottage cheese, American cheese, apple	15
Pizza, beer	15
Haddock, potato chips	16
Tuna fish, hot dog, eggs, pie, spaghetti	18
Candy bar	25
Chocolate pudding or cake	30
Hamburger	45

NOTE: These figures are based on average portion size, average body weight, and jogging at 6 miles per hour.

ically adjust to keep them in balance. In Chapter 1, we discussed the caloric expenditure of various forms of exercise (see Figure 1–9). You can easily create your own formula balancing the calories you eat against the calories you burn. Figure 4–2 can help get you started with this by showing how much exercise you'll need to "run off" some of your favorite foods.

At first glance this may be a bit discouraging, for it is surely much faster and easier to gain weight by overeating than it is to lose weight by exercising. In fact, since the average energy cost of walking or jogging is 100 calories per mile, you would have to walk thirty-five miles to burn off the calories in just one pound of fat.

Don't take off your jogging shoes and head for the pantry — it's not as bad as it sounds. What you need is the big picture. Exercise, like diet, is a lifelong proposition, and the reward of fitness is a longer (and fuller) life. Patience and persistence are the key elements. Let's assume that you really get into your fitness program and that you gradually build up your exercise level to the equivalent of twenty miles per week. Even if your diet does not change a bit, this moderate level of exercise will take off thirty pounds in a year.

Another point to keep in mind is that regular aerobic exercise may actually suppress your appetite. It is not clear how this happens. Some studies have shown that exercise increases the hormones that increase the blood sugar, thus eliminating one hunger signal. Or the changes may be behavioral. Some scientists even believe that the body contains a control center, which adjusts your appetite so that your weight will stay constant. According to these theories, the only way to reset this control mechanism to a thinner target is to exercise regularly. Whatever the reason, exercise tends to decrease rather than increase your appetite — so you will tend to take in fewer calories while burning off more.

Remember that the most important thing about weight reduction is not how fast you take it off, but how long you keep it off. For sustained weight control, a reduction of no more than one or two pounds per week is considered ideal.

With time and patience, exercise will help provide weight control. Moreover, exercise will decrease your percentage of body fat. This benefit occurs above and beyond weight reduction, and will help you look trim faster than diet alone. You'll feel better too. Finally, exercise will help motivate you to follow a sound diet so that you will establish a lifelong pattern of exercise and diet, which together will lead to ideal body weight

and fitness. A regular exercise program will teach you an all-important lesson: you have control over your body. As your physique and your fitness improve, you will naturally begin to exert control over your diet as well. In this way, too, exercise and nutrition will work together in your total fitness program.

CARBOHYDRATES

Bread is the staff of life, and carbohydrate is the fuel of exercise.

The central importance of carbohydrate and the impact of dietary carbohydrates on athletic performance has been one of the most important nutritional discoveries of sports physiology. In fact, in this area sports medicine has led the way to a reevaluation of much of our traditional nutritional "wisdom." Western society in general and Americans in particular tend to be disdainful of carbohydrates. In part, this attitude results from cultural and economic prejudice, for carbohydrates such as rice, corn, wheat, and other grains are the dietary mainstays of most of the world's people. Because carbohydrates are inexpensive sources of energy, more expensive foods such as steak have become the prestige items in the American diet. "What costs most must be best for you," the reasoning seems to go. Whatever the reasons, carbohydrate-rich foods have been maligned as fattening sources of "empty calories."

Carbohydrates are organic compounds containing carbon, hydrogen, and oxygen, nothing more than various sugar combinations. Complex carbohydrates such as starches are made of many sugar molecules put together, whereas simple carbohydrates are just that, individual sugar molecules. But all digestible carbohydrates are broken down in the gastrointestinal tract and are absorbed into the bloodstream as simple sugars. The only exception is fructose (fruit sugar), which can be absorbed as is — but even fructose must be converted into glucose before the body can make use of it.

To understand the importance of carbohydrates for an active, healthy life, you have to understand a little bit about energy sources and metabolism. Like all tissues and organs, muscles require energy to do their work. But unlike other tissues, the energy demands of muscle increase tremendously during exercise (see Chapter 2). Where does this energy come from?

Muscle can use either fat or carbohydrate for fuel; at rest, both are burned equally, but as the intensity of exercise increases, muscle becomes increasingly dependent on carbohydrates. When you are working all-out, you rely entirely on carbohydrate for energy. Muscles store energy in the form of a sugar compound called glycogen. The liver also stores glycogen, which can be converted to glucose (simple sugar) and transported in the blood to muscle.

Unfortunately, your body's supply of glycogen is quite limited. As you can see in Figure 4–3, all of the muscles in your body contain only enough glycogen to provide 480 calories, less than enough to keep you running for an hour. Liver glycogen can help out, but a maximum of 280 calories are stored in the liver. The blood itself contains glucose at all times, but these 80 calories are a minor contribution to energy stores.

All of these glycogen-glucose stores together contain only enough energy for twelve hours at rest, and for hardly more than one hour of maximal exercise. Does the body have a perpetual energy crisis of its own? Not if you are healthy and well nourished. As you can see in Figure 4–3, body protein contains much more energy. Although protein can be burned to give energy, this is a last resort for the body because the protein has other jobs to do. Much more abundant energy stores are available in the form of adipose tissue, or fat. Fats are broken down into free fatty acids, which are carried in

the blood to muscles. But fat is a much less efficient fuel for muscles than carbohydrate is, and fat cannot be used for maximal effort.

Clearly it would be nice to increase the amount of glycogen stored in your muscles so that they would have plentiful supplies of efficient fuel. And it can be done. This is where dietary carbohydrates come in: carbohydrates are to plants what glycogen is to man — the storage form of glucose, and hence energy. By manipulating your carbohydrate intake, you can actually change your muscle glycogen stores. In this respect, at least, you truly are what you eat.

Athletes should have a high-carbohydrate diet. Remember our theme: we are all athletes. In point of fact, high-carbohydrate diets are more healthful for sedentary people as well as for athletes in training. At the present time, the average American obtains only about 45 percent of his calories from carbohydrates. We believe this figure should be closer to 60 percent — to enhance performance for the athlete and health for everyone.

Are carbohydrates "empty calories"? It is true that refined sugars and other sweets provide concentrated calories without other nutrients. "Natural" sweets such as honey are no more nutritious than processed or refined carbohydrates such as white sugar. Sugar is sugar — refined carbohydrates are not harmful (except for your teeth, for they do promote tooth decay) but they do give you calories without other nutrients. And sad to say, our current American diet is very high in sugar content, to the detriment of optimal nutritional balance.

One additional problem of refined sugars is that they add calories without bulk. If you are overweight, this can be a problem, since your body will lack an important signal that you have had enough, and you may go on eating. For example, a cookie has about 100 calories, as does an apple. Try eating six apples!

Fortunately, the "empty calorie" thesis does *not* apply to complex carbohydrates, such as starchy foods, which can be excellent sources of nutrients. Are complex carbohydrates fattening? Carbohydrates contain 4 calories per gram, as do proteins, but fats contain more than twice as many calories, 9 per gram. The fact is that a six-ounce potato contains only 150 calories, whereas a six-ounce steak contains 600 calories and potentially harmful fats.

You cannot live on potatoes alone. However, because many foods are rich in carbohydrates, a high-carbohydrate diet can be nutritionally balanced and varied enough to appeal to most people. *Pasta* is an

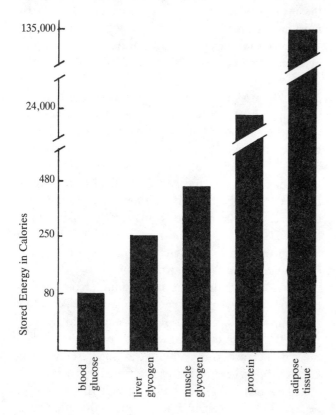

FIGURE 4–3: YOUR BODY'S ENERGY STORES

excellent source of carbohydrate, and many enriched spaghetti and noodle products contain important vitamins and minerals. *Potatoes* provide iron, vitamins, and fiber or "roughage" as well as carbohydrates. Obviously, baked or boiled potatoes are a much better nutritional "bargain" than fried potatoes, which have additional fat and calories. *Grain products*, such as breads and cereals, are also good sources of carbohydrates. Look for whole wheat products because they provide needed vitamins and bran (roughage). Avoid sugar-coated cereals. The added sugar will provide calories without nutrients, and can promote tooth decay. *Rice* is another good source of carbohydrate, as are *peas* and *beans*, which also provide protein and minerals. *Fruits* and *vegetables* provide fiber, vitamins, and minerals in addition to carbohydrates. Moreover, they provide the flavor, variety, and fun, which are essential to maintaining a high-carbohydrate diet. Finally, *skimmed milk products* are very healthful foods that will give you some of the carbohydrates you need for athletics while also providing protein, calcium, and other nutrients. Yogurt is an excellent example. You can find out more about the carbohydrate content of specific foods from the sources listed in the Appendix.

Even granting the benefits of a high-carbohydrate diet, is there anything more the competitive athlete can do? The answer is yes — dietary manipulations called "carbohydrate loading" can further increase muscle glycogen levels and improve endurance. This technique is not recommended for all athletes, since it will benefit only those who actually need extra muscle glycogen. Marathon runners, cross-country ski racers, long-distance bike racers and others who engage in high-intensity work for prolonged periods are in this category. But even these athletes are advised to reserve carbohydrate loading to the three or four most important contests each year.

As early as 1939, Scandinavian scientists showed that high-carbohydrate diets improve endurance. For example, in one study, trained athletes fed a low-carbohydrate diet could exercise vigorously for only 80 minutes before exhaustion set in, whereas a high-carbohydrate diet extended endurance to 210 minutes. More recent studies have revealed that this extended endurance is directly related to pre-race muscle glycogen levels. Finally, it has been demonstrated that muscle glycogen stores can be increased to 45 grams per kilogram of muscle — more than twice the normal levels — if carbohydrate loading is preceded by a phase of carbohydrate depletion.

Here is how it works. Six days before the big event, the athlete exercises strenuously — using the same muscles as he will in the race. For example, a marathoner will take a long, hard "depletion run" to reduce muscle glycogen stores to very low levels. Then for three days the runner eats a low-carbohydrate, high-fat–protein diet to keep muscle glycogen stores low. Most of us find this to be sheer torment — fatigue, muscle aches, and a grumpy disposition regularly accompany the depletion phase. But then bliss — three days of high-carbohydrate feedings prior to the race itself. Only light exercise should be performed during this period, so that muscle glycogen levels stay high. As muscles gain glycogen, they also gain water. This has good effects and bad effects: body weight increases, which means extra work for the racer, but as the glycogen is burned during the race, the water is returned to the circulation when it is needed most to prevent dehydration.

Some sample menus for carbohydrate loading are provided in Figure 4–4. Frequently the loading phase can be an enjoyable social event, with informal "pasta parties" the night before the race. You may want to give it a try, but you should undertake these dietary manipulations with caution and common sense.

Clearly carbohydrate loading is an elaborate ritual with somewhat limited application. How about the time-honored, widespread practice of eating candy or other sources of sugar for "extra energy" before an athletic event? The results of some recent studies may surprise you: sugar intake prior to exercise actually *reduces* the amount of energy available to your muscles. The reasons for this are a bit complicated. In brief, when a large amount of sugar reaches your bloodstream at one time, your pancreas responds by secreting extra amounts of the hormone insulin. Insulin in turn has three effects: (1) the blood glucose is lowered; (2) the ability of the liver to convert its glycogen stores into energy is reduced; and (3) the ability of adipose tissue to release free fatty acids for the muscles to burn is impaired. All three factors reduce the amount of energy available to muscle. In fact, Dr. David Costill of Ball State University estimates that taking sugar before exercise may reduce endurance by up to 19 percent.

You should avoid sugar intake for two to four hours before you compete athletically. But how about sugar during a race itself? For most athletic events, sugar is not helpful, and may be harmful to performance. In addition to the effects discussed above, sugar will delay the absorption of fluids from the stomach and intestines. Bloating may result, and you may get dehydrated if the fluids you need stay in your stomach instead of entering your bloodstream. However, sugar may be helpful for one very special type of exercise — very prolonged, high-intensity work such as marathon and ultramarathon running, cross-country ski marathons, and long bike races. In these rather extreme conditions of human performance, blood sugar may decline, and this hypoglycemia can produce mental fatigue and muscular exhaustion (see Chapter 2). So participants in these events should take glucose while they exercise. But even here, frequent small feedings are best.

We've taken away your candy bars — how about the last cup of coffee before you exercise? Dr. Costill's research has provided some surprising answers about coffee as well. It turns out that caffeine will improve endurance. The reason goes back to your muscles' two basic energy sources, glycogen and fat. Remember that the name of the game is to prolong the supply of muscle glycogen. Early in exercise, a "glycogen burst" occurs in which a disproportionate amount of glycogen is burned up. This wasteful overutilization of glycogen can be prevented by caffeine. Caffeine makes more fat available to muscle at the start of exercise, thus allowing the muscle to save its glycogen stores for when they are needed most in endurance events — at the end. Approximately 300 milligrams of caffeine (about two cups of coffee) taken one hour before you start exercising seems optimal. Of course, if caffeine produces heartburn, nervousness, rapid heart action, or tremors, you would best avoid this final way to manipulate your carbohydrate balance.

Needless to say, carbohydrates are only one element of a balanced diet. But they are a crucially important element — both to provide energy for exercise and to provide nutrients for health. Complex carbohydrates should provide 60 percent of your caloric needs, whether you are just starting your fitness program or have already progressed to competitive athletics. If 60 percent carbohydrate seems a lot, just remember that two of the world's finest endurance athletes adhere to the Pritikin *80 percent* carbohydrate diet: for more than six years both Robert de Castella, who has the fourth fastest marathon in history to his credit, and David Scott, winner of Hawaii's grueling Iron Man Triathlon, have been on diets that are very high in carbohydrate and very low in fat. We won't promise that a high-carbohydrate diet will make you a world-class athlete — but you will have more energy for sports and a better diet for health.

PROTEIN

In the fifth century B.C., Greek athletes concluded that the best way to build muscle was to eat muscle — and

---

FIGURE 4–4: SAMPLE MENUS FOR CARBOHYDRATE LOADING

	Depletion Phase (optional) Days 6 through 4 prior to the race	Loading Phase Days 3 through 1 prior to the race
Breakfast	Eggs	Cereal
	Cheese	Pancakes with syrup
	Cottage cheese with artificial sweeteners	Bread, muffins
		Fruit juices
Lunch or Dinner	Meat or fish	Yogurt
	Lettuce, green beans, celery	Pasta
	Cheese	Potatoes
	Soft drinks with artificial sweetener	Peas, carrots, squash, corn
	Breads and cakes	Fruit
Snacks	Hard-boiled eggs	Sherbet
	Cheese	Fruit
	Celery	Candy and cookies

so the high meat diet for athletes was born. We don't know if these ancient competitors benefited from this diet. But for twenty-five hundred years, training tables have groaned under platters of steak and eggs. More recently, countless thousands of dollars have been spent purchasing pills, powders, or potions with high-protein contents; these dietary supplements are said to provide greater power and energy for the athlete. Even non-athletes have succumbed to this media blitz, and steak has become the number-one prestige food in America.

Are the claims for protein valid? The best available evidence suggests that they are *not*, and that protein supplementation constitutes one of the greatest myths in sports nutrition. Put another way, it seems quite clear that the athlete's training table should be set with spaghetti and yogurt instead of steak and eggs.

Having said that, we must hasten to point out that protein is essential for human performance and, in fact, for health and life itself. Moreover, both the quantity and quality of dietary protein are crucial. However, once your metabolic requirements are satisfied, *extra* protein will just provide extra calories instead of extra power and muscle bulk. And many of the favorite sources of animal protein, such as steak, provide relatively large amounts of animal fats, which can be harmful.

The protein requirement of healthy, active adults is .36 gram of protein per pound of body weight. For a 150-pound person, this amounts to two ounces of protein per day. Put in everyday terms, this amount of protein is contained in any of the following foods: nine ounces of poultry, meat, fish, cheese, or peanut butter; two cups of cottage cheese, nine eggs, three pints of milk, or four cups of beans. Since protein contains 4 calories per gram, the minimal daily protein requirement would provide 225 calories per day. As a rule of thumb, approximately 15 percent of your daily calorie intake should come from protein sources.

Proteins are the backbone of all human tissues. As we said earlier, proteins are essential to the structure and function of our bodies. Protein can also be broken down to provide energy, and can even be converted to glucose for this purpose. However, carbohydrates and fat are much better energy sources. The body does not store extra protein — since all of the body's proteins are at work, they will be burned for energy only under condition of starvation, when all the carbohydrate and fat stores are exhausted.

Protein requirements are increased in circumstances that require the body to produce or repair its tissues. Examples of these conditions are growth and the re-

covery from injury, illness, and surgery. But if athletes do not need protein for energy, do they need extra protein to build up their muscles?

To answer this question, we must first consider the issue of the quality of the protein you eat. Although you could fulfill your *quantitative* protein needs by eating four cups of beans a day, this would be nutritionally unwise because you would still be *qualitatively* deficient. This may seem paradoxical, but the explanation is simple: we really don't require protein *per se*, but rather amino acids. Amino acids are the building blocks of the protein in your food and of the protein in your body's tissues.

Before it can be put to use in your body, the protein you eat must be broken down into its constituent parts, the much smaller and simpler amino acids. Dietary proteins are first digested in the stomach and intestines. Amino acids are liberated by this process of digestion. After being absorbed into your bloodstream, the amino acids are carried to your body tissues where they are put back together into the proteins that your body needs.

Of the twenty amino acids in nature, eight are considered "essential." The body cannot synthesize these eight amino acids, so they must be obtained from the food you eat. The remaining twelve amino acids can actually be put together in the body if the proper raw materials (nitrogen and energy sources) are provided.

The best dietary proteins are those which contain an ideal mix of amino acids. This can be expressed in terms of a score, the so-called biologic value of proteins. Animal foods such as milk, eggs, and meat are the best source of protein. But vegetable sources such as soybeans and other legumes, peanuts and other nuts, grains, and seeds are also good protein sources. Vegetable proteins have a lower score than animal proteins only because they are each low in one or more essential amino acids. However, if you eat a mixture of vegetable proteins, you can get all the amino acids you need. And remember that there are many factors in addition to amino acids that should influence your protein choice. Egg white is the only "pure" protein (albumin) source in food — you get other items in all other foods. In the case of red meat, the price you pay for its excellent protein and iron content is large amounts of saturated animal fat, which adds calories and may contribute to hardening of the arteries. All in all, poultry, fish, skimmed milk products, and legumes appear to be the most healthful sources of protein.

Fit, active people do need extra sources of energy, which should be obtained from carbohydrates. Do athletes need more protein, different proteins, or amino acid supplements? Despite two and a half millennia of tradition and thousands of dollars in expense, the answer is no. Obviously, athletes do need more protein if they are recovering from major tissue injury. But to build muscle strength and bulk, they need exercise plus calories, not extra protein. If you follow the 15 percent rule, you will get plenty of protein. As you exercise more, your caloric needs will rise and, with a balanced diet, your protein intake will keep pace as well. Finally, natural proteins from healthful food sources are much better than commercial dietary supplements. These potions, pills, and powders promise energy and power, but they provide only expense. And that is one supplement athletes don't need.

FATS

Dietary fat intake is one of the few areas of nutrition in which athletes have not generated their own misconceptions. Instead, athletes are subject to exactly the same misconceptions that affect the rest of Western society.

There is no doubt that fats are an essential component of our diet. Fats are the carriers for the so-called fat-soluble vitamins A, D, E, and K. Fats are critical in the structure of many human organs and tissues. They are the body's major form of energy storage, and are an important source of energy for muscles (particularly at low or moderate workloads). Even cholesterol itself, the archvillian of cardiovascular disease, is vital for health as the building block for various hormones, including cortisone and the sex hormones.

However, fats are also a major cause of human disease. The prime example, of course, is atherosclerosis, which can lead to heart attacks, strokes, and peripheral vascular disease.

Chapter 1 discusses the value of exercise in reducing the risk of atherosclerosis, and Chapter 3 examines the importance of stress reduction. What about the role of dietary fats in modifying cardiovascular risk factors? As in many areas of medical research that depend heavily on large, long-term population studies, there is some controversy here. There is no doubt that elevated blood cholesterol levels are linked to atherosclerosis. And there is good evidence that dietary restrictions can lower total cholesterol levels. The controversy exists only because there is no *proof* that dietary changes can directly affect the incidence of heart attacks. However, since diet affects blood cholesterol and cholesterol affects the heart,

it is highly likely that this link exists, and an increasing amount of medical evidence supports this hypothesis.

As we pointed out in discussing exercise and heart disease, physicians often have to make recommendations before the final facts are in. But you need to know what type and amount of exercise is best for you *now*, not fifteen years from now. So it is with diet. It will take years to settle all the debate, but we agree with the American Heart Association and recommend prudence in dietary fat intake *now*. There is much to gain and little to loose — the only "side effects" of a low-saturated-fat diet are the economic problems of the meat and dairy industries.

The average American consumes eleven gallons of ice cream, 261 eggs, and seventy-nine pounds of beef each year, totaling more than 40 percent of his daily calories from fat. We recommend that this figure should be much closer to 25 percent. A reduction in total fat intake will help with weight control, since fat, as we mentioned, has 9 calories per gram — more than twice the amount found in carbohydrates and protein. And the type of fat you eat is just as important as the amount of fat you eat. Aside from minute amounts of an essential fatty acid (found in vegetable oils), the body does not have a requirement for any particular fat. Hence, the prudent diet stresses a relative increase in unsaturated or vegetable fats and a decrease in saturated or animal fats.

Most dietary fats are in the form of triglyceride, a combination of glycerol and fatty acids. Fatty acids are composed of chains of carbon atoms to which hydrogen atoms are linked. Saturated fatty acids are those in which all the available carbon atoms have hydrogens attached. Unsaturated fatty acids are those with some "empty" carbons — i.e., not all carbon atoms have hydrogen atoms attached. If you are more comfortable in the kitchen than in the laboratory, you know that saturated fats come from animal sources and tend to be solid at room temperature, whereas unsaturated fats derive from vegetable source and are liquid at room temperature.

Cholesterol deserves special mention. Although it is technically not a fat but a sterol, cholesterol has been identified as the major culprit in arteriosclerotic heart disease. All animal tissues contain cholesterol — in fact, the human body can make all the cholesterol it needs without having any dietary sources. It seems prudent, therefore, to limit dietary cholesterol intake. This does not mean the elimination of all animal products, but does mean a change in food to keep dietary cholesterol intake to about 200 milligrams per day, less than is found in a single egg yolk.

On the other side of the coin, the healthful fats are the *poly*unsaturates — fatty acids in which many carbon atoms lack their full quota of hydrogens. No more than one-third to one-half of daily fat intake should be in the form of saturated fat; the remaining one-half to two-thirds should come from unsaturated fats, particularly the polyunsaturates. Vegetable oils such as corn, soybean, safflower, peanut, and cottonseed oil are good sources of unsaturates; beware, however, of coconut and palm oils, which are highly saturated. Figure 4–5 and the Appendix can guide you to more detailed information about the fat and cholesterol content of specific foods.

Whereas vegetable oils have been popular sources of

FIGURE 4–5: FATTY ACID AND CHOLESTEROL OF COMMONLY CONSUMED FOODS

FATTY ACID COMPOSITION
(as percentage of total fatty acids)

Food	Saturated	Monounsaturated	Polyunsaturated
Butter, cream, milk	65	30	5
Beef	46	48	6
Bacon and pork	38	50	12
Lard	42	45	13
Chicken	33	39	28
Fish, shellfish	29	31	40
Coconut oil	92	6	2
Palm kernel oil	86	12	2
Cocoa butter	63	34	3
Olive oil	15	76	9
Peanut oil	20	48	32
Cottonseed oil	27	20	53
Soybean oil	16	24	60
Corn oil	13	26	61
Sunflower seed oil	11	22	67
Safflower seed oil	10	13	77

CHOLESTEROL CONTENT

Food	Amount	Cholesterol (mg.)
Brains	3.5 oz. (100g.)	>2,000
Kidney	3.5 oz.	375
Liver (beef)	3.5 oz.	300
Egg yolk	1	252
Shrimp	3.5 oz.	150
Crab	3.5 oz.	100
Lobster	3.5 oz.	85
Cheddar cheese	3.5 oz.	84
Chicken	3.5 oz.	67
Beef	3.5 oz.	65
Clams, oysters	3.5 oz.	50
Flounder	3.5 oz.	50
Scallops	3.5 oz.	35
Milk, whole	1 cup	14

unsaturated fatty acids for years, nutritionists are just now turning to another excellent source: fish. The average American eats only thirteen pounds of fish a year; Greenland Eskimos eat *far* more and have far *less* heart disease. It turns out that fish contains two special polyunsaturated fatty acids that are not found in vegetable oils: eicosa-pentaenoic acid (EPA) and docosahexaenoic acid (DHA). EPA and DHA can actually *lower* your blood cholesterol and triglyceride levels, and will also make your platelets less sticky. This should lower the risk of atherosclerosis; without disputing the traditional assertion that fish is "brain food," we can suggest that fish is heart food.

Although all fish contain EPA and DHA, oily or dark-flesh fish have larger amounts; examples are tuna, salmon, bluefish, sardines, and mackerel. Shellfish were long considered to have harmful amounts of cholesterol, but new analyses suggest that clams, oysters, scallops, and mussels are actually quite low in cholesterol. Lobster and crab have intermediate cholesterol contents, and even shrimp has no more cholesterol than meat.

One final reminder before you head off to your fish store: smoked fish has a very high salt content, which can raise your blood pressure; many canned and processed fish also have added salt. Fish packed in water rather than in oil will have fewer calories, but breading and frying will also add calories.

While there is general agreement that saturated fats are harmful and *poly*unsaturated fats are healthful, there is still uncertainty about *mono*unsaturated fats, which are plentiful in olive oil and, to a lesser extent, peanut oil. Monounsaturated fats have traditionally been regarded as health "neutral," but new studies suggest that they may compare favorably with polyunsaturates in lowering LDL or "bad" cholesterol levels while preferentially preserving HDL or "good" cholesterol counts. More studies will be needed, but for now there is certainly no reason to restrict the amount of olive oil in your diet.

The American Heart Association's prudent diet calls for a reduction in the intake of animal fats including red meats and hard cheese (which have more than 75 percent of their calories as fat), egg yolks, whole milk, cream, ice cream, butter, and so forth. You don't have to avoid all meat, but you should choose lean cuts, trim the fat, and bake or broil instead of frying. Get your unsaturated fats from vegetable oils and your protein from fish, poultry, and skimmed milk products.

We have stressed the blood lipids and their effect on

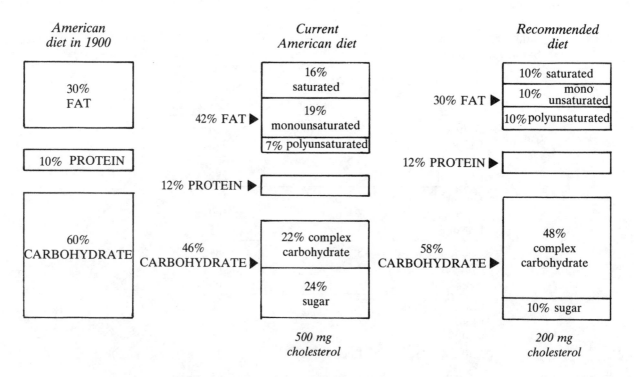

FIGURE 4–6: COMPARISON OF AMERICAN DIETS

the heart and blood vessels. But fats are also important for good health. They carry vitamins and are important in cell structure and function. They provide insulation against the cold. They are the body's major energy storage depot, and provide fuel for exercising muscles. They can even be aesthetically desirable. But the trick is to have the right amount of the right type of fat in the right places. Proper exercise and a prudent diet should help you keep saturated fat out of your blood vessels and still enable you to store up enough unsaturated fatty acids to fuel your exercise.

WATER

Water is unquestionably the single most important nutrient for the athlete, before, during, and after exercise. And yet the vital role of water is frequently overlooked or, worse, misunderstood.

Nearly two-thirds of the human body's weight is composed of water. Obviously water is indispensable for life and health. Because water is an integral participant in all the body's processes, the amount of water in the body and its distribution in our various cells, tissues, and fluids is very closely regulated. How is this precise control of body water achieved?

The central element in fluid regulation lies in one of the brain's most important control centers, the hypothalamus. Within the hypothalamus there are a group of cells called osmoreceptors. If the body lacks water, the blood becomes more concentrated and saltier, triggering the receptor cells in the hypothalamus to give up some of their own water to the blood. This causes the cells to shrink, which in turn has two very important effects: a sensation of thirst, and secretion of a hormone called ADH or "antidiuretic hormone," which causes the kidneys to conserve fluids by putting out smaller amounts of more concentrated urine. When you drink enough water to dilute your blood, the opposite reaction occurs: the osmoreceptor cells in the hypothalamus take up a tiny bit of this excess water, which causes them to swell. Once again, the results are twofold. First, you feel less thirsty so your intake of fluids stops. Second, the secretion of the hormone ADH stops, so your kidneys put out large amounts of dilute urine, rapidly ridding your body of excess water.

These rather complicated and completely involuntary mechanisms control the amount of water in your body. People's water needs vary widely, depending on body size, climate, and exercise. On the average, you need about a quart of water for each 1,000 calories you burn. In rough terms, the average adult takes in about two quarts of fluids daily — about two-thirds of this is in the form of the fluids you drink, while the remainder is contained in the food you eat. To stay in balance, the same amount of water must leave the body. About two-thirds of this fluid is excreted in the urine. The other types of water loss are less obvious but are very important, particularly when we consider the water needs of athletes. Even in cool weather when you are unaware of perspiring, about one pint of water is lost each day in the form of sweat. Finally, about a half-pint of water is lost each day in water vapor carried away from the lungs in the air you exhale.

If the body's fluid control mechanisms are so precise and so automatic, why discuss fluids at all? The answer is simple: the wisdom of the body often exceeds the wisdom of coaches and trainers. There are many misconceptions about water and exercise. Athletes are often cautioned against drinking water because fluids are rumored to cause bloating, excess weight, or sluggishness. Cramps and fatigue are erroneously attributed to drinking before or during competition. And in extreme cases, dehydration is actually encouraged to "build character" or "toughness." In fact, all of these common dictums are entirely wrong — appropriate fluid intake *prevents* fatigue, cramps, and weakness, while dehydration impairs performance and can even lead to life-threatening illness.

Dehydration or "sweating it out" is a common way for wrestlers, boxers, and lightweight crew members to "make weight." Nor is the athlete alone in these misconceptions. Fluid restriction is recommended in various crash diets, and some physicians even prescribe diuretic medications for weight reduction. These practices are to be deplored — dehydration is safe for "making weight" *only* if it is modest in degree and is substantially corrected before exercise. And dehydration has no place in long-term weight control.

To understand the importance of fluid replacement and the dangers of dehydration, we need only consider the water requirements of exercise. All exercise produces heat. At peak exertion, trained athletes can generate up to fifteen times more heat than the body produces at rest. Unless this heat is dispelled, body temperature would rise to disastrous levels — less than an hour of jogging, for example, produces enough heat to increase body temperature to over 110°F. We are not broiled with each hour of exercise because the body is able to get rid of excess heat through two major mechanisms.

First, heat is lost through the skin surface by simple radiational cooling. But when environmental temperatures are high or when muscular activity generates lots of heat, the second mechanism becomes crucial: sweating.

You can produce truly prodigious amounts of perspiration when you exercise. Aesthetics notwithstanding, this perspiration is very beneficial, because as sweat evaporates it takes heat away from the body. In fact, a quart of sweat will, if fully evaporated, remove all the heat generated in an hour of jogging so that body temperature remains normal. In our fastidious culture, such volumes of perspiration may seem unthinkable, but in reality the body can shed over two quarts in an hour of vigorous exercise, especially if the weather is hot and humid.

We are all aware of fluid loss during warm-weather exercise, but winter sports can also result in significant fluid losses. If you dress properly for cross-country skiing, skating, or winter jogging, you will stay quite warm, and as you exercise all those layers of clothing will become saturated by sweat. An additional factor is the dryness of winter air — substantial amounts of water vapor can be lost from your respiratory passages while you exercise in the dry, cold winter atmosphere.

So fluid losses accompany exercise in all seasons. What are the hazards of falling behind in your fluid replacement? The first effect is impaired athletic performance; you will tire more easily and have less strength and endurance if you become dehydrated. Moreover, fatigue and irritability can persist for hours after you stop exercising if fluids are not replaced. If dehydration is allowed to become pronounced, some very serious illnesses can result. A fall in blood pressure is one such problem. A second consequence may be damage to kidney function. Finally, in warm weather, heat exhaustion and even heat stroke can be triggered off by dehydration during exercise.

Unfortunately, you cannot rely on your body's automatic fluid regulation system to tell you how much to drink during exercise. The fluid shifts that accompany exertion begin very early in exercise, and thirst lags quite far behind. And even when you begin to feel thirsty, the other physical and mental sensations of sports competition may well distract you from thirst and cause you to underestimate seriously your fluid needs. Chapter 7 will provide the practical details of fluid replacement for sports. For now, we have a simple but very important message: drink early and drink often.

MINERALS

At least fifteen mineral compounds must be provided by the diet to insure good health. Most of these minerals are required in trace amounts only. A well-balanced diet will provide all the minerals you need, so that supplements are not necessary except for menstruating women, who may require extra iron, and postmenopausal women, who may need calcium supplements. Other athletes do not need extra minerals.

Sodium (Salt)

One of the great paradoxes of sports nutrition is the underuse of water and the overuse of salt. The fact that huge volumes of sweat are lost during exercise has led to the widespread belief that athletes need extra salt. Even today, salt tablets are often recommended to make up for the sodium lost in sweat. This practice is unnecessary and may well be harmful.

Extra salt is unnecessary because a normal diet supplies more than enough to compensate for the athlete's sodium losses. Although sweat is salty, it actually contains a much lower concentration of sodium than does the blood. Moreover, the sodium content of sweat decreases as you acclimate to the heat. Since you lose relatively more water than salt in sweat, the blood sodium concentration may actually rise during exercise. Hence, your body needs water, not salt. If your body begins to fall behind in salt, it has compensatory mechanisms that allow the kidneys to conserve salt very efficiently. So the salt provided in a normal diet will allow you to catch up very nicely.

Extra salt may be harmful because a high-sodium diet can contribute to high blood pressure (hypertension). It has been estimated that more than twenty-three million Americans — 15 percent of our adult population — have hypertension. Although there are many causes of hypertension, the excessive salt content of the average American diet is a contributory factor in many cases. An average adult needs only one to three grams of sodium daily (one to three level teaspoons of table salt), yet the dietary intake may easily be *many* times higher.

Unfortunately, we have been conditioned to like high-salt foods from childhood onward. In fact, until recently even baby foods had extra salt added. Many of the "fast foods" and processed foods that sell so well contain enormous amounts of sodium; for example, just ten potato chips contain as much salt as twenty-five *pounds* of potatoes. Salty foods must be strictly avoided by people with hypertension and heart disease, and should be used sparingly if at all even by healthy individuals. Unfortunately, the term "junk foods" is well deserved — you should read food labels and develop an awareness of the salt content of your diet. The Appendix can direct you to sources listing the sodium content of selected foods. The same restraints apply to the ubiquitous saltshaker. Even healthy people should learn to avoid table salt, and to cook with as little salt as possible.

Are there any circumstances in which fit, active people should seek extra salt? The answer is a qualified yes. Vigorous exercise in warm climates is a reasonable excuse for *temporarily* using the saltshaker or having some bouillon, pickles, cold cuts, or other salty food. As you acclimate to the heat, you will have less justification for these indulgences. Salt tablets are almost never needed. All in all, a normal diet will provide plenty of salt, and nutritional planning should strive for a lower sodium intake, even for athletes.

Potassium

Most commercial replacement solutions for athletes contain potassium, reflecting the widespread belief that exercise leads to potassium depletion. As with so many other traditions of sports nutrition, there is startlingly little scientific evidence for this belief. Only small amounts of potassium are lost in sweat. Potassium is lost in the urine; while the body can limit this potassium loss to some degree, the kidneys cannot conserve potassium as well as they can retain sodium. Even so, studies have shown that the body's potassium stores remain normal even during vigorous exertion on consecutive days in warm weather. All that is needed is a normal diet. Many foods, including vegetables, dairy products, and meat, contain potassium, but citrus fruits and bananas are particularly rich in potassium.

Far from being necessary, potassium supplements can actually be harmful. Unlike sodium, most of the body's potassium is stored within cells instead of in the free fluids such as blood and tissue fluid. Muscle cells have a high potassium content. Vigorous exercise can cause muscles to transfer some potassium to the blood. The acid condition that can accompany anaerobic exercise also tends to raise blood potassium levels. Finally, dehydration impairs the kidney's ability to excrete potas-

sium. All three factors, then, tend to raise blood potassium levels during exercise. The last thing you need during exercise is extra potassium, since very high blood levels can be dangerous to the heart.

All in all, a normal diet will give the athlete plenty of potassium, and a good fluid intake will help avoid the dangers of high blood potassium levels. Once again, the basics of sound nutrition are much more healthful then expensive supplements.

Iron

Iron is an essential component of the hemoglobin molecule in red blood cells, and a deficiency of iron will lead to anemia. Anemia in turn can produce fatigue, weakness, and impaired athletic performance. Although some competitors take iron to aid performance, there is not a shred of evidence that extra iron will improve athletic skills unless you are anemic. Hard work, rather than iron, is what you need to build muscles of steel.

Iron is one of the few nutrients that may actually be deficient in the average American diet. Iron is present in many foods, but the absorption of iron from the intestinal tract can be erratic, averaging about 10 percent. Red meat is the best dietary source of iron. But if your fitness program is turning you away from a high-meat diet, you will have to rely on other foods to provide your iron. Deep green vegetables (spinach, kale, beet greens), beans, peanuts, and raisins are examples of iron-rich foods. However, even these natural foods may not provide enough iron. As a result, iron is now added to many grain products such as breads and cereals. The iron content of these "fortified" or enriched products is listed on their labels.

The amount of iron you need depends on your age and sex. Growing children have relatively high iron needs, but these needs are invariably met by a healthful diet. However, even a good diet may not provide enough iron for pregnant or lactating women, so obstetricians routinely prescribe iron supplements for their patients.

Adult men require no more than 10 milligrams of iron daily, and this amount is readily available in the average diet. Women need nearly twice as much iron; since they lose blood with each menstrual period, extra iron is required to produce new red blood cells. Women should make a conscious effort to get about 18 milligrams per day of dietary iron. Fortified breads and cereals may do the trick. But if there is any doubt, have your red blood cell count checked (hemoglobin or hematocrit test). This should be part of your regular medical evaluation in any case. If you have iron deficiency anemia despite a good diet, your physician will prescribe iron supplements to correct the situation.

Other Minerals

Calcium is the major mineral in bones and as such constitutes nearly 25 percent of the body's weight. Calcium is also important for nerve conduction, muscle contraction, and other vital functions. Calcium may help prevent high blood pressure and adequate calcium intake may even have a role in protecting against colon cancer. Healthy adults require about 800 milligrams of calcium daily; this requirement is increased by 5 percent in adolescents and in pregnant or lactating women. Postmenopausal women should be particularly careful to get enough calcium, because calcium deficiency can contribute to osteoporosis (thin bones) and fractures. Calcium supplements are generally advisable for postmenopausal women. Athletes do not require additional calcium. Dairy products are the best dietary sources of calcium, but green vegetables and soy beans also provide calcium. Vitamin D is necessary for optimal absorption of calcium.

Phosphorus is bound to calcium in bone and is crucial for many other functions. Almost all foods have at least some phosphorus, and it is hard to imagine a dietary deficiency of this element.

Iodine is important for the function of the thyroid gland. Iodine is present in many foods and in water. Because the iodine content is low in some inland regions, iodine is added to salt. But even if you limit your salt intake, you should get plenty of iodine in a normal diet. Iodine is one of the few nutrients that has not, to our knowledge, been inappropriately recommended as a supplement for athletes.

A number of other metals are necessary for health. For adults the recommended daily dietary intake for *magnesium* is 350 milligrams, for *zinc* 15 milligrams, and for *copper* and *manganese* about 3 milligrams. Trace amounts of *chromium, cobalt, molybdenum,* and *selenium* are also required. However, a normal diet will provide all these elements without any difficulty. Supplements of these minerals are entirely unnecessary and could even be troublesome if excessive.

The minerals required for fitness are no different from those required for good health. The average American diet will provide the right balance of minerals with just three exceptions: the usual diet often has too much salt

for everyone, and may have too little iron for menstruating women and too little calcium for postmenopausal women.

VITAMINS

Whereas many aspects of nutrition are debatable, none is more heatedly debated than vitamins. And if vitamins are controversial, megavitamins are megacontroversial.

We believe there is enough scientific evidence to warrant three clear-cut conclusions about vitamins: (1) a well-balanced diet provides all the vitamins required for optimal health; (2) supplementary vitamins do not enhance either health in general or fitness in particular; (3) in moderate doses, supplementary vitamins are safe, though expensive. Self-confidence is an important element in sports and in most other human endeavors. If you feel better taking vitamins, there is no reason for us to discourage you from doing so, providing the dosage is not excessive.

In a sense, we have started at the finish line by giving you our conclusions about vitamins. Let's go back to the starting blocks and look at the reasons for these statements.

Perhaps the only fact about vitamins that is universally agreed upon is that vitamins are essential to health, and indeed to life. Vitamins are organic chemicals that the body cannot make for itself, but that are required for innumerable metabolic processes. Despite the importance of vitamins, only tiny amounts of these substances are needed by your body. The question is not if you need vitamins (you do), but if you need extra vitamins in pill form.

Vitamins fall into two broad groups. The fat-soluble vitamins (A, D, E, and K) are true to their name — they are eaten with fat-containing foods, are absorbed into the body along with fat, and are stored in the body's adipose tissue. This storage capacity means that you do not need to ingest these substances each day because your own tissues contain large reserves. That's the good news. The bad news is that if you take too much of these vitamins, you can gradually store up toxic amounts, especially of vitamins A and D.

The water-soluble vitamins (vitamin C and the eight B vitamins) are not stored by your body to any appreciable degree. So you need these substances at frequent (if not daily) intervals. Excessive cooking can remove these vitamins from foods, but balanced diets contain such generous amounts that deficiencies of these vitamins rarely develop unless serious underlying diseases are present. Because these vitamins are not stored up in the body, supplementary doses are safe. But for exactly the same reason, large amounts of these vitamins are no more beneficial than small amounts — once the body's needs are filled, the excess vitamins are simply spilled out in the urine (where large doses of vitamin C can sometimes cause the formation of stones). People who take vitamins may not be healthier than those who don't — but they certainly have more expensive urine.

Let's briefly consider the individual vitamins:

Vitamin A is important for healthy skin and mucous membranes, and for vision in dim light. Deficiencies of vitamin A produce "night blindness" and skin disorders. Adults require an average of 5,000 units of vitamin A daily. Vitamin A is found in yellow and green vegetables, in liver and other meats, and in fortified dairy products. Overdoses of vitamin A (more than 20,000 units per day) can cause headaches due to brain swelling, skin and eye disorders, and liver damage. A derivative of vitamin A is being used experimentally to treat severe cases of acne.

Thiamine (B_1) is important for the utilization of carbohydrates. Deficiencies of thiamine produce disorders of the nervous system and heart (beriberi). Adults require up to 1.5 milligrams of thiamine daily. Thiamine is found in many foods, including vegetables, meats, and grain. Although cooking can substantially lower the thiamine content of foods, deficiencies are rare in Western society, except in alcoholics.

Riboflavin (B_2) is also important for the body's metabolism. Deficiency of riboflavin can cause lesions of the lips, tongue, and cornea. Adults require up to 1.7 milligrams daily. Riboflavin is widely distributed in many foods, including leafy vegetables, meat, and fish. Hence, deficiency states are most uncommon.

Niacin (B_3) also functions in the body's metabolism. Deficiencies cause disorders of the tongue, diarrhea, and mental changes (pellagra). Adults require up to 19 milligrams of niacin daily. Niacin is widely distributed in meat, fish, poultry, legumes, whole grains, enriched bread, and other foods, so that deficiencies are rare. Niacin can be used medically to treat elevated cholesterol levels but may cause flushing, headaches, and other side effects in these large doses (300–2,000 milligrams daily).

Pyridoxine (B_6) is important for proper function of the nervous system, for red blood cells, and for other metabolic functions. Deficiencies can cause anemia, neurologic disorders (including decreased sensation or seizures), and other problems. Adults require 2 milligrams daily. Pyridoxine is present in meat, whole grains, soy beans, peanuts, and many vegetables, so that deficiencies are rare. Oral contraceptive pills increase the requirements for B_6, but dietary sources are still sufficient to fulfill these needs. Large doses of B_6 (more than 500 milligrams per day) can cause nerve damage.

Cobalamin (B_{12}) is important for the formation of blood cells and for the proper function of the nervous system and gastrointestinal tract. Deficiencies of B_{12} produce pernicious anemia. Adults require perhaps 3 milligrams of B_{12} daily. B_{12} is found only in animal products, so strict vegetarians should take supplementary doses of B_{12}. The only other people who need extra B_{12} are patients with pernicious anemia, disorders of intestinal absorption, or certain infections. The B_{12} shot is one of the most abused treatments in medicine, since it is of no proven benefit except in these special circumstances; the many testimonials to B_{12} stem from psychological factors. Fortunately, supplementary B_{12} appears to be harmless.

Pantothenic acid is another of the B vitamins, which functions in metabolism. Deficiencies may result in neurological damage and impaired ability to fight infection. The recommended daily intake for adults is 4 to 7 milligrams. Meat, egg yolks, members of the cabbage family, and whole grains contain pantothenic acid, as do other foods. Deficiencies are rare except in undernourished alcoholics.

Biotin is a member of the B complex that is presumed necessary for man. A deficiency syndrome has not been defined. The daily requirement for biotin is not known with certainty, but 100 to 200 milligrams is recommended. Biotin is so widely distributed in foods that deficiency is extremely unlikely and supplementary doses are surely unnecessary.

Folic acid is unlike other water-soluble vitamins, in that substantial amounts are stored in the liver. Folic acid is important for the formation of blood cells, and deficiencies can produce anemia as well as disturbances of the gastrointestinal tract. The daily requirement for adults is .4 milligram. Folic acid is present in green vegetables, legumes, yeasts, liver, and other foods. Deficiencies, however, can occur in alcoholics and other malnourished individuals, and in patients taking certain antiseizure medications. High doses of folic acid (many times the normal dietary intake) can on occasion mask vitamin B_{12} deficiency.

"*Vitamin B₁₅*" is not a bona fide vitamin. In other words, there is no known human requirement for this substance. The promotion of "vitamin B₁₅" as an aid to athletic performance and health is a prime example of nutritional exploitation based on misinformation, avarice, or both.

Vitamin C (ascorbic acid) has many roles in the body, including the normal function of blood vessels and wound healing. A deficiency of vitamin C results in scurvy. Citrus fruits and vegetables contain vitamin C, and true deficiencies are quite uncommon. The daily requirement for vitamin C is 60 milligrams. Larger doses are sometimes used medically to suppress urinary tract infections. Vitamin C is one of the most widely used vitamins, and many claims are made for ascorbic acid, including prevention of the common cold. Unfortunately, there is no scientific evidence to support these claims, and substantial information has accumulated refuting some of them. Whereas modest doses of vitamin C appear safe, large doses (more than several grams per day) can interfere with the action of vitamin B_{12} and can cause diarrhea or kidney and bladder stones.

Vitamin D is one of the fat-soluble vitamins, and is essential for the regulation of the body's calcium stores and for the health of the skeletal system. Vitamin D is available in fortified milk and in other foods such as egg yolk, liver, and fish. Vitamin D can also be produced in the skin as a result of the sun's action. The recommended daily allowance for adults is 400 units. Although deficiencies of vitamin D cause significant problems in bones, excessive amounts of the "sunshine vitamin" (more than 50,000 units twice a week) can also produce serious disorders related to high blood calcium levels. In a sense, vitamin D is an object lesson for nutrition in general and vitamins in particular: the fact that a little is good does not necessarily mean that a lot is better.

Vitamin E serves a variety of important roles in the body but does not, unfortunately, possess the miraculous properties claimed for this fat-soluble vitamin. Deficiencies of vitamin E can contribute to anemia and other problems. The recommended daily allowance for adults is 30 units (about 10 milligrams). Your requirement for vitamin E increases as your fat intake increases, but fats such as vegetable oils and margarine, as well as other foods, provide plenty of vitamin E for your needs. Vitamin E is currently one of the most fashionable vitamin supplements. Industrial doses of vitamin E are recommended for many purposes, including athletic performance and sexual prowess. Although vitamin E accumulates in the body, even fairly large doses (ten times the daily requirement) appear to be relatively safe. At the present time, the major side effects of vitamin E supplementation are headaches and nausea in a few people and disappointment in many.

Vitamin K plays a crucial role in blood clotting. Deficiencies of vitamin K are uncommon except in occasional newborns and in patients with diseases that impair the absorption of fats. The administration of antibiotics can also lead to vitamin K deficiency. The daily requirement for vitamin K is estimated at 70 to 140 micrograms. Leafy green vegetables and members of the cabbage family contain vitamin K. This vitamin is also made by the bacteria in the human intestinal tract, so that deficiencies are very rare except in the special medical conditions outlined earlier.

All of these vitamins are crucial for health. A normal diet will provide more than enough vitamins to prevent deficiency diseases, but will higher doses enhance either health or athletic performance? With regard to performance, the answer is no. Four of the B vitamins (B_1, B_2, B_3, and pantothenic acid) are necessary for the body's metabolism to generate energy. Athletes need more energy than people who are not fit, but a normal diet provides a superabundance of B vitamins, so supplements are not necessary.

As for health, there is only one area in which higher than usual quantities of vitamins *may* be helpful — but it is an important area indeed: cancer. There is some evidence that vitamin A may help reduce the risk of cancer. The evidence is still very preliminary, and in fact, a recent study showed that cancer patients and healthy people had identical levels of vitamins A and E. A study of supplementary carotene, which is converted by the body into vitamin A, in twenty thousand healthy volunteers (all physicians, we may note) is under way, but the results won't be available for years. Until then, the best advice is that of the American Cancer Society: eat lots of vegetables, especially yellow and dark green ones that are high in carotene and vitamin C, but don't bother with vitamin pills. And while we are on the subject, the best ways to reduce your cancer risk are to stop smoking, limit your intake of alcohol, high-fat foods, and smoked or salt-cured foods, eat lots of fiber, and avoid exposure to known carcinogens.

If sufficient vitamins are provided by a normal, well-balanced diet, why then are vitamins so popular? The answer is as complicated as human nature itself. We are all looking for ways to improve the quality of life and prevent illness. Vitamins provide a seductively simple solution — it's easy to take them and easy to believe in them, so the faith is spread.

Vitamin enthusiasts may be perfectly sincere and honest, but their subjective endorsement really cannot be given the weight of fact. And athletes are no less susceptible than the rest of us. In fact, because of their fierce desire to find a competitive edge, athletes may actually be *more* prone to believe in vitamins. Fifty percent of all competitive athletes take vitamins; the half who don't take them, however, perform just as well as the half who do.

Sad to say, another incentive may also explain the vitamin craze: Americans spend more than two billion dollars annually on vitamins, and the profit motive surely plays a role in the widespread promotion of vitamin supplementation.

The great majority of people who make vitamins, sell vitamins, and take vitamins are neither foolish nor greedy. They genuinely believe that supplementary vitamins contribute importantly to health and well-being. Although we cannot discern a scientific basis for this belief, neither is there any medical reason to interdict vitamin supplements in moderate doses (such as one or two multiple-vitamin pills daily). So if you feel better taking such vitamins, go right ahead. But keep three facts in mind: (1) Natural vitamins are no better than synthetic vitamins, and costly vitamins are no better than inexpensive preparations. Your body simply cannot tell the difference. (2) Excessive doses of vitamins can be toxic. (3) Vitamins alone do not insure good nutrition. Even the most "high potency" multiple-vitamin-mineral preparation does not provide the carbohydrate, protein, fat, or calories that you need. Vitamins cannot replace missed meals and should not be used as substitutes for sound nutrition.

FIBER

In most areas of nutrition, the athlete's requirements are identical to those of other healthy individuals. When the athlete has special needs, they are generally for increased nutrients: more calories, more carbohydrates, and more water. But when it comes to fiber, the athlete may be best advised to use *less,* at least on the day of an important competition. What are the pros and cons of dietary fiber for health and for sports?

Ten years ago, the medical profession was cautioning patients with diverticulosis to avoid roughage in their diets. We have now done an about-face: fiber is in fashion to treat and even to prevent this common disease of the colon. This change of heart may at first seem like good reason for you to ignore all medical advice about your diet. But in fact, it should have the opposite effect. The "low roughage" recommendations were based on time-honored teachings and traditions that had no medical data behind them. When the question was finally examined scientifically, surprising results emerged. The moral is to remain skeptical about nutritional dogmas based only on tradition or testimonials, and to favor advice based on sound scientific information.

The new look at fiber began with epidemiologic studies, which suggested that the incidence of diverticulosis began to rise in Western society with the widespread use of refined foods. Moreover, it was shown that there is a much lower incidence of diverticulosis and constipation in cultures that have retained high-fiber diets. The third step was to try high-fiber diets on patients in the United States. The results have been encouraging, and there is widespread agreement that dietary fiber is an important way to prevent and treat diverticulosis and constipation.

But in our quest for a dietary cure-all, the enthusiasm for fiber may have gotten a little ahead of the data. The same studies that showed a reduction in diverticulosis among people who eat lots of fiber showed also that these groups have a lower incidence of many other conditions including hernias, hemorrhoids, varicose veins, gallstones, bowel cancer, diabetes, and even atherosclerosis; one type of fiber, oat bran, even lowers serum cholesterol levels. The problem is that most of these diseases stem from a complex group of genetic and environmental causes. Fiber is only one factor among many, and it is premature to assume confidently that a high-fiber diet will protect you against all of these diverse disorders.

Fiber, or "roughage," is a group of plant carbohydrates including cellulose, pectin, and gum. But unlike the dietary carbohydrates that are digested and absorbed to provide energy, these carbohydrates have no caloric value. Because it cannot be digested in the stomach and intestines, fiber passes into the colon, where it acts to pull water into the stools. The results are bulkier, softer stools and more frequent bowel movements, with better emptying of the colon.

None of this sounds particularly appealing. American society has been trained to favor refined foods which are low in fiber. But we urge you instead to develop a taste for high-fiber foods, including root vegetables, raw unskinned fruits, and whole grain or bran. The average American diet contains only 10 to 30 grams of fiber, whereas high-roughage diets may contain up to three times more fiber. You can find more information about the fiber content of various foods from sources listed in the Appendix.

If fiber is so beneficial, why deny athletes these benefits? There is no reason to do so, and we do recommend generous amounts of dietary fiber to competitive athletes, with only one qualification. As with most good things, there are potential problems with fiber. Some people develop abdominal bloating, gas, and even cramps from high-fiber diets. Obviously, a bloated belly will slow you down, so you should avoid eating too much fiber on the day of competition.

FACT OR FANTASY: SELECTED NUTRITIONAL CONTROVERSIES

Alcohol

Is alcohol a nutrient or a drug? Both. As a nutrient, alcohol is metabolized as a carbohydrate. Alcohol contains 7 calories per gram, putting it just below fat as a concentrated source of calories. But as a nutrient, alcohol is a classic example of the "empty calorie," for you get no nutritional benefits from alcohol apart from the calories. Moral? Alcohol is fattening.

As a drug, alcohol has some potential benefits. For centuries alcohol has been used for relaxation and celebration. These social benefits cannot be overlooked, and are widely utilized by athletes from the locker room to the tap room. Alcohol has also been suggested by physicians over the ages as an aid to circulation or digestion. Although there are a few situations in which alcohol is a useful medication (methanol poisoning, premature labor), the testimonials to alcohol's medicinal benefits cannot be substantiated. However, recent studies do suggest an improvement in the blood lipid profile and a decreased incidence of heart attacks as a result of about two drinks per day. More studies will be needed to confirm these findings.

Even if alcohol in modest doses is shown to have some long-term benefits, it will be difficult for most physicians actually to prescribe the fruit of the grape.

This is because excessive doses of alcohol can have devastating effects. Acute intoxication is a major source of motor vehicle accidents and other severe injuries. Chronic use can lead to addiction, with terrible personal and social consequences. Anyone who reads the sports pages regularly will be able to name star athletes from all sports who have gone public with their alcoholism. And if untreated, alcoholism can produce grave damage to the liver, stomach, nervous system, and blood-forming organs.

All in all, there is nothing wrong with a little alcohol — it may even be good for you. But be careful: excessive amounts of alcohol are very hazardous.

Is the athlete any different vis-à-vis alcohol? Not really. Alcohol does not give special energy and has no benefits for strength or endurance. Alcohol can impair coordination, judgment, and "reflexes," and is therefore best consumed after competition rather than beforehand.

Caffeine

Like alcohol, caffeine is a drug, and is so widespread in various beverages that it is often considered only as a food. Caffeine is present in coffee and tea and in drinks made from cocoa beans and kola nuts. Coffee contains about 100 milligrams of caffeine per eight ounces, the other drinks half as much.

We have already noted that caffeine may be useful for some endurance athletes by improving glycogen utilization. These benefits are small, and although caffeine is a stimulant it does not seem to assist strength or speed. Some people do feel more alert and confident and may play better after a cup of coffee or two. Others note unpleasant effects such as rapid heartbeats and even fine tremors; obviously they should avoid caffeine prior to sports.

Caffeine does have some medical uses. It is present in many over-the-counter painkiller combinations; although caffeine itself is not a painkiller, it can increase the potency of the aspirin or acetaminophen in these pills. Caffeine can also be used to fight asthma; whereas caffeine itself is rarely used for this purpose, chemically related drugs are very helpful for asthmatic patients.

Efforts have been made to link coffee with various diseases ranging from heart attacks to fibrocystic disease of the breast to cancer of the pancreas. There is really not enough data to support any of these associations at present. Caffeine may increase blood cholesterol levels and can elevate blood pressure, so it should be used sparingly by people with hypertension or heart disease. Caffeine may have a slight role in producing birth defects; though it's too early to be sure, pregnant women should be cautioned against excessive use of caffeine. If you have a tendency toward ulcers, palpitations, or insomnia you should avoid caffeine. Otherwise you "pay your money and take your choice": caffeine consumption is a matter of personal preference.

"High-Energy" Foods

We have already discussed the merits of a high-carbohydrate diet in general and the demerits of concentrated sweets prior to exercise. But the athlete's desire for a shortcut to success is so great that numerous foods are commercially promoted as aids to performance. Examples include wheat germ, bee's honey, protein supplements, amino acids, lecithin, and so forth. Save your money.

Fasting

The current interest in fasting is one of the minor mysteries of mankind. Short-term fasts have a role in various religious experiences and are medically safe for healthy people. Long-term fasts are occasionally useful in political protests and civil disobedience but are medically very dangerous. No form of fasting will "purify the system" or aid health or athletic performance. Save your zeal.

Natural Foods and Food Additives

The jury is still out on food additives. It is easy to sympathize with an instinctive preference for the natural and an aversion for the artificial. Indeed, some food additives have been shown to be harmful to laboratory animals or man. Quite properly, these additives have been banned, and continued testing and vigilance is obviously mandatory. But other food additives have been used for years and are perfectly safe; examples of safe additives include calcium proprionate, which is added to baked goods to retard spoilage, and lecithin, which is added to margarine, baked goods, and ice cream for texture and consistency. Remember, too, that vitamin D, which is added to milk to prevent rickets, and iodine, which is added to salt to prevent goiter, are additives that have been very helpful to society.

The best advice we can give you is to consider food additives individually — some may be harmful, some are helpful, and most are medically neutral but economically helpful to manufacturers and aesthetically helpful to consumers who want flavor and color in their foods. Don't confuse additives with contaminants —

we share your concern about dangerous insecticides such as DDT and EDB, which have accidentally contaminated grain products in the past, but this has no bearing on well-studied, safe products such as calcium proprionate, which is intentionally added to grain products. Don't be turned off by all chemicals in food — all foods are made up of chemicals, and some of the most "natural" substances — such as salt — can be among the most harmful chemicals in your diet. Finally, don't go to the other extreme and assume that any food that is "fortified" or "enriched" with added vitamins and minerals is automatically good for you — no amount of vitamins can alter the fact that sugar cereals and other "junk" foods are just that — junk.

What about "organic" foods? Unfortunately, this term has no precise legal definition; it usually signifies foods that are grown without fertilizers and insecticides, but these claims are hard to substantiate. The same is true for "natural" foods — the Agriculture Department requires only "minimal" processing and no artificial flavoring, coloring, or preservatives for any food that is labeled "natural."

"Natural" or "organic" foods have no special attributes other than expense. And synthetic fertilizers and insecticides have had enormous agricultural benefits, which provide some help in keeping food prices down and in feeding the hungry. To be sure, some of these chemicals are unsafe and have been appropriately banned. In a climate that opposes government activism it is important to keep an open mind and to support further objective study. Save your outrage.

The Vegetarian Diet

Whereas the "casual" vegetarian can easily slip into unhealthful dietary patterns, the well-informed vegetarian who plans meals carefully can have a nutritious and healthful diet. There are several forms of vegetarian diets: pure vegetarians eat plant foods only, lacto-vegetarians eat dairy products in addition to plant foods, and lacto-ovo-vegetarians add egg products as well. In other less formal variations, some individuals eat fish but not meat. Because vitamin B_{12} is found only in animal products, vegetarians need supplementary B_{12}. With careful planning, a vegetarian diet can provide all the other nutrients needed if a variety of fruits, vegetables, beans, nuts, and grains is included. The addition of dairy products greatly simplifies the vegetarians' major problem, which is the need for high-quality protein.

Numerous claims are made for the virtues of a vegetarian diet. The only clear-cut advantages of these diets are their low saturated-fat content and their high fiber content. As a result, vegetarians do tend to have less obesity, lower blood lipid levels, and less diabetes than their omnivorous peers.

A vegetarian diet is neither helpful nor harmful to athletic performance. A number of highly successful athletes have been vegetarians. The assertion that vegetarian athletes lack assertiveness or competitiveness is laughable. Save your scorn.

Nutritional Difference Between Male and Female Athletes

This is yet another area of nutrition that has generated more heat than light. Feminists and chauvinists notwithstanding, the only differences are the higher iron needs of menstruating women, the higher calcium needs of postmenopausal women, and the higher caloric requirements of men. Save your slogans.

The Pre-game Meal

No area of sports nutrition is more embroiled in myth, misconception, and dogma than the pre-game meal. Most athletes develop a series of rituals before competition, which may include the ingestion of a bewildering variety of foods, ranging from raw meat to wheat germ, as well as an equally diverse selection of fluids, from bottled water to bottled beer.

The best advice we can offer about the pre-game meal is to skip it. During the two hours prior to exercise, you should avoid eating solids. A light snack three or even four hours before competition is a good idea. We usually suggest complex carbohydrates such as toast or yogurt, but the choice is up to you. However, you should avoid roughage, spicy or heavy foods, high-fat foods, and concentrated sweets. You can and should continue to drink fluids right up to the game time; we particularly recommend six to eight ounces of water fifteen minutes before the start. Save your appetite until after the game, when you can really indulge it.

CREATING A BALANCED DIET

Good nutrition for fitness is good nutrition for health.

Throughout this chapter, we have explained the principles of sound nutrition by breaking your requirements down into their component parts so that we could review those individual elements one at a time. But you can't put "protein" on your shopping list or order "poly-

unsaturated fats" at a restaurant. Let's now put the individual nutrients back together to outline a balanced diet for fitness and health. The nice thing about this overall plan is that you do not have to weigh, measure, and analyze each item you eat or drink. Unless you are on a special therapeutic diet (very low salt, fat, or calorie, for example) you can stick to those basic principles and the details will take care of themselves.

Eating for fitness requires both overall balance in your diet and weight control; let's look first at the balanced diet and then at the problem of weight reduction.

Most people know that a balanced diet requires daily portions of each of the four "food groups": dairy products, fruits and vegetables, cereals and breads, and meat, fish, or legumes. There is nothing wrong with this credo (as long as you use skimmed milk products and modest portions of lean meat to reduce your cholesterol intake), but modern nutrition is a good deal more sophisticated. We can now outline eleven principles of a balanced diet:

1. *Eat a variety of foods.* Here's where the concept of the four food groups comes in. It is not necessary to select foods from each group at every meal, but it is a good idea to eat a varied menu. If you get in the habit of choosing a broad range of foods, you will get all the nutrients you need and you will also minimize your chance of being overexposed to unforeseen contaminants in any given food product. In addition, variety will make eating for fitness enjoyable and satisfying.

2. *Maintain ideal body weight.* People who are in the appropriate weight range are healthier and live longer than do people who are very over- or underweight. We'll tell you how to assess your own weight and how to combine exercise and diet for weight control.

3. *Reduce your intake of saturated fats.* Figure 4–6 shows you the traditional composition of the American diet with regard to fat, carbohydrate, and protein — as well as the distribution which we recommend. As you can see, our recommendations are not a radical new scheme, but a return to the good old days. Your fat consumption should not account for more than 25 percent of your daily caloric intake. Moreover, the majority of your dietary fat consumption should be in the form of unsaturated fat. Choose low-fat milk and

dairy products. Sharply limit your intake of high-cholesterol foods, such as eggs, butter and cream, and organ meats. Avoid hydrogenated margarine and coconut oil. Favor fish and fowl over red meat; select lean cuts of meat, and trim off all the fat you can. Whenever possible, broil or bake foods instead of frying. You should also avoid overcooking meat and should limit your intake of charcoal-broiled foods — not because of their fat content, but because of a possible cancer risk.

4. *Eat plenty of complex carbohydrates.* "Spaghetti," said Sophia Loren, "is a psychological necessity." Without debating the point, we would add that complex carbohydrates — pasta, grains, unrefined cereals, breads, and so forth — are a physiological necessity. These foods should make up the majority of your caloric intake; in addition to energy, they will give you fiber, nutrients, and enjoyment.

5. *Avoid too much sugar.* Simple sugars and refined carbohydrates give you calories without nutrients. If weight is no problem, you can indulge yourself a bit — but for most of us, calories do count, and sugary foods are the first things you should restrict. "Natural" sweets such as brown sugar, honey, or molasses are no more healthful than white sugar. And all sweets increase your risk of tooth decay.

6. *Obtain adequate fiber in your diet.* High-fiber foods are filling, help regulate bowel function, and reduce the risk of a variety of diseases. Bran, unrefined grain products, and raw fruits and vegetables are excellent sources of dietary fiber.

7. *Eat lots of fresh fruits and vegetables.* In addition to providing carbohydrate, fiber, and vitamins, there is preliminary evidence that this may reduce your risk of cancer. Avoid overcooking vegetables so that you don't boil nutrients away.

8. *Avoid excess sodium (salt).* One to three grams a day will give you *more* than enough sodium in your diet; if you have high blood pressure or certain heart, liver, or kidney problems you may have to restrict yourself to much less. Use as little salt as possible in cooking and take the saltshaker off the table. Be particularly wary of processed foods: potato chips, pretzels, salted nuts, many condiments and sauces, canned soups, pickled foods, and sandwich meats are particularly salty.

9. *If you drink alcohol, do so in moderation.* We hate to be party-poopers, but from a medical viewpoint, you should average no more than two ounces of hard liquor or two portions of beer or wine per day.

10. *Distribute your meals wisely.* There is some scientific evidence that your mother is right: a good breakfast is helpful to nutrition and weight control. Three moderate meals a day makes good sense. In particular, avoid snacks if you are watching your weight. And if you do snack, try to avoid processed foods, which are often high in salt or fat. Unfortunately, most of the typical snack foods really do belong in this "junk" category.

11. *Read food labels.* This is really the only way you know what you are eating. With careful reading, you can determine the caloric, fat, salt, and carbohydrate content of your foods. Remember that when salt or sugar head the list, you may want to change your menu. Be wary of simple terms such as "organic," "natural," "fortified," "enriched," "low-calorie," "dietetic," and "sugarless" — all of which can be very misleading. Foods proudly designated as having "no cholesterol," for example, may nevertheless contain saturated fats, which can be just as harmful to people on low-cholesterol diets. Similarly, foods boasting "all vegetable" fat content may contain palm or coconut oils, which are highly saturated fats that can raise blood cholesterol levels. "Sugarless" foods have no sucrose (table sugar) but can have other sugars like sucrase, fructose, glucose, or sorbitol, which are just as caloric and no more healthful. "Dietetic" foods are those intended for *any* special dietary use — the term itself does not imply a low-calorie content. Even terms as specific as "low-calorie" can be misleading — a low-calorie designation means only that the food has fewer than 40 calories per "serving," whereas "reduced-calorie" foods need only have 40 percent fewer calories than the original food with which they are being compared. But if you read them carefully instead of skipping the fine print, food labels can give you lots of

nutritional information. Labels also list additives and will give you an expiration date.

Clearly these eleven guidelines for a balanced diet can't tell you everything there is to know about nutrition. But in combination with the charts and tables in this chapter, you'll have plenty of food for thought. You can get lots of additional information at your library or book store or from excellent publications by the U.S. Department of Agriculture and the Food and Drug Administration.

WEIGHT CONTROL

Dieting is a way of life in America. It's hard to go through a full day without meeting someone who is "on a diet." A diet manual is almost always on the best-seller list. Magazines and newspapers are full of diet schemes. Weight-loss clinics abound. Numerous medications are sold to reduce weight, and many types of "spot reducing" gadgets are available. All in all, dieting is a hundred-million-dollar business.

We don't believe in diets. Obesity is a serious problem, but there is just no quick fix or magic cure. Almost any diet will work at first — but the pounds return with amazing speed. What we have been advocating throughout these pages is life-style modification to achieve lifelong fitness, a program combining exercise with sound nutrition to attain and maintain your best weight in the context of optimal health.

But because diets are so popular, we would like to give you a few tips:

1. *Get a medical checkup before you begin a weight-reduction program.* As a rule, obesity is the result of taking in more calories than you burn up, but in a few cases a metabolic disorder may be responsible. Be sure you are not that exception.
2. *Do not take drugs to lose weight.* Most "diet pills" are related to the amphetamines — speed. They will raise your blood pressure and heart rate and have only a mild and transient effect on your appetite. We are currently prescribing amphetamines to only one patient, who has narcolepsy. The drugs prevent him from falling asleep uncontrollably — but have not prevented him from getting rather fat.
3. *Do not participate in extreme diets.* Diet schemes are almost as numerous as dieters. Some plans involve severe calorie deprivation. Some allow you to eat all you want of one or two foods, depending on monotony to curb your appetite. Some require liquids only. Some allow you to eat only once a day. All such radical schemes are doomed to failure — you will probably lose weight at first, but will invariably regain it. And drastic diets can be harmful. We won't review specific weight-reducing diets, but we would like to mention two broad categories of diets which are in widespread use. "Protein-sparing" diets are low-calorie diets that provide mainly protein to eat. These diets do work, but they have two problems. The first problem is the familiar one of compliance and relapse. These diets are hard to stick with. The second problem is that you may develop metabolic disturbances on these diets, so you can get sick. Even on a "protein-sparing" diet, therefore, we think it is very important to eat some carbohydrate and fat.

   At the other end of the spectrum are the high-carbohydrate, low-protein, very low fat programs, of which the Pritikin diet is the best-known example. We have advocated a dietary mix of 55–60 percent carbohydrate, 25–30 percent fat, and 15 percent protein for fitness. The Pritikin diet aims for 80 percent carbohydrate, 10–15 percent protein, and only 5–10 percent fat. This is a very restrictive diet, and is very hard to follow. It does have a logical basis, and may be useful for patients with high blood lipids and heart disease who are under medical supervision. At the present time, we have glowing testimonials but no long-term scientific data.
4. *Calories do count.* Count them. The only way to lose weight is to take in fewer calories than you burn up. Period.
5. *Exercise does help.* Do it. Exercise will help by burning up excess calories. Your body's metabolism will also continue to burn up calories faster for hours after you stop exercising. Exercise may help reduce your appetite and improve your eating habits. Each pound you lose from diet alone will be 75 percent fat and 25 percent lean tissue, but a pound lost by combining exercise with diet will be 95 percent fat.

6. *Take a long-range view.* You should aim for a slow, steady weight loss of one to two pounds per week. Don't be disappointed by small setbacks — weight control is a lifelong goal.

7. *Pick a diet you can stick with.* Your menus should be varied and nutritionally sound. You should not start a diet unless you can plan a long-term maintenance phase once you have achieved your ideal weight.

8. *Don't waste your time trying to "spot reduce."* Various exercises to build muscle tone will help you to look better but will not remove adipose tissue in a particular area. Muscle tone is important, but don't neglect endurance exercises, which develop cardiopulmonary fitness and burn calories.

This is a fitness book, not a diet book. We are encouraging exercise and nutrition as tools to fitness, and weight control is only one aspect of fitness. But if weight control is important to you, make it part of your balanced fitness program: a total program will succeed better than the individual parts would alone.

SELF-ASSESSMENT

As with the three other facets of fitness, you need to know your starting point in order to plan your program for nutritional fitness. Some of the information must come from your doctor: your blood pressure will help determine your salt tolerance, your cholesterol level will help establish how much fat you can eat, and your blood sugar level can tell you if you need to restrict calories and concentrated sweets.

Even without this information, your own self-assessment will go a long way toward establishing your game plan. First, chart out exactly what you are eating each day. Fill out a three-day food diary, using sheets based on Figure 4–7. Most people are amazed by what they

---

Date_____

FIGURE 4–7: FOOD DIARY

	Food Item	*Portion Size*	*Calories*
Breakfast			
Lunch			
Dinner			
Snacks			

FIGURE 4–8: IDEAL WEIGHT (IN POUNDS)

MEN

Height Feet	Inches	Small Frame	Medium Frame	Large Frame
5	1	112–120	118–129	126–141
5	2	115–123	121–133	129–144
5	3	118–126	124–136	132–148
5	4	121–129	127–139	135–152
5	5	124–133	130–143	138–156
5	6	128–137	134–147	142–161
5	7	132–141	138–152	147–166
5	8	136–145	142–156	151–170
5	9	140–150	146–160	155–174
5	10	144–154	150–165	159–179
5	11	148–158	154–170	164–184
6	0	152–162	158–175	168–189
6	1	156–167	162–180	173–194
6	2	160–171	167–185	178–199
6	3	164–175	172–190	182–204

WOMEN

Height Feet	Inches	Small Frame	Medium Frame	Large Frame
4	8	92– 98	96–107	104–119
4	9	94–101	98–110	106–122
4	10	96–104	101–113	109–125
4	11	99–107	104–116	112–128
5	0	102–110	107–119	115–131
5	1	105–113	110–122	118–134
5	2	108–116	113–126	121–138
5	3	111–119	116–130	125–142
5	4	114–123	120–135	129–146
5	5	118–127	124–139	133–150
5	6	122–131	128–143	137–154
5	7	126–135	132–147	141–158
5	8	130–140	136–151	145–163
5	9	134–144	140–155	149–168
5	10	138–148	144–159	153–173

Modified from data of the Metropolitan Life Insurance Company

	Small Frame	Medium Frame	Large Frame
Wrist size: Men	6½″ or less	6¾″–7¼″	7½″ or more
Women	5½″ or less	5¾″–6″	6¼″ or more

actually take in. You will probably be surprised also about *when* and *why* you eat — habit, social situations, boredom or stress may account for almost as many calories as legitimate hunger and valid nutritional needs. Compare what you are eating now with the eleven-point guidelines for balanced nutrition — and make the appropriate changes. Repeat a three-day food diary in eight to twelve weeks to see if you are really changing your long-term eating habits.

You'll also need to know if your weight is right. First, determine your body build using your wrist measurement (see above).

Next, weigh and measure yourself.

Figure 4–8 provides a chart listing ideal body weight according to height and body build. These time-honored normal values from the Metropolitan Life Insurance Company are just averages, but they have been very useful. For years it has been known that obesity is linked to a shorter life expectancy because of a variety of medical complications, including high blood pressure, diabetes, and heart disease. But in the popular mind, these facts lead to the belief that the less you weigh, the more healthy you will be. Bear in mind, however, that life expectancy is also decreased in underweight people. All in all, ideal body weight seems to be just that — ideal.

As useful as the ideal body weight concept is, it does not tell the whole story. For one thing, as you can see from Figure 4–8 the normal values span a rather large range. In addition, the athlete faces special problems because muscle is dense and weighs more than fat. Because of an increase in lean body mass, a muscular athlete checking himself on the ideal body weight chart might mistakenly conclude that he is overweight, even though he has very little fat and is a paradigm of fitness.

To get around these problems, nutritionists have learned that the best determination of whether you weigh too little or too much is the percentage of your body which is fat. Unfortunately, a precise measurement of fat percentage depends on the determination of density by displacement of water. Although this is an ancient concept and a simple measurement, it requires an elaborate apparatus and is not readily available. But there

are some easy ways in which you can estimate whether or not too much of your body weight is fat:

1. *The "mirror test."* This test is very simple — but even though no needles are involved it can be very painful. Just strip down and have a look. Although the mirror test can be very revealing, it has two problems. First, objectivity and reproducibility. The eye of the beholder can play funny tricks. Second, with increased age even healthy lean tissues can sag, so you may err on the side of an unjustly harsh verdict.

While the mirror test is done in private, the other two tests require help:

2. *The "pinch test."* The back of the arm is the best place for this test. Pick a spot over the triceps muscle halfway between the shoulder and the elbow. Pinch a fold of skin, and measure what you've got. For young adult males, a measurement of less than 7 millimeters indicates a lean build, between 7 and 13 millimeters is the average range, and values above 13 millimeters reflect obesity. Because women normally have a higher percentage of fat, you can add 1 to 2 millimeters in each range for women. And give yourself a millimeter or so if you are over thirty-five and another one or two if you are above fifty.

3. *Skin fold calipers* allow precise measurements of skin fold thickness and hence the percentage of fat. Figure 4–9 illustrates the use of calipers. For a single measurement the triceps fold used in the pinch test is best, but measurements below the shoulder blade and at the side of the waist are also helpful. An increasing

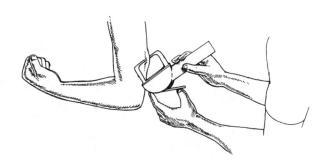

FIGURE 4–9: *Skin Fold Calipers*

number of doctors and other health care professionals who are interested in fitness have these calipers along with tables that will determine your percentage of body fat based on age, sex, and skin fold measurement. Figure 4–10 shows the percentage of body fat in athletes from various sports. You can compare these values with your own results if you have your skin folds measured.

Well, with the help of a scale, a mirror, and a pinch you can find out where you stand in terms of body weight and body fat. And you know where you should be for optimal fitness and athletic performance. How can you get there? Part II will take you from theory to practice — the tactics of fitness.

FIGURE 4–10: REPRESENTATIVE VALUES FOR RELATIVE BODY FAT

	Men	Women		Men	Women
Body build:					
Very thin	7–9.9	14–16.9	Bicyclists	8–10	11–19
Thin	10–12.9	17–19.9	Basketball players	8–12	12–16
Average	13–16.9	20–26.9			
Plump	17–24.9	27–30.9	Skiers		
Obese	above 25	above 31	cross-country	8–12	15–21
			downhill	10–14	17–23
Athletes			Gymnasts	6–10	6–10
Runners					
long-distance	4–8	6–10	Tennis players	12–16	15–20
sprinters	14–16	16–19	Baseball players	12–16	14–18
Swimmers					
long-distance	8–12	10–14			
sprinters	6–10	8–12			

NOTE: Values are for body fat as a percentage of body weight. The normal ranges are for young adults; percentage body fat normally increases above age 35, so that at age 65 an average man has 30% body fat, and an average woman 44%.

II

THE TACTICS OF FITNESS

Practical Instructions for Constructing Your Own Balanced Program

5

Collaborating with Your Physician for Fitness and Health

If we have done our job in Part I of this book, you should now understand the scientific basis of fitness. To facilitate that understanding, we divided fitness into four fundamental facets, devoting a chapter to each. In each area, we've provided self-assessment tests so you can find out just where you stand. And in two areas, psychological fitness and nutritional fitness, we've given you some guidelines to begin progressing from self-assessment to self-improvement. But now it's time to put these facets of fitness back together. Now it's time for you to begin a balanced program to achieve total fitness.

Exercise is the cornerstone of total fitness. We hope we've already made believers of you — but we don't want you to slam this book closed so you can hurriedly wax your old skis, dust off your tennis racquet, or dash to the store to buy some running shoes. Sports are indeed an ideal way to achieve fitness — which is why we've devoted Part III of this book to a detailed explanation of the demands and benefits of a wide range of sports. We hope you'll choose to play sports to stay fit, but it is not necessary for you to do so. In fact, it is best for you to get into shape *before* you turn to sports seriously — if you use a balanced fitness program to get into shape for sports, you'll play better, have fewer injuries, and you can then use sports to maintain your hard-earned fitness. And if your choice is fitness without sports, you can use this balanced program as an end in itself, to maintain fitness for health, appearance, and self-confidence without the competition of sports.

We've already said that exercise is the key to total fitness, but in reality things are just a little more complex — there are actually three very different types of exercise that are important for complete fitness and health. Perhaps the most important type is *aerobics;* aerobic training is the basis of the cardiovascular conditioning, which is crucial for health. *Flexibility* exercises are important to keep your joints and muscles supple and healthy, and flexibility training will also improve your coordination and gracefulness. Exercises for *strength* round out the program, not because we should all pump iron competitively, but because strong muscles are healthy muscles.

These three forms of exercise are important for fitness and health — and they are also important for sports. Aerobics will give you endurance and stamina. Flexibility training will give you reach and range. Strength work will give you power, and will combine nicely with flexibility training to prevent injuries. Whereas these three forms of exercise are sufficient for fitness and health, a fourth type — speed training — is also important for sports.

In Chapter 6 of this book, we'll explain aerobics, flexibility, and strength training in detail, and we'll also outline the basic principles of speed or anaerobic training. And in Chapter 7 we'll put these exercises together into a simple balanced fitness program called FAS(S): Flexibility, Aerobics, Strength, and Speed (which is optional). But as important as fitness is, it's only part of your total health needs. Let's start, then, by briefly reviewing some of the ways in which you can collaborate with your doctor to be sure your overall health is optimal for your fitness program.

MEDICAL EVALUATION

Like most fitness books, this one has already told you to "get a checkup" before you begin to work out. Unlike most fitness books, however, we'll tell you what to expect from your doctor — what tests and procedures you should request, and which you should avoid.

First, of course, you have to find the appropriate physician for you. Your choice of a doctor will depend on many factors, some of which are highly personal. But certain objective criteria should influence your choice. Pick a physician who is well trained and who is affiliated with a good hospital. Your doctor should be available on short notice if problems or emergencies arise, and should have a sound coverage system to fill in during absences. Your doctor should be willing to answer questions and explain recommendations. He or she should be willing to arrange a second opinion if you are faced with major decisions but are uncertain about the right choice. Above all, your doctor should be someone you like and trust. And last but not least, we hope that he or she will be someone who understands and believes in exercise and other aspects of health enhancement, preventive medicine, and life-style modification.

How often should you see your physician? If you are injured or ill, the answer is simple: if you don't respond to simple first aid and home remedies, or if your problem seems unusual or severe, you should call and/or visit your physician. But what if you are perfectly healthy? How often should you get a "routine" physical?

In our opinion, even young, apparently healthy athletes should have periodic medical evaluations (see page 21). At a minimum this should include a review of your medical history and current symptoms, as well as a physical exam. Most athletic programs require a blood count and urinalysis as part of the initial screening for athletes. Although not required for athletics, blood-cholesterol testing can be very beneficial, even in young people who feel well. Whereas this is sufficient for apparently healthy people, more detailed evaluations should be performed if you have any warning symptoms (see page 23) or if you have any cardiac risk factors, such as a positive family history, high blood pressure, a nicotine habit, diabetes, or obesity. Finally, if you are just starting to get into shape after being sedentary, or if you're

above age forty, more detailed studies are probably indicated. These studies might include blood chemistries such as blood sugar and kidney function determinations. A chest X ray can screen for lung disease and enlargement of the heart, but because this involves exposure to radiation, it should not be done indiscriminately, or repeated unnecessarily.

The electrocardiogram (ECG) is another important screening test. ECGs are not needed routinely in healthy young athletes, but they can be helpful in the older age groups. Unfortunately, the ordinary ECG may be perfectly normal even in the presence of heart disease. For this reason your doctor may order an exercise ECG or stress test, particularly if you have experienced symptoms or if you have cardiac risk factors. If you have a stress test, you will be asked to exercise on a treadmill or bike while your ECG is recorded continuously and your blood pressure is checked periodically. In some cases your doctor may order a simultaneous heart scan. The goal is to get your heart working hard in order to provoke abnormalities under carefully controlled conditions. In addition to looking for coronary artery disease, these tests enable an estimation of your level of fitness and therefore they can be extremely useful in preparing an exercise prescription.

Although exercise tests are safe, they are time consuming and expensive. Whereas stress tests are very important if there is reason to suspect heart disease, they should not be taken indiscriminately by everyone who exercises. In fact only 17 percent of middle-aged physician-runners had stress tests done on themselves before they began marathon training. Although there is room for debate, we generally recommend stress tests only if risk factors are present, if there is a clinical suspicion of heart disease, or for people beyond age fifty who are embarking on exercise training for the first time.

All of these tests may make you think that your doctor is primarily responsible for preventing heart complications of exercise. This is not the case. All tests are imperfect; even the highly touted stress test can have both false positive and false negative results. So in the last analysis, even in this age of modern medicine and sophisticated tests the ultimate responsibility for spotting signs of trouble and taking care of your heart rests squarely with you. This is not as formidable as it sounds. A few commonsense guidelines and elementary precautions are all that you should need; we'll set out these guidelines when it is time for you to construct your own exercise program.

MEDICAL CARE AND FOLLOW-UP

We have just pointed out the importance of a checkup with appropriate screening tests *before* you embark on exercise training. After this initial evaluation, however, it is the person who chooses *not* to exercise who is most in need of routine medical care, since an active fitness program and healthful life-style will help protect you from many problems. But even the most active and fit individual can benefit from "routine" checkups in the absence of symptoms. How often should you see your physician?

We certainly feel that everyone should have a complete history and physical at the point of entry into an adult health care system, sometime between ages fifteen and twenty. If no health problems are detected, routine checkups at five-year intervals seem highly reasonable up until age thirty-five. We usually recommend two checkups between ages thirty-five and forty, and repeat evaluations at one- or two-year intervals between ages forty and fifty. Beyond fifty, an annual checkup seems reasonable. Needless to say, if any health problems are detected, more frequent visits will be necessary. Even life-style problems without overt illness may merit more frequent visits to the doctor; we ask certain patients to return annually simply to be reminded about the importance of smoking cessation, good nutrition, stress reduction, exercise, and so forth.

What should you expect at the time of your "routine" checkups? One of the most important elements is a careful medical history. You should have a chance to sit down with your doctor and review all the health-related events that have occurred since your last checkup; at the time of your initial checkup, you should also provide a detailed family medical history.

A second element of a periodic health examination is a careful physical exam, including your blood pressure and weight as well as a head-to-toe physical. Your physical should include a rectal exam in both men and women above age forty (including a test for occult blood in a stool specimen). Women should also have a pelvic exam and pap smear at regular intervals.

How about tests and treatments? The only immunization that is recommended routinely in adults is a tetanus immunization booster shot, which should be administered every ten years. This is particularly important for athletes who may sustain cuts, which could cause problems if their boosters are not up to date.

Another simple test we recommend below age thirty-five is a skin test for tuberculosis. We also recommend a routine complete blood count and urinalysis at the time of each checkup. Blood tests to determine your cholesterol (both HDL and LDL), blood sugar, and kidney function are also worthwhile. Your stool should also be checked for traces of blood.

More fancy (and more expensive) laboratory tests are somewhat controversial. We generally obtain a "baseline" chest X ray at about age forty and request repeat films at ten-year intervals. Whereas the recommendations for chest X rays are decreasing, however, recommendations for breast X rays are increasing. The American Cancer Society now recommends a baseline mammogram at about age forty, with annual breast X rays above age fifty. The idea of a baseline study followed by periodic repeat tests also applies to the electrocardiogram. We generally order the first ECG at about age forty; if the first test is normal and there are no signs or symptoms of problems, repeat ECGs need not be obtained until age fifty and beyond.

All of these examinations and procedures can be done by your general physician, internist, or gynecologist. A few other checkups may require specialists, such as eye screening for glaucoma, which is important for people over forty. And let's not forget the value of routine dental checkups and care.

Needless to say, all of these recommendations are only guidelines, which should be modified depending on your particular health situation, your own beliefs and desires, and the opinions and practices of your doctor. But even the most frequent and thorough health checkups should not lull you into a false sense of security, for no matter how often you see your doctor, the ultimate responsibility is yours. We have already stressed time and time again the importance of good health habits. It is also very important for you to listen to your body so that you will be able to detect early symptoms of potentially serious disease; women should also perform regular breast self-examinations. If warning symptoms occur, don't bury your head in the sand — it's up to you to report potential problems to your doctor promptly so that appropriate tests and treatments can be undertaken. Remember, too, that if you have any uncertainty about your doctor's recommendations, a second opinion is always sound advice. And through all this, you should keep careful health records of your own, for yourself and for each member of your family.

The best way for you to protect your fitness is to be an intelligent, informed health consumer. Medicine is a rapidly changing field, and you should be alert for new developments and breakthroughs as they appear in newspapers and magazines. You should develop a comfortable, trusting, working partnership with your doctor, both for routine health maintenance and for the diagnosis and treatment of any problems that may arise.

LIFE-STYLE MODIFICATIONS: THE BEST PREVENTIVE MEDICINE

To be fit, you have to be healthy. And even in this age of medical sophistication, the most important elements are the simple rules of a healthful life-style: exercise, good nutrition, stress reduction, and avoiding abuse of tobacco, alcohol, and drugs. This book is devoted to the first three principles; before going into more details, however, let's look briefly at the other life-style factors which are so important to your health.

SMOKING

Let us suppose for one awful moment that despite reading 98 pages of this book, you are still an overweight, sedentary, highly stressed cigarette smoker. And, to continue the nightmare one step farther, let's suppose that you could change only one of these bad health habits. Which of these cardinal sins of preventive medicine should you give up? In our minds the answer is clear: smoking.

You may be surprised that we'd put smoking cessation ahead of regular exercise, sound nutrition, and stress control. Needless to say, we do believe very strongly in all of these life-style modifications. But smoking is so hazardous to your health that smoking cessation surely deserves first place on our list.

In 1964 the United States Surgeon General established beyond a scientific doubt that smoking is an important cause of lung cancer. In the two decades that have followed, this link has been confirmed again and again in more than thirty thousand scientific publications. Cigarettes are the number-one cause of premature death in the United States, accounting for over 350,000 deaths each year — nearly a thousand deaths each day. More Americans die each year from smoking than died in all of World War II (292,131). It may be hard for you to relate such large numbers to your individual situation, but looked at from an individual's point of view the toll of cigarette smoking is no less ominous. If you are twenty-five years old and smoke two packs per day, your life expectancy is 8.3 years less than that of a twenty-five-year-old nonsmoker. The message is clear: the more you smoke, the shorter your life expectancy.

Virtually everyone is aware of the fact that cigarettes cause lung cancer, but you may be surprised to learn about the many other serious diseases that can be caused by cigarette smoking.

Heart Disease

Cardiovascular disease is the number-one killer in the United States; cigarette smoking accounts for about 30 percent of all heart disease deaths, and is the number-one preventable cause of heart disease. Smoking will elevate your blood pressure and increase your heart rate, so that your heart works harder just at the time when your blood carbon monoxide levels are highest. A single cigarette will raise your pulse by 15 beats per minute for at least fifteen minutes; a pack of cigarettes will force your heart to pump an extra hundred gallons of blood. Smoking also contributes importantly to other serious vascular diseases, including strokes and peripheral vascular disease.

Cancer

Cancer is the second most frequent cause of death in the United States, and tobacco accounts for about one-third of our cancer deaths. Cigarette smokers have cancer death rates that are two times greater than nonsmokers. Smokers have a ten times greater risk of dying from lung cancer than do nonsmokers; many other forms of cancer are also much more common in tobacco users, including cancer of the larynx or voice box, the mouth, the tongue, the esophagus (food pipe), the bladder, and the pancreas.

Other Health Hazards

Tobacco abuse contributes to many other health problems. Emphysema, chronic bronchitis, pneumonia and other respiratory infections, and ulcers are much much more common in smokers. Cigarettes even contribute to tooth loss, and smoking during pregnancy is a major cause of stillborn and premature babies.

Athletic Performance

Hopefully, we've convinced you by now that smoking is terrible for your health. Despite all these facts, many people, particularly teenagers and young adults, have a hard time believing that they are vulnerable to smoking-related diseases, which are admittedly more common in the older age groups. By the time these young people reach their forties and fifties, their perspective may change — but it may also be too late for at least some of them. Even vigorous young athletes who believe they will live forever should be impressed with the fact that smoking impairs lung function and, hence, athletic performance. Many of us remember the bad old days when professional athletes appeared frequently on television advertising cigarettes. This clever advertising tactic may have given you the false impression that smoking and athletics were compatible. In fact, just the reverse is true — smoking will clearly undo your hard efforts to improve in sports. Smoking and fitness are mutually exclusive.

All of these problems would be distressing enough if they were confined to the people who choose to run the risk of smoking. Unfortunately, however, the hazards of tobacco abuse can extend even to nonsmokers. The loss of many lives in a fire is an obvious example of the way in which nonsmokers can suffer along with smokers, but even being in a room with smokers can cause health problems. Many studies have shown that so-called passive smoking can increase carbon monoxide and nicotine levels in the blood of nonsmokers. In fact, nonsmokers with heart or lung disease can develop chest pain or shortness of breath simply from being in a room where tobacco smoke is present; allergies and bronchitis can also be aggravated in these circumstances. Finally, all of us nonsmokers have to bear the tremendous economic costs and increased insurance rates attributable to tobacco abuse. Smokers have 35 percent more work absenteeism and 50 percent more hospitalization than nonsmokers.

Quite obviously we are reciting all these grim statistics because we believe that everyone should stop smoking. But is there another alternative? Are low-tar and -nicotine cigarettes any safer?

In our opinion, low-tar, low-nicotine cigarettes are one of the greatest frauds ever perpetrated on the public. The tar and nicotine content of the tobacco in these cigarettes is no different from that in ordinary cigarettes. The only difference is that "low-tar" cigarettes have a series of holes around the filter so that more of the smoke goes directly into room air and less into your lungs. In theory at least, you will get less tar and nicotine from smoking these cigarettes, but the measurements you see advertised are made with smoking machines, not with people. If you hold your "low-tar" cigarette so that your fingers block the holes in the filters, you will get a full dose of smoke. Moreover, studies have shown that people who buy "low-tar" cigarettes tend to smoke more, so that their total exposure to toxins is reduced little if at all. To make things even worse, some "low-tar" cigarettes have additional chemical additives, which could produce heretofore unrecognized health problems. The effects of "safe" cigarettes are summarized best by the words of Great Britain's Health Education Council: smoking low-tar cigarettes is "like jumping from the 36th floor instead of the 39th."

Smoking cessation is not easy, but it is possible. Some thirty-four million Americans have stopped smoking, though about fifty-five million still smoke, to the tune of about four thousand cigarettes per year for each adult in this country. Can quitting make a difference even if you've smoked for many years? The answer is a resounding yes. If you stop smoking before you have contracted a smoking-related disease, your risks of becoming ill will gradually return to the lower risk of nonsmokers over a seven- to ten-year period. In fact, your risk of developing a heart attack will take just two years to diminish to normal levels. And if you have a smoking-related illness, you can still benefit from smoking cessation. For example, smokers who have had a heart attack will reduce their risk of a second heart attack by 25 percent if they stop smoking. And if you are working your way toward fitness, you'll find that kicking the habit will give you a tremendous boost in energy, stamina, and "wind."

Quitting can be difficult but it is possible for everyone. We advise our patients first to try quitting on their own, preferably by stopping abruptly (cold turkey). But if you have trouble quitting on your own, many forms of help are available. The local chapter of your Cancer Society, Heart Association, or Lung Association will be glad to give you helpful literature. And they can also refer you to professional help, ranging from hypnosis to group education and aversive conditioning programs. Ideally your physician will also help by providing education and advice, or in some cases by prescribing chewing gum containing nicotine for the hard-core smoker. Remember, if at first you don't succeed, quit, quit again; statistics reveal that most people who succeed in licking the nicotine habit require two or three attempts before they finally succeed.

Even if you don't smoke yourself, you should contemplate the great social cost of smoking. Smoking is everyone's problem. In the years since the Surgeon

General's report, some six million Americans have died needlessly. Tragically, this tobacco-holocaust has been abetted to some degree by our own government's tobacco subsidies, export programs, and so forth. Tobacco is an eighteen-billion-dollar industry, which spends more than one billion dollars annually on advertising alone. Tobacco has one of the highest profit margins of any U.S. industry, and profits have risen in nearly every year since the 1964 Surgeon General's report.

If three jumbo jets crashed every day, you'd never fly in one, and they would be permanently grounded. Yet cigarettes kill just this many people in the United States each day. All of us who wish to make health our business must act together to put smoking in its place. Get off your butt to help others get off their butts. Improved health and fitness will be our reward.

ALCOHOL AND DRUGS

Our final life-style modification advice concerns one of the most worrisome problems in our country today: substance abuse. Alcohol is a drug that has addictive properties and many serious side effects. In small doses, alcohol can actually be good for you; the equivalent of two drinks per day seems to reduce the risk of heart disease by raising your blood high-density lipoprotein cholesterol ("good cholesterol") levels. But don't assume that just because a little is good, more is better. In fact, quite the reverse is true. People who average just four to five drinks per day have significantly higher mortality rates from a wide variety of diseases, including cirrhosis of the liver, cancer, intestinal bleeding, and pneumonia. Alcohol can also be an acute toxin, causing death by poisoning if excessive amounts are taken over a short period of time. Last but not least, alcohol is a major contributor to accidental deaths; more than half of the nation's fifty thousand annual highway fatalities are alcohol-related.

Whereas our life-style advice regarding alcohol urges moderation and caution, our advice concerning "recreational" drugs is even simpler: avoid them. Like alcoholism, drug abuse is present in all segments of society, and causes untold harm in both social and medical terms. It's no secret that many highly visible athletes abuse alcohol and other drugs, often with tragic results. This is one area in which you certainly cannot hold up the athlete as a positive example. Instead, the numerous examples of impaired athletic performance, personal, financial, and legal problems, illness, and death related to drugs should serve as a cautionary tale.

6

FAS(S): The Building Blocks of Fitness

It is now time for you to discover the athlete within, and to construct a comprehensive fitness program to turn you into that athlete. Being fit is being able to withstand stress. To make your body fit enough to withstand stress, you have to *apply* stress — exercise training involves the application of progressive workloads in a manner that will allow your body to adapt to that stress, to grow stronger and more fit so that you can rise to the challenge of ever greater demands. But to get the benefits of training without risk and regret, you have to apply the stress of conditioning properly: slowly, predictably, and intermittently so that your body will have time to adapt, recover, and then progress to new plateaus. At its best, training is stress and gain without injury or pain — but it is work. To plan your own fitness program, you need to know what point you are starting from, what your total health status is, and what your goals are. And you have to reevaluate your results periodically and refine your plans as your fitness program progresses.

You've had your medical checkup and are cleared to begin exercise training for fitness. If you're like most people who have not yet experienced the rewards of fitness firsthand, your attitude toward exercise may be somewhat akin to St. Augustine's view of sin — a strong desire to give up the sin of sloth but "not yet, oh Lord, not just yet." You're probably not a saint, so don't delay any longer. It's time to prepare your exercise prescription.

Prescriptions are given out by doctors to improve health; training schedules are given out by coaches to improve athletic performance. Your prescription for fitness will cover both aspects.

A balanced exercise program contains three elements: flexibility training, aerobic or endurance training, and strength training. For fitness, you won't need the fourth type of exercise, but for those of you who are looking ahead to sports as well, we'll conclude with an overview of speed training.

FLEXIBILITY TRAINING

It's no accident that "F" is the first letter in FAS(S). While aerobics is the central element for fitness, health, and sports, flexibility is the essential starting point. Stretching exercises are the cornerstone of the warm-up period that begins every workout, and they are also important in the cool-down, which concludes each FAS(S) training session. Flexibility is very important to avoid injuries — with it, you will be able to train for aerobics, strength, and speed, but without it, injuries are likely to interrupt your fitness program. Flexibility is also important for daily life: you will stand taller, move more gracefully, look better, and have many fewer musculoskeletal aches and pains.

Although some people are inherently more limber than others, flexibility is an acquired trait. Like the other aspects of fitness, you can improve and develop your flexibility by regular exercise training. Stretching exercises are the way to flexibility.

Your own stretching program will depend on your starting point (review your flexibility self-assessment test in Chapter 2). Equally important are your goals; as your fitness program evolves, you will have to review and modify your stretching routine to help you prepare for various aerobic and strength exercises as well as for specific sports. In fact, the stronger your muscles become, the more you'll need to stretch them to prevent tightness from developing. Everyone interested in fitness should understand the facts about stretching.

There are two basic types of stretching exercise. *Static* stretches, many of which are derived from yoga routines, involve maintaining a single position or posture until the desired stretching effect is accomplished. *Dynamic* stretching exercises have much in common with certain calisthenic and dance routines; they involve moving your body repeatedly through a range of motions. Static stretching is gentler and can be adjusted more precisely to a given degree of tightness. Dynamic stretching can be overdone, producing muscle pulls, but has the advantage of adding a little aerobic and endurance work to your flexibility training. In addition, dynamic stretching tends to be a bit better for large muscle groups.

Each type of stretching has its advocates. But you don't have to choose sides: both static and dynamic stretching should be part of your flexibility program. For beginners, or for muscles or joints that are very tight, do static stretches until you start to limber up — then add dynamic stretching. Begin each warm-up or flexibility session with static stretches and then gradually switch to dynamic exercise; reverse the order during your cool-down, saving static stretching for last.

Flexibility is a means to an end (injury-free participation in aerobic, strength, and speed training), but it is also an end in itself. As you progress with your stretching, you will find that your muscles and joints feel much better. Stretching is relaxing — for your muscles and your mind. Most people who stretch regularly look forward to it and enjoy it. Your FAS(S) training schedules (see Chapter 7) call for you to stretch during warm-ups and cool-downs at first, and then to add specific flexibility sessions. But you may want to stretch at other times as well. Stretching is a good way to start your day each morning, and is likewise very relaxing at bedtime. Stretching for a few minutes during your workday will help dissipate muscular and mental tension. Stretching can help take the edge off travel. You don't need a mat and gym clothes to stretch — find a discreet corner or a corridor and do a few subtle standing, stretching exercises whenever you need them during your day.

GENERAL PRINCIPLES

In general, as we mentioned, you should begin with static stretching and then progress to dynamics. Start with your most limber muscles and joints, and then work on tight areas. Start with exercises you can do while standing and then move on to mat exercises. As a rule, save your back for last.

When you begin to stretch, you will have to follow the directions carefully. At first, it can be a bit tricky to translate words into actions. Have a friend read you the directions and watch you perform the stretch, to see if you are getting your body where you want it.

Work out a routine. Plan a series of stretches that meets your needs, learn each thoroughly, and perform them in the same order each day. Within a week or two it will be second nature and you will no longer need to refer to the directions each time.

Stretching exercises call for soft floor coverings. Mats are good, but so is the bedroom rug. Health clubs provide mirrors and ballet barres, which will help you realize how far you have to go before you can try out for the Rockettes. But even without the objective view a mirror offers, you can effectively stretch anywhere, any time, using your own sense of what feels tight or comfortable.

Get used to thinking in terms of angles so you can record your gains in flexibility (see page 44). Remember to test your left and right sides separately — most people have a dominant side, which is stronger and tighter. If you are tighter on one side, you'll have to stretch it more diligently and more carefully until it catches up in flexibility. Your goal should be to gain flexibility gradually. Don't try to recover from twenty years of inactivity in thirty days of hard work. To gain optimal flexibility, a full year of progressive daily stretching may be necessary. Do it slowly, do it steadily, do it regularly.

Always listen to your body. Stretch to the limits of tightness but not to the point of pain. This is particularly important with dynamic stretching — never bounce or push yourself to the point that muscle pulls are a risk.

FLEXIBILITY EXERCISES

A general, basic flexibility program will systematically stretch your body's key areas: calves, Achilles tendons, hamstrings, quads, groin, lower back, and shoulders. The primary exercises are described and illustrated here, but you will want to emphasize any areas that are particularly tight (see your self-assessment tests from Chapter 2). In addition to the basics, we've included more advanced stretches, including some from yoga routines.

The basic program below uses only static exercises. All of them are within the capability of most people, although most of us will not be able to achieve the full range of flexibility at first. Hold the stretch at least 10 seconds and work up to 30 seconds. Take a deep breath and hold it during the stretch. Concentrate; focus on the muscles being stretched. Details will be found with each figure.

1. Calf and Achilles tendon stretches (Figures 6–1 and 6–2)
2. Hamstring stretch (Figure 6–3)
3. Quadriceps stretch (Figure 6–4)
4. Hip stretch (Figure 6–5)
5. Groin stretches (Figures 6–6 through 6–8)
6. Anterior thigh (Figure 6–9)
7. Hip stretch and spinal twists (Figure 6–10)
8. Lower back stretches (Figures 6–12 through 6–13)
9. Shoulder stretch (Figure 6–14)

This set of exercises should take five to ten minutes once you've learned the sequence. When you're through, you will have stretched the muscles of all the major body areas. But beyond this basic regimen, there are many more flexibility exercises that will supplement your routine depending on what your goals are.

We've added a few more, relatively easy ones here in a supplementary section (Figures 6–15 through 6–19), but all of the dynamic ones are included in the section on calisthenics (Figures 6–74 through 6–95).

ADVANCED YOGA-STYLE STRETCHES

Even when you've attained your flexibility goals, you'll have to keep stretching to maintain your flexibility. But you may well want to go beyond the basics to new goals. Advanced stretching, especially when combined with relaxation techniques, as in yoga, is a rewarding and enjoyable form of exercise in its own right. Certainly, some yoga-style postures will accomplish major gains in flexibility beyond what you might need for sports, especially for your back and pelvis.

Hatha yoga, a series of postures held for varying periods of time, is the basis for many of the stretches incorporated into these advanced stretches. Eight advanced stretches are worth considering, though all are difficult: (1) the plough (Figure 6–20); (2) the seated and lying warrior (Figure 6–21); (3) reaching for the sun (Figure 6–22); (4) head to shin (Figure 6–23); (5) the stork (Figure 6–24); (6) the bow (Figure 6–25); (7) the cobra (Figure 6–26); and (8) the trunk rotation (Figure 6–27).

While yoga is ideal for flexibility, it cannot stand alone: yoga provides no gains in aerobic capacity, muscular strength, or endurance. As such, it needs supplementation by a good aerobic program and by good muscular strengthening and endurance training.

NEUROMUSCULAR FACILITATION

Physical therapists and athletic trainers have learned to use the stretch and motion receptors to facilitate stretching of large, tight muscles. When a muscle contracts, there is a reflex relaxation of its opposing antagonist muscle (see page 36). This allows the contracting muscle to move the limb against minimal opposing muscle forces. A secondary reflex then helps relax the contracting muscle so that the return motion can be accomplished. You can use these reflexes to advantage by actively contracting the muscle being stretched for five seconds or so, then performing a slow stretch again. Try it. Lie on your back and have a friend carefully raise your straight leg as far as it can go. Then, push down against your friend's hands, consciously contracting the hamstring without moving it. When you relax, your friend will be able to gain another 5 to 15 degrees of motion for your hamstring. This maneuver leads to a reflex relaxation of the muscle and an improvement in its stretch. Physical therapists use similar "neuromuscular facilitation" techniques to help athletes recover from sports injuries. You can use this method to help stretch your larger, stronger muscles, particularly if they are tight or sore. In particular, practice this alternating contraction and stretch with your groin, hamstring, and quad stretches.

BASIC STRETCHES (FIGURES 6–1 THROUGH 6–14)

Figure 6–1: Calf Stretch

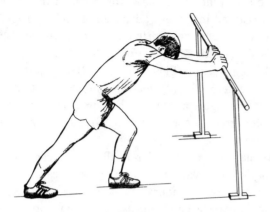

Structures: The gastrocnemius muscles of the calf

Instructions: Stand about 3 feet away from a wall with your feet pointing straight forward. Step forward with one foot but keep your back knee straight. Lean forward as far as comfortable, keeping your heel firmly on the ground. Hold for 10 to 20 seconds. Repeat for the other side. As you improve, step farther away from the wall to allow yourself a greater stretch. Try to get to the point where your ankle will make a 45-degree angle with the floor.

Figure 6–2: Achilles Tendon Stretch

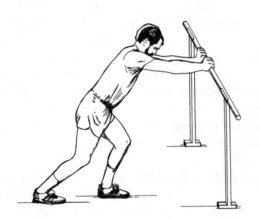

Structures: Soleus muscle of the calf and the Achilles tendon

Instructions: Assume the same posture as the previous exercise. Step forward with one foot, keeping your other foot back while allowing your knee to bend. Lean forward as far as comfortable. You will feel the stretch farther down your calf and into the Achilles. Hold for 10 to 20 seconds. As you become more flexible, stand farther away from the wall. You will have about 5 to 10 degrees more flexibility with your knee bent than with your knee straight, since when you bend your knee it shifts the stretch down toward your Achilles tendon and soleus muscle.

Figure 6–3: Hamstring Stretch

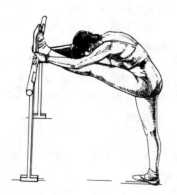

Structures: Hamstring muscles

Instructions: Stand and place one leg in front of you, on a low chair or stair. Make sure your leg is fully straight. If this is difficult or painful, use a lower foot support. Slowly lean forward, extending your hands toward your foot until you feel a pull along the back of your leg. Hold the stretch for 10 to 30 seconds. Repeat with your other leg.

With each stretching session, try to bend farther until you can grab your ankle, then your foot. At this point, change to a higher foot support, until, after a period of time, your extended leg is at a right angle (90 degrees) to your supporting leg.

Figure 6–4: Quad Stretch

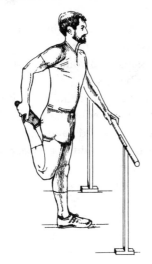

Structure: Quadriceps muscle

Instructions: This is done while standing, and you may need to support yourself initially. Stand on your left foot. Bend your right leg and grab your right ankle with your hand. Try to pull your right foot tight against your buttock. Hold for 10 to 20 seconds and then relax. Repeat on the other side. Eventually, to improve your balance, try to do this exercise while standing on one foot and with your free hand stretched straight up in the air.

Figure 6–5: Hip Stretch

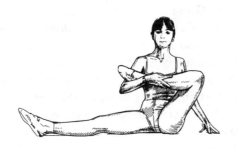

Structures: Various hip muscles, ligaments, and tendons

Instructions: Sit on the floor with your legs in front of you. Bend one knee, point your foot inward, and grab your ankle. Then rotate your leg upward as far as you can comfortably. Hold for 20 seconds and then switch sides.

Figure 6–6: Seated Groin Stretch

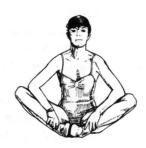

Structure: Groin

Instructions: Sit on the floor with your feet together and your knees bent out to the side. Your legs will form a V-shape with respect to the floor. Place your elbows on the inner aspect of your knees, and put a small amount of pressure on your knees, helping to force them gradually to the floor. Hold this stretch for 10 to 20 seconds and then relax.

Comment: You can increase the effect of the stretch by bringing your feet closer to your body. You can also help lower-back flexibility by leaning forward during this stretch. The ultimate goal is to be able to get your legs almost flat against the floor.

Figure 6–7: Seated Leg Spread

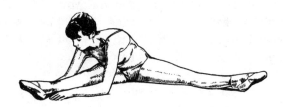

Structures: Groin, hamstring muscles, and lower back

Instructions: Sit on the floor with your legs spread as far as possible and your knees straight. Lean forward with your back straight, first over one leg and then over the other, reaching out with your hands to try to touch your toes. Hold the position over each leg for 10 to 20 seconds and then straighten up. Then lean toward the middle, between your legs. The goal is to get your chest down to your leg or to the floor while keeping your knees straight.

Figure 6–8: Starter Stretch

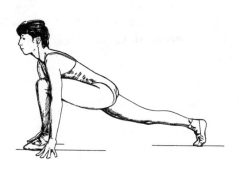

Structures: Groin and anterior thigh

Instructions: Get in position on the floor with one knee on the ground and the other foot flat in front of you with that knee bent. Place your hands on the floor parallel to your forward foot. Extend your back leg until it is straight and you are on the toes of that foot. Gradually lower your body down until you feel the stretch along the anterior thigh and groin muscles. Hold that stretch for 10 to 20 seconds and then switch sides. The key to this exercise is to try to keep your forward knee directly above your forward foot.

Figure 6–9: Lying Anterior Thigh Stretch

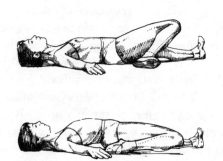

Structures: Anterior thigh and iliopsoas muscle

Instructions: Lie face-up on the floor. Bend your right leg so that your foot is lying toward the outside of your hips. Your knee will be up off the floor and your back somewhat arched. Try to bring your knee down toward the floor while pressing your back down flat. Hold for 10 to 20 seconds and then relax. Repeat on the other side.

Figure 6–10: Hip Stretch and Spinal Twist

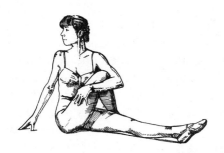

Structures: Spinal muscles, particularly thoracic spine, and the lateral aspects of the hip

Instructions: Sit on the floor with your legs straight in front of you. Bend your right leg and place your right foot on the outside of your left knee on the floor. Keeping your upper body rigid, twist your torso to the right side, bracing yourself by putting your right hand behind you. Place the elbow of your left arm against the outer side of your right knee and use pressure there to help push your body around farther. You should feel this stretch along your upper back and along the outer aspect of your hips. Hold the stretch for 10 to 20 seconds and then repeat on the other side.

Figure 6–11: Static Toe Touches

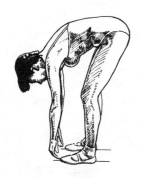

Structures: Lower back and hamstring muscles

Instructions: Do these as you would conventional repetitive toe touches, but when your hands reach the floor, hang there carefully trying to round your back and allowing your muscles to relax. Keep your knees slightly bent. Then slowly roll back up again. Remember, this exercise is not for those who have back problems.

Figure 6–12: William's Exercise

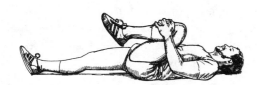

Structures: Lower back and hip extensors

Instructions: This exercise can be done with one leg at a time or with both legs. It is a basic exercise for stretching out sore back muscles and can be done by people who have had back trouble. Lie comfortably on your back with your knees bent. Bring your knees up to your chest; you should ultimately be able to bring your knees to your chest comfortably, but you may find it difficult at first. Hold the posture for 5 to 10 seconds and then relax. Repeat this four or five times.

Figure 6–13: Cat's Back

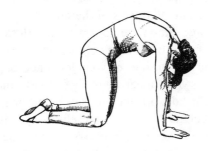

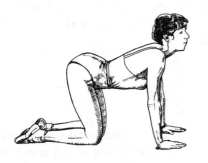

Structure: Lower back

Instructions: This is a more advanced stretching exercise for your lower back, designed to provide you with increased limberness and flexibility. Position yourself comfortably on your hands and knees. Then arch your back up as a cat does when frightened. Put your head down and create a smooth curve from your neck all the way to your lower back. Then slowly reverse the position, holding your head up and trying to allow your back to sway. Slowly alternate these positions four or five times, but avoid strain.

Figure 6–14: Shoulder Stretch

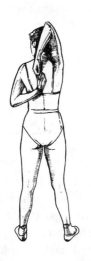

Structures: Rotator cuff and anterior deltoid muscles with the arm in the down position; latissimus with the arm in the up position.

Instructions: With one arm reaching from above and the other from below, try to clasp your hands behind your back. If you can't do this, use a towel to bridge the gap. Gradually pull up on your lower arm, gently stretching the shoulder muscles. Hold for about 20 seconds and then reverse your arm positions. Don't force the stretch.

Comments: Most of us will find that the dominant side (the right side in right-handed people) will be very tight when that arm is reaching up from underneath. The stretch is primarily for the shoulder of the arm reaching from underneath. You should eventually improve your range of motion sufficiently so you can do without the towel.

SUPPLEMENTARY STRETCHES (FIGURES 6–15 THROUGH 6–19)

Figure 6–15: Warrior's Posture

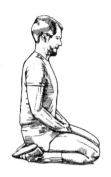

Structures: Anterior tibial muscles

Instructions: Kneel on the floor with your legs and feet straight behind you. Place your hands on the floor to support part of your weight. Then gradually lower your weight onto your heels, slowly forcing your feet down to the floor. Be careful not to put too much pressure on your feet. Hold for 10 to 20 seconds.

Figure 6–16: Straight-Leg Raising

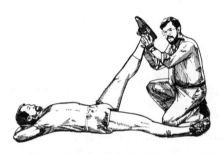

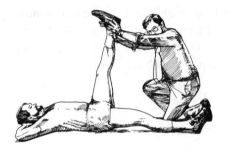

Structures: Hamstring muscles

Instructions: Lie on your back. Keeping your knee straight, raise one leg until it is as high as it will go. Try to achieve a 90-degree angle with the floor. Hold for 10 to 20 seconds and then repeat on the other side.

Comments: This exercise can be helped greatly by a partner alternately assisting the stretch by pushing gently up on your leg, and then resisting when you try to push your leg downward. This is an example of neuromuscular facilitation techniques (see page 103).

Figure 6–17: Leaning Chest Stretch

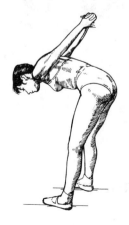

Structures: Pectoral and anterior deltoid muscles

Instructions: Clasp your hands behind your lower back, gradually raising your arms away from your back. Lean forward to help. You should feel this stretch in your shoulders and down across the side of your chest. Hold for about 20 seconds.

Figure 6–18: Lateral Side Bend

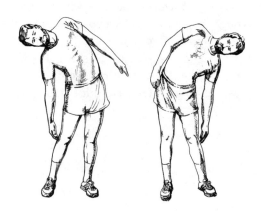

Structures: The upper torso muscles

Instructions: Stand with your feet slightly wider than your shoulders and lean to your left, holding your right arm stretched over the top of your head. Hold the stretch for about 20 seconds, then reverse and stretch the other side.

Figure 6–19: Neck Stretch

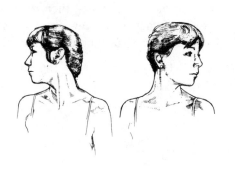

Structures: Neck and upper back muscles

Instructions: Put your head in each of the six positions shown, first with your chin forward, then with each ear to your shoulder, trying not to shrug your shoulder, then with your chin on each shoulder, and finally with your head fully back. Hold each position at its maximum for about 10 seconds.

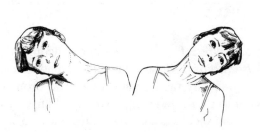

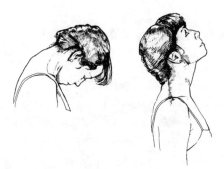

ADVANCED, YOGA-STYLE STRETCHES (FIGURES 6–20 THROUGH 6–27).

Figure 6–20: The Plough

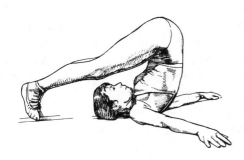

Structures: Hamstrings, lower and upper back

Instructions: Lie on your back with your arms next to your body to support yourself. Raise your lower back, lifting your legs over your head and supporting your weight on your shoulders and arms. Try to bring your legs and feet as far down to the floor as possible, keeping your knees straight. As you gain proficiency and balance, you'll find that you can eventually lower your feet to the ground behind you. This exercise provides the maximal amount of hamstring and back flexibility. Do not attempt this exercise if you have back problems.

Figure 6–21: Seated and Lying Warrior

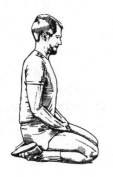

Structures: Anterior tibial, quadriceps, and anteror thigh muscles

Instructions: This is similar to Figure 6–15, except that the goal is to get your feet completely straight and then to extend this exercise by lying backward. Sit on your heels until you can rest comfortably without supporting your weight on your hands. At that point, extend this exercise by lying straight back until your torso is on the floor.

Figure 6–22: Reaching for the Sun

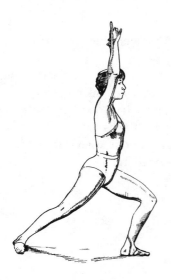

Structures: Groin, lower and upper back

Instructions: Stand with your legs spread wide apart. Point your right foot outward and twist your torso so that you are facing right. Bend your right knee, keeping your left leg straight. Raise your arms above your head and stretch upward. Gradually bend your right knee farther, lowering yourself until your right thigh is parallel to the floor. Hold this posture for 30 seconds or more. Repeat on the other side.

Figure 6–23: Head to Shin

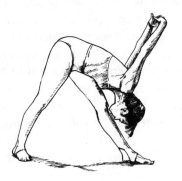

Structures: Hamstring muscles, chest, upper and lower back

Instructions: Stand with your legs apart and your right foot facing outward. Place your arms behind your back and rotate your torso until you face your right foot. Bend at the waist, trying to place your forehead on your knee while raising your arms behind your back. Hold for 30 seconds or more. Repeat on the other side.

Figure 6–24: The Stork

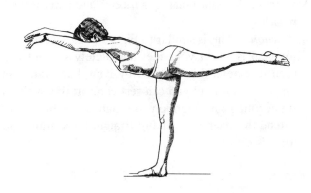

Structures: Back and hamstring muscles

Instructions: Stand with your arms straight above your head. Bend over at the waist until your torso is parallel to the floor with your knees straight. Then lift your left leg behind you while standing on your right leg. Eventually you should be able to keep your left leg parallel to the floor in a straight line with your upper body while balancing on your right leg. Repeat, standing on your left leg.

Figure 6–25: The Bow

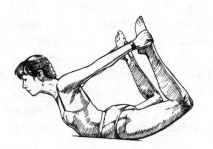

Structures: Abdomen, chest, shoulders, anterior thigh, and back

Instructions: Lie on your stomach. Bend your knees and grab both your ankles behind your back. Lift your head and pull up on your feet so that your upper body and your thighs are off the floor and you are resting only on your stomach. Hold this stretch for 30 seconds or more.

Figure 6–26: The Cobra

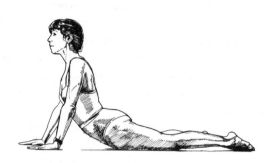

Structures: Abdomen, chest, shoulders, mid back

Instructions: Lie face-down on the floor. Raise your upper body off the floor so that your chest and upper abdomen are completely clear. You can use your arms for support. Hold this position for 30 seconds or more.

Figure 6–27: Trunk Rotation

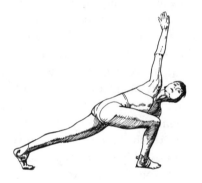

Structures: Trunk, abdomen, back

Instructions: Stand with your feet spread apart and your right foot pointed outward. Keep your torso erect and turn to face right. Bend your right knee so that your thigh is parallel to the floor. Hold your arms out to the sides and then twist your trunk to the right, bringing your left hand down to your right foot, and right hand straight up above your head. Look upward at your right hand and hold this posture for 30 seconds. Repeat on your other side.

AEROBIC TRAINING

Doctors call it "aerobic power"; horse trainers call it "foundation"; baseball players call it "legs"; runners call it "base"; tennis players call it "wind." Whatever you call it, it's the ability to play hard and fast and to recover from strenuous exertion quickly.

Aerobic or endurance exercises are those in which large muscle groups are used in rhythmic repetitive fashion for prolonged periods of time. Examples of dynamic or aerobic exercises include brisk walking, jogging, swimming, biking, cross-country skiing, and aerobic dance. In aerobic exercise the heart rate increases substantially but never reaches its maximum level. Your heart is always able to deliver sufficient oxygen-rich blood to your muscles so that they can derive energy from fat and glycogen aerobically. Aerobic exercise builds stamina for sports and it also is the most important form of exercise for your health, since it increases the efficiency of your heart, your circulation, and your muscles. Aerobic exercise is the keystone of fitness.

The first element in your aerobic exercise prescription is a careful *warm-up,* which is important both for your muscles and your heart. Stretching exercises and calisthenics are ideal for your warm-up. Walking is also an excellent warm-up because it will raise your heart rate gradually; jogging can replace walking at the conclusion of your warm-up regimen. Don't skimp on your warm-up period. At least ten minutes of warm-up exercises is a wise investment of your time; you will be repaid many times over in terms of safety for your heart, fewer injuries to your muscles and joints, and smoother play.

After you are warmed up, you can begin a period of *sustained aerobic exercise.* Your conditioning program should take account of three elements: the *intensity, duration,* and *frequency* of exercise. In terms of *frequency* it takes three to four workouts per week to get really into shape. If you are just getting started, it's best to do your aerobics only every other day, so that your muscles will have forty-eight hours to recover. When you're in better shape, you can exercise daily, but even then it is advisable to alternate hard workouts with gentler sessions so that you won't overtax your muscles, ligaments, and joints. The lower-intensity days are ideal for extra stretching exercises and calisthenics. If you go beyond fitness to competitive sports, you should taper down your strenuous workouts in the days preceding an important event, while increasing your stretching exercises. Although recreational athletes will rarely work out more than once a day, competitive athletes often work out two or even three times per day. Even at this level it's important to alternate hard and easy workouts, and to vary the exercise schedule so that speed, strength, and endurance workouts are never attempted during the same session.

The *duration* of each exercise session will also increase as you get into shape. If you are just starting out, you should aim for fifteen minutes of aerobic work in addition to your warm-up and cool-down. At first you will probably have to include some low-intensity exercise, such as walking, in a fifteen-minute aerobic period. As you get into shape, you will be able to increase the amount of high-intensity work and decrease the lower-level exercise. For example, if you are using running as your aerobic exercise, you may start out alternating two minutes of walking with one minute of jogging. Over a period of several weeks you should be able to change the ratio so that you walk for one minute and jog for two minutes. The next step will be to eliminate the walking entirely, so that you can jog for an uninterrupted fifteen minutes. Once you have achieved this plateau, it is merely a matter of extending the duration of aerobic exercise. These same principles of slow progression and alternating more intense effort with less strenuous recovery periods apply to all aerobic training,

whether you are walking or jogging, or using a stationary bike or rowing machine. We'll detail the major aerobic training techniques shortly. For all programs, you should aim for gradual improvement, lengthening your exercise sessions by 10 percent per week until you can sustain a full thirty minutes of uninterrupted exercise. A thirty-minute workout four times per week plus warm-ups and cool-downs each session will give you an excellent exercise regimen for health and endurance.

If you are using aerobics to build stamina for sports, you may want to go even farther. Again the theme is gradual progression. The rules are the same for the accomplished athlete as they are for the beginner — you should continue to warm up gradually, stretch regularly, and alternate hard and easy days. No matter what first motivated you to exercise, the chances are very good that once you reach this level you'll find that you enjoy jogging, biking, rowing, swimming, cross-country skiing, or aerobic dance for its own merits. Nor do you have to confine yourself to any one of these activities. In fact, optimal fitness can be built with a balanced program mixing these sports; chances are you'll feel better and play each sport better. Most people come to enjoy aerobic sports; the first few months are slow and discouraging, but gradually the work gives way to fun. Once you reach the twenty- to thirty-minute plateau, you will probably find a great deal of satisfaction and enjoyment from aerobic exercise. There are many theories that attempt to explain this feeling of relaxation and well-being (see Chapter 3).

It's easy to gauge the frequency of your exercise by the calendar and the duration of your exercise by the clock, but how do you measure *intensity?* This is the most difficult thing for you to do, but it is also the most important element of your conditioning program.

There are two simple ways to monitor the intensity of exercise: measuring the heart rate and measuring the respiratory rate. You can estimate the latter quite easily. When you cross the anaerobic threshold, your muscles develop an oxygen debt and build up acids. The increased acid production in turn leads to an increased carbon dioxide (CO_2) production. To get rid of the CO_2, you have to breathe more rapidly. All this may sound very complicated, but it is very simple for your body and is entirely automatic. You will know when you cross the anaerobic threshold because you'll suddenly find yourself breathing very rapidly, and you'll feel breathless or winded. You can be sure you're in the aerobic range by preventing this — work hard enough to break

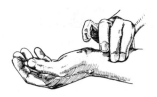

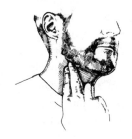

FIGURE 6-28: *How to Take Your Pulse (see text for details)*

into a sweat but not hard enough to feel short of breath. You can use the "talking pace" as a guide; if you are exercising aerobically, you should have enough wind in reserve to carry out at least a limited conversation with a companion.

The talking pace will prevent you from getting anaerobic, but you may well err on the side of too much talking and not enough working. In other words, you may not push yourself hard enough to get the full benefits of aerobic exercise. Because of this, heart rate is a much more precise guide to endurance training. You'll have to do three things to use your heart rate as a guide to the intensity of exercise.

1. *Learn to take your pulse.* Each heartbeat pumps blood through the arteries; thus your pulse rate equals your heart rate. Your pulse is easiest to feel in the radial artery on the thumb side of your wrist or in the carotid artery in your neck just below your jaw. Figure 6-28 shows you how to feel these pulses. Practice until you can feel and count your pulse easily at rest. Then practice taking your pulse immediately after exercise, which will be a bit harder since your heart is beating faster. It is important to take your pulse immediately after you stop exercising because your heart rate slows down rapidly when you rest. Use a wristwatch with a second hand and count your pulse for ten seconds. Then multiply by six to get your heart rate per minute. Most people can learn to count their pulse quite accurately. If you can't, but you still want to use your heart rate to guide your exercise intensity, you may want to look into a portable pulse meter. A number of these gadgets are available. They are cute, accurate — and expensive.

2. *Know your maximum heart rate.* If you've had an exercise tolerance test, your maximum heart rate has been measured on a treadmill or bike, so your doctor can give you the number. If you haven't had a stress test, you can estimate your predicted heart rate based on your age: just subtract your age in years from 220 and you'll have your maximum heart rate.

3. *Know your target heart rate.* Remember that the idea of aerobic endurance training is to work hard, but not all out. This translates to a target heart rate of 70 to 85 percent of your maximum rate. If you are out of shape or in the older age groups, you should initially

FIGURE 6-29: YOUR TARGET HEART RATE

Age	Maximum Heart Rate	Target Range (beats per minute)		10-Second Pulse Count	
		Low (70% max.)	High (85%)	Low	High
20	200	140	170	23	28
25	200	140	170	23	28
30	194	136	165	22	27
35	188	132	160	22	26
40	182	128	155	21	26
45	176	124	150	20	25
50	171	119	145	20	24
55	165	115	140	19	23
60	159	111	135	18	23
65	153	107	130	17	22

aim for the lower end of your target range; if you are young and athletic, you can push toward 85 percent of your maximum rate.

Your goal should be to keep your heart rate in this target range throughout your entire aerobic exercise period. To make it easy for you to figure out your target range, Figure 6–29 shows you your age-related range in beats per minute and in counts per ten-second interval. We can give you the target, but you'll have to do the work yourself. As you get into shape, you'll discover a remarkable change in how well you do. Although your target range remains the same, you'll find yourself working harder and harder to stay on target, because your work capacity will increase with conditioning.

You've warmed up for ten minutes and exercised aerobically for fifteen to thirty minutes. But don't head for the showers just yet. The third phase of your exercise prescription is just as important as the first two — spend a final five minutes *cooling down*. Medical studies have shown that the levels of adrenaline in your blood continue to rise *after* you stop exercising. If you stop abruptly, your heart rate will fall rapidly; rising blood adrenaline levels could cause irregularities of the heart's rhythm that might be very serious indeed. Protect yourself by changing gears gradually: after you finish your intensive training, walk for three minutes to let your heart cool down slowly. Then do some stretching exercises (see pages 104–113). Now — finally — you can take your shower, but even here a little thought is in order. Don't follow the macho advice to take a "bracing" shower in ice-cold water. A cold shower after exercise could trigger irregular heartbeats, so you should always allow your body the luxury of relaxing in nice warm water. Because warmth is pleasantly relaxing, many health clubs offer saunas, hot tubs, or steam rooms for use after exercise. These don't add to your fitness, and should never be used as substitutes for your cooldown routine, but if they add enjoyment, go ahead with them — after you've spent at least five minutes walking and stretching. But be sure to avoid dehydration and don't let yourself get overheated, especially if you have cardiovascular problems.

SPECIFIC AEROBIC TRAINING TECHNIQUES

One of the nice things about aerobic training is that you can achieve your fitness goals in many different ways. Any activity that uses large muscle groups in a rhythmic, repetitive fashion for periods of at least twenty minutes at an intensity sufficient to raise your heart rate to 70 to 85 percent of its maximum will build your aerobic power and cardiovascular fitness. You will also develop endurance and stamina in the specific muscles you are training.

We prefer to use lifesports to build aerobic fitness: walking and running (Chapter 8), swimming, rowing, aerobic dance, biking, and cross-country skiing (Chapter 9) are all excellent aerobic activities. You can also use certain competetive or team sports (Chapter 10) for aerobic fitness, but these are most useful as maintenance workouts for people who are already fit.

But what if you are not interested in sports, or if logistics prevent you from participating in these activities? Can you get fit in the comfort and privacy of your home?

The answer is yes. You can start your aerobic program at home or at a health club by using various training devices ranging from a one-dollar clothesline jump rope to a five-thousand-dollar treadmill. These devices will all build cardiovascular fitness, and by alternating among them you can build endurance in most of your major muscle groups. If you train at home, you'll have an initial financial investment, but your fitness program will then be free. You'll also have total flexibility in choosing the best time for your training, and you'll have complete privacy as well. If you want companionship, motivation, or instruction you can use these devices at a health club. For a modest fee, health clubs will also give you access to a variety of high-quality, expensive training machines. And since many hotels offer health clubs, you will be able to continue your exercise-machine fitness program even when you travel.

With all these advantages, why not recommend exercise machines for everyone's fitness program? The major problem with all of these devices is motivation. Too often, the stationary bike can be characterized as an excellent device for aerobic fitness which has two pedals, one wheel, and no rider. None of these machines will help unless you use them regularly and properly. But if you keep a log to chart your progress (see page 167) and work out frequently enough to feel all the benefits of fitness, you should be motivated to continue. Many people listen to music or watch TV while they use an exercise machine. Another trick was discovered by our patient Edward Harderer. We prescribed aerobics for fitness and blood pressure control, but Mr. Harderer found that home exercise was the only thing he could fit into his busy schedule. A stationary bike did wonders for his blood pressure, but boredom threatened his compliance — until he discovered that he could enjoy large-print books and newspapers while pedaling his way to fitness.

Exercise machines can give you all the benefits of sports without many of their problems. A treadmill will enable you to walk or jog without worrying about rain or dogs. You can bike in your bedroom without wearing a helmet or watching out for cars. You can row without water, ski in July, and jump your way to fitness even if aerobic classes are closed.

Which of these techniques is best for you? As in choosing your sports, personal preference, specific fitness needs, and overall goals will determine your choices. Each device will build cardiovascular fitness. If you need to build up your arms or back, you should choose a rowing machine. If your goal is skiing, a cross-country ski machine is the thing for you. If your aim is overall fitness or leg strength, use a stationary bike, treadmill, or jump rope. Figure 6–30 compares the benefits of these approaches.

As you can see, by combining these activities you can get a comprehensive aerobic workout. Add flexibility and strength training, and you'll have total fitness. Use these machines to get into shape for sports, as alternates when climate, injury, or travel keep you off the roads, or as fitness ends in themselves.

Let's look at these techniques individually.

Stationary Bikes

Stationary bikes are the most commonly used home-exercise devices. They all work the same way: by pedaling you turn the wheel; by adjusting the resistance of the wheel, you can adjust the amount of work it takes to pedal. You can convert your ten-speed bike to home use by mounting it on special rollers or by attaching a windmill-like device to your rear wheel to provide resistance. But if you are serious about using an exercise bike for fitness, buy a stationary model for home or use one at your health club.

Stationary bikes vary in price from under $100 to over $2,000. You don't always get what you pay for. What should you look for in a stationary bike?

· *Sturdiness.* Choose a bike that is built to last; fitness, after all, is a lifelong commitment.
· *Comfort.* Your bike should have an adjustable seat and handlebars so that your hips and back are comfortable. One-piece pedals with stirrups are comfortable and convenient.
· *Variable resistance and easy-to-use controls.* As you improve, you'll be increasing the resistance; choose a model with good calibration and accessible controls. The least expensive bikes use rollers to provide resistance, but these tend to be noisy and may be jerky and uneven. Caliper wheels are quieter and more accurate, but a flywheel and belt system is the best of all. One model, the Schwinn Air-Dyne, uses air displacement to generate the workload; a cooling breeze is a pleasant side effect of this device, which also features movable arm levers so that you can use your arms and legs simultaneously or independently.
· *Smooth pedaling action.* The key here is not the pedals, but the flywheel. Flywheel momentum prevents jerky pedal movement; the heavier the flywheel, the smoother the action; a sixty-pound

FIGURE 6–30: A COMPARISON OF AEROBIC EXERCISE MACHINES

| | CARDIO-VASCULAR FITNESS | MUSCLE ENDURANCE | | | | | FLEXI-BILITY | COORDI-NATION |
		calf	quads	hamstrings	back	shoulders and arms		
Treadmill	+	+		+				
Stationary bike	+	+	+					
Rowing machine	+		+		+	+	+	
Nordic skier	+			+		+	+	+
Rope jumping	+	+	+		+		+	

flywheel will provide smoother resistance than a twenty-pound wheel, but will cost more.

· *A rigid frame.* A rigid frame permits smooth riding, whether on a stationary bike or on a ten-speed. In both cases, flimsy frames will flex, which interferes with efficient biking.

Don't skimp on these essentials when you select your bike; you can get a sturdy, reliable machine for about the price of a super-deluxe tennis racquet, and you'll never have to pay for court time. But if you want to spend a little more, look for a model that will allow you to calibrate your work output in watts. Speedometers, odometers, and timers are nice, but are not necessary because you'll be using your heart rate and a clock to measure the intensity and duration of your aerobic workout. You may enjoy using fancy computerized bikes that allow you to monitor your pulse automatically and program in "hills," but let your health club pay for these expensive extras and stick to the essentials at home.

Like all aerobic workouts, stationary biking should be preceded by a warm-up and followed by a cool-down. We'd suggest you use the stretching and gentle calisthenics outlined on pages 104–113, but you can also use leisurely pedaling at low resistance for this purpose.

If you are new to exercise in general, or bicycling in particular, get your legs used to pedaling by free-wheeling without resistance three times weekly for a week or two, beginning at fifteen minutes and building to twenty minutes a session. After you can pedal for twenty minutes without too much soreness the next day, add the smallest increment of resistance available on your bike. Pedal for as long as you feel comfortable, but for at least fifteen minutes.

From here on, you should progress by varying resistance and time. As you increase the resistance, you will probably have to decrease the time you can bike. During the first week or two at the higher resistance, you'll be able to build back up to twenty to thirty minutes. At first, you'll be limited by quad strength and will have to be very empirical as to how much resistance to use. Later, the limit will be your cardiovascular and muscular endurance and fitness, and there we can be more precise. Use your target rate to calculate how hard you are working. As you increase the resistance, your pulse will increase and you will tire faster. As you improve at any given resistance level, you will find that your pulse slows and you can pedal longer without fatigue; gradually this will lead to your fitness goal.

There are really very few drawbacks to exercycles. They are good for people who are very overweight, since they don't penalize you for your excess weight. If you push too hard too soon, you can get typical overuse injuries, such as chondromalacia or bursitis and tendinitis of the knee (see Chapter 12). Finally, unless you wear lightweight clothing you can get overheated, since you'll be burning 300 to 500 calories per hour without a cooling breeze.

Bicycling for aerobic fitness, as well as quad strength and endurance, is an ideal complementary exercise to running, cross-country skiing, and skating. And, as you can see, it is also an excellent method of conditioning in its own right.

Rowing Machines

Rowing machines are the latest rage in indoor fitness devices — but this is one fad that has really earned its reputation.

Rowing machines give you all the advantages of aerobic training, convenience, and freedom from injury, but they have an extra feature: unlike stationary bikes, rowing machines will build endurance in your shoulders, arms, and back as well as in your legs.

When you "row" on a machine, you'll be pulling on handles or "oars" against resistance. Just as in stationary biking, variable resistance is the key to your graded exercise program. In most home rowing machines, the resistance is provided by adjustable hydraulic pistons, but the more expensive machines use flywheels. Piston machines are less expensive ($100–$350) and more compact, but flywheel models ($600) are more precise and are much closer to real rowing. These rowing ergometers can also be used to measure strength, power, and work output. In fact, when Harry Parker, the legendary Harvard crew coach, was holding preliminary trials for the 1980 U.S. Olympic team, the first cut among candidates was based not on technique and fitness but on raw strength and power as measured by the ergometer. Although the rowing machine you use at home will generally lack this sophisticated calibration and measuring equipment, it will get you just as fit if you use it properly. All good machines allow you to push against foot rests as you row, so that your legs and lower back will share the work with your arms. A sliding seat is the final essential ingredient. Look for sturdiness, comfort, smooth action, and convenient controls when you select your rower.

Use your rowing machine just as you would your

stationary bike: start with low resistance and gradually add resistance and time as you improve. Don't forget to warm up and cool down; incorporate flexibility exercises for your shoulders and back (see pages 107–108) with warm-up and flexibility routines to prevent overuse injuries.

Rowing machines can be used for total fitness or can nicely complement activities such as biking and jogging, which lack upper-body exercise.

Treadmills

A treadmill will allow you to walk or run indoors. You'll get all the benefits of these praiseworthy sports (see Chapter 8) without the worries about climate, competition, and accidents. You can use a treadmill to get your fitness program started at a beginner's level, and you can continue training right up to competitive running. You can even adjust the incline on most treadmills so you can train "on hills."

The best treadmills have motors that will drive the tread at varying speeds; set the speed according to how fast you want to run. Unfortunately, motorized treadmills are so expensive and bulky that they are suitable for your club but not your home. Nonmotorized treadmills depend on your stride to move the belt; they can be used to develop cardiovascular fitness and calf and hamstring endurance at home, but they are not as smooth as the motorized models.

Except for considerations of climate and terrain, a treadmill program is just like an ordinary walking or jogging program — see Chapter 8 for guidelines.

We are less enthusiastic about treadmills than we are about stationary bikes or rowing machines. Price ($500–$5,000), bulk, and the potential for running injuries explain our bias. Moreover, you can simply jog in place at home to get many of the benefits of a treadmill without requiring a machine. Be wary, however, of little trampolines for stationary jogging; you'll get much less of a workout, because the springy rubber will be doing much of the work.

Cross-Country Ski Machines

Cross-country skiing is an ideal aerobic fitness activity (see Chapter 9), but climate limits its value for most of us. Ski-simulators, however, are now bringing skiing to the Sunbelt.

To ski without snow, you'll strap your feet on to short "skis" that rest on rollers. Instead of holding poles, you'll pull on cables. The net result will be a smooth gliding action. But since you're not going cross-country, you'll need to work against resistance in order to work at aerobic intensity; an adjustable device provides all the resistance you'll need to work as hard as your exercise prescription permits, and you can vary the resistance for your arms and legs independently to get the work your body needs most.

Cross-country ski simulators have it all: aerobic training, which you can do at your own intensity level, and endurance training for your arms and legs. You'll also help develop flexibility and coordination on these machines. And injuries are really quite rare. Ski machines cost about $500; they are used mostly by dedicated cross-country skiers who want to stay in skiing shape all year long, but they are excellent fitness devices for nonskiers as well.

Rope Jumping

Rope jumping is the best-kept secret of physical fitness.

It is hard to know why rope jumping hasn't become more popular in today's fitness boom. Perhaps it is because there are no commercial interests to encourage this activity; all you really need to jump rope is a clothesline and a pair of good athletic shoes. Or perhaps the obscurity of rope jumping is due to the fact that there are no adult competitions and hence no glamour or sex appeal. Finally, many of us may mistakenly associate rope skipping with only preteens in pigtails or punch-drunk pugilists. Whatever the reasons, rope jumping does not deserve the obscurity it suffers from at present, for jumping can be a truly excellent fitness activity.

Rope jumping has many advantages. It is inexpensive and requires very little equipment. It is highly portable and hence is an ideal activity so you can stay fit during a trip. You can jump rope in privacy indoors or you can take the rope outside on good days and enjoy fresh air. You can jump in the morning or the evening, and can even use your lunch hour to jump rope at work. You can jump in solitude or in company. You can jump in silence, you can jump while watching TV or listening to the news, or you can jump in time to rhythmic music.

Rope jumping is an excellent aerobic activity that can provide high-level cardiovascular conditioning. Rope jumping will also help develop your coordination and balance. You will develop strength and endurance in the muscles of your legs, particularly your calves; you will also build forearm strength. Jumping does not improve flexibility, however, so you will need supplementary stretching exercises. Finally, because jumping is so strenuous, you can pack a lot of benefit into a short period of time. Fifteen minutes of vigorous rope jumping will give you the same endurance and metabolic benefit as two and a half miles of jogging. So if you jump vigorously (but jog slowly), you may be able to get as much benefit from fifteen minutes of jumping as you would from twenty-five to thirty minutes of jogging.

The first thing you need, of course, is a rope. A piece of ordinary clothesline will do the trick — if you don't have any handy around the house, go to your hardware store and buy an appropriate length of number-ten sash cord. Although the rope is simplicity itself, it is important to cut the cord to the right length. To measure your rope, stand with the rope running under both feet; the rope should be long enough to run up your legs and body on both sides to the level of your armpits, so most ropes are seven to ten feet long. If you find that you enjoy rope jumping and intend to stick with it, you may want to buy a specially made rope; these ropes are usually made of rubber, have lightly weighted handles with comfortable grips, and often have ball bearings so that the rope will swivel smoothly. Some ropes also have counters in the handles so you can record precisely the number of times you jump.

Although rope jumping doesn't require a special setting, it does require a smooth, level floor; a resilient or forgiving surface will also help by decreasing your impact and thus reducing stress and injury. A high ceiling is a must, and adequate ventilation is a big plus. The only other equipment you'll need is a pair of good athletic shoes. When you jump vigorously, you land on the balls of your feet and transmit a great deal of stress to your feet and legs. To avoid injuries, pick a well-fitting shoe with good forefoot stability and lots of cushioning. Aerobic dance shoes are best, but good tennis shoes can do the job. Running shoes are a third choice; since runners land on their heels, running shoes emphasize rear foot stability rather than forefoot control.

Although we've all seen tiny girls execute elaborate rope-skipping patterns on street corners with apparent ease, the technique of skipping may be a bit tricky at first. Unless you retain jumping skills from your youth, we'd advise that you get started slowly and methodically. Begin by practicing jumping without the rope. Jump with both feet at once, trying to get your body only two or three inches off the ground at first. When you can jump comfortably 100 times without tiring, you're ready to take up the rope. Even before you start jumping over the rope, however, you may want to practice your coordination: double the rope over and swivel it in one hand to the side of your body, so that you can practice your timing by jumping every time the rope slaps the floor.

Next you can start full jumping (Figure 6–31). Hold the rope in both hands and place the loop behind your heels. Swing the rope up behind your back, over your head, and down under your feet as you jump up with both feet together. Keep your upper arms in close to your chest with your elbows flexed at 45 degrees, so that your hands are at the level of your belly button. Your knees should be bent slightly so that you can jump rhythmically and comfortably. Your first goal should be to get over the rope smoothly, so you shouldn't try to jump more than one to three inches in the air. Begin at a modest pace of perhaps one turn per second. As you improve, you can progressively jump faster and longer.

Since rope jumping is quite strenuous, you should always begin with a warm-up period. We'd suggest stretching exercises for your lower back, hips, and particularly your calves and ankles as illustrated on pages 104–108. You may want to do some brisk walking, slow jogging, or running in place before you actually start jumping. Jump slowly at first; when your breathing is comfortable and your rhythm is smooth, you can pick up your pace.

Most people find rope jumping very tiring, so they jump in intervals or sets. When you are starting you should aim for 60 to 70 turns per minute. Depending upon how fit you are, keep this pace up for one to two minutes and then rest for thirty seconds. Be sure to check your heart rate after your first set of jumps. You

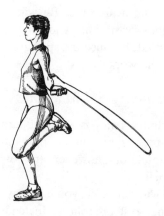

FIGURE 6–31: *Jumping Rope*

may be surprised at how quickly you reach or even exceed your target heart rate; you may even have to cut back on the intensity or duration of your jumping until you get fit. As your fitness improves, you can add additional one- to two-minute sets, still allowing yourself thirty seconds of rest between each series of jumps. When you can do five or six sets, it is time to decrease the rest period. If you jump every day or every other day, you should be able to improve steadily so that after a month or so you can jump for five minutes continuously. When you can jump continuously for five minutes at 60 to 70 turns per minute, you can begin jumping faster, at perhaps 100 turns per minute. When you can jump 500 times within five minutes, extend the duration of your jumping, adding thirty seconds to a minute at a time. Even with this gradual progression, you may find that your legs get tired and you may choose to maintain thirty-second rest periods between five-minute sets. If you find yourself gettting bored with ordinary jumping, you can try skipping one foot at a time or even using fancy arm work in the best street-corner traditions.

What should your goals be? Remember that rope jumping is quite strenuous. Even at a modest 60 turns per minute you can burn up 575 calories in an hour of jumping; at 100 turns per minute you can consume 850 calories, which is equivalent to running eight to nine miles in an hour. If rope jumping is your sole fitness activity, you may want to build to a total of two to three hours a week of jumping. However, because jumping is so strenuous, it takes a fit athlete to be able to jump for as much as thirty minutes. For ordinary people, fifteen minutes of jumping is an excellent workout, which can serve as a terrific supplement to other fitness activities, rather than as a complete program in and of itself.

As with other strenuous forms of exercise, you should cool down gradually after jumping. If you jump vigorously, you'll find that you'll sweat copiously, so good fluid intake is important.

Jumping is an excellent aerobic conditioning activity for your heart and circulation, and it will also develop your leg strength and overall coordination. But as we said, jumping will not enhance flexibility; so you should always add stretching exercises (see pages 104–113) to your jumping. Similarly, jumping will not do much for your trunk and arms — for balanced fitness, supplement your jumping with upper-body strength exercises (see pages 128–139) or add swimming or rowing. For variety, running and biking are excellent substitutes for jumping.

Jumping does stress your feet, lower legs, and hips so even with good shoes and a smooth wooden floor, you may develop injuries to these areas. Although most rope-jumping injuries are relatively mild, if you neglect them you can develop more serious problems. Chapter 11 details the common leg injuries that you may experience from rope jumping or other sports.

There are no medals for rope jumping — yet. Since there are still plenty of people who like to watch televised exercise from a recliner on Sunday afternoon, there may someday be awards for jumping speed, endurance, or style. Until then, you'll have to jump for fitness or to improve your legs and your coordination for running, tennis, or team sports.

You can be justifiably proud of yourself if you build up to fifteen minutes of jumping. But if jumping is your thing, you can set your own goals for jumping longer or faster. Are there limits? Perhaps. But the limits are extraordinary. In Australia, Tom Morris skipped rope for 1,264 miles. In Japan, Katsumi Suzuki jumped for nine hours and forty-six minutes. And closer to home, Geoff Smyth skipped through the San Francisco Marathon in four hours and fifteen minutes. Suit yourself — you can jump for fitness, jump for style, jump for sports, jump for records — or just jump for joy.

Aerobic training is the most healthful form of exercise and is the physiological key to cardiovascular fitness. Flexibility and stength training round out your program for total fitness.

STRENGTH TRAINING

Good muscle tone and strength are important goals of your fitness program and are also necessary requirements for successful participation in aerobics and sports.

There is only one way to make your muscles strong: exercise them. The exercises in this section are organized according to the areas of your body and your major muscle groups and joints. We have also included two extensive charts (Figures 6–32 and 6–33) so that you can relate these exercises to your previous self-assessment tests, to the sports you want to concentrate on, and to your ultimate fitness goals.

GENERAL PRINCIPLES

Muscular fitness has two components as we've discussed: strength and endurance. Both can be developed by training, but different techniques are required. Strength will be built by exercises that require muscle power: high-resistance, low-repetition work. Endurance will be built by exercises that require stamina: low-resistance, high-repetition work.

We will focus on the three basic methods for muscular training: exercise machines, free weights, and calisthenics. Whereas all three techniques may help with both strength and endurance, the first two are best for strength, while calisthenics (and aerobic exercises, too) are best for endurance.

As with any fitness training, strength work must be done regularly. One month of inactivity can undo many months of strength training. The moral is simple: you must work out regularly to maintain your gains.

Before you begin using any strength exercises in this

FIGURE 6–32: BODY REGIONS, MUSCLE GROUPS, AND SPORTS USAGE

Region	Muscle Group	Sports Usage
Shoulders	Deltoids (first, lateral, rear), rotator cuff	Throwing Lifting Pushing
Upper arms	Biceps (front), biceps brachials (rotational)	Pulling Throwing
	Triceps (rear)	Pushing
Forearms	Wrist flexors (palm side), wrist extensors (back side)	Throwing Grasping
Chest	Pectorals	Pushing
Upper back	Trapezius, latissimus dorsi (lats)	Pulling
Lower back	Spinal erectors, paravertebrals	Throwing Hitting Lifting Twisting
Hip flexors	Iliopsoas, rectus femoris	Sprinting Kicking
Abdomen	Rectus abdominus	Twisting Bending Sprinting
Buttocks	Gluteus maximus (hip extension), gluteus medius, tensor fascia lata (hip abductors)	Running Jumping Skating
Front thighs, knees	Quadriceps (quads)	Running
Back thighs	Hamstrings (hams)	Running
Inner thighs, groin	Hip adductors	Skating Kicking
Calves	Gastrocnemius (gastrocs), soleus	Swimming Jumping
Shins	Tibialis anterior	Running Kicking

book, review the principles in Chapter 2, where we discussed the anatomic and physiologic basis for muscular strength. Muscular power depends primarily on fast-twitch, anaerobic muscle fibers. Muscle power increases by exercising these fibers against high resistance. This increases their mass and increases the number of fibers that are recruited during a given activity. High-resistance exercises are, by necessity, low repetition, because muscles fatigue rapidly at these levels of activity. They are performed in "a set" of exercises ranging from eight to twelve (in some cases more) repetitions. We recommend doing only *one set* of each exercise per session, but advanced programs utilize two or three sets and other techniques.

A second principle of strength training is that muscles are developed concentrically — that is, when lifting a weight — and eccentrically — that is, when setting it down again while resisting the force of gravity. All exercise regimens require as much care in lowering a weight as in lifting it. In practice, this means carrying out both phases in a slow, controlled manner.

Third, regardless of the method by which resistance is supplied — whether it is free weights (barbells and dumbells), machines using cams, weights, pulleys, or hydraulics, or your own body weight (calisthenics), the training effect is the same — the muscles exercised are the only muscles strengthened, whatever the modality used.

WEIGHT TRAINING, WEIGHT LIFTING, AND BODYBUILDING

The resistance exercises you choose depend on your goals. If you want to look better, feel firmer, be able to handle your snow shovel and your tennis racquet without strain and injury, "weight *training*" is the activity for you. A general weight-training program will firm up most of the major muscle groups, and, especially if supplemented with some specific exercises, will allow you to play your sport better and with less risk. Such a program is the thrust of the material in this section.

"Weight *lifting*" is a competitive sport in which you develop to the maximum your ability to lift weights in certain well-defined routines. "Power lifting" is similar but uses somewhat different routines. The goal in weight lifting, as with most sports, is competitive, whether you compete against yourself or in matches against opponents. Maximum power requires techniques that are much more intense than weight training. It is important to remember that weight and power *lifting* will only

incidentally help your tennis, whereas weight *training* may help a great deal. On the other hand, successful weight lifting requires the same intensity of training, concentration, skill, and coordination as any other sport. It also benefits from good aerobic training, and lifters run and bike as supplementary exercises. Contrary to popular belief, lifting, when done properly, leads to increased rather than decreased flexibility. Techniques and training for this sport are beyond the scope of this book. And once a participant moves beyond the beginning stages, knowledgeable coaching is very important.

The goals of "*bodybuilding*" are altogether different. Here, the athlete uses variations of weight training to increase the muscle mass of selected muscle groups in an effort to sculpt his or her body. The regimen involves intense and specialized techniques and, in fact, more muscles are used and trained than in power and weight-lifting programs. Unfortunately, the use of anabolic steroids in bodybuilding is very widespread because they enhance muscle bulk, even if they don't increase strength. As we've noted before, the health effects of steroids are adverse, and their use has tainted an otherwise legitimate sport. Bodybuilding has become a woman's sport as well. Despite the fact that muscle mass increases to a smaller degree in women as compared to men, muscle definition is enhanced, allowing women to achieve the desired "sculptured" look but with less muscle bulk. Bodybuilding requires literally hours of exercise per day to achieve and maintain the desired look.

The distinction between weight lifting and bodybuilding seems to be one of degree and emphasis, since most people who "pump iron" are interested in its effect on their appearance as well as on their strength. It is fair to say that for weight lifters, form *and* function play a joint role, while bodybuilders focus primarily on form.

For most, though, the purpose of resistance training is increased strength, a firm, confident-looking body, and the reduction of injuries from playing sports or other physical exertion. That, also, is our perspective. The rest of this section will focus on these goals and restrict the discussion to *weight training*.

Weight Training for Strength

Weight training calls for *progressive* resistance in a series of well-defined exercises or lifts. Gradually, you add repetitions of a given lift until you reach your goal, then add about 2½ to 10 pounds more, reduce the number of repetitions, and gradually build up again. For

FIGURE 6–33: STRENGTH AND ENDURANCE TRAINING BY REGION AND MUSCLE GROUP

UPPER BODY

Muscles	Resistance Exercise	Calisthenics	Endurance	Flexibility
Shoulders, upper back	Bent-over lateral raises Bent rows Front lateral raises Clean and press Military press Nautilus press machine	Push-ups	Swimming Rowing machine	Windmills Shoulder stretch
Chest	Lying lateral raises Bench press Clean and press Nautilus fly machine Various press machines	Pull-ups	Swimming	Swimming
Latissimus dorsi	Various pull-down machines Lying pull-overs	Pull-ups	Cross-country skiing Swimming Cross-country ski machine Jumping rope	Lateral side bends
Triceps	French press Military press Clean and press Various press machines	Push-ups	Cross-country skiing Cross-country ski machine	—
Biceps	Arm curls	Pull-ups	Rowing machine	—
Forearms	Reverse arm curls Wrist curls Reverse wrist curls	—	Hand strengtheners	—

LOWER BODY

Muscles	Resistance Exercise	Calisthenics	Endurance	Flexibility
Calves	Toe-ups with barbell Sitting toe-ups with barbell	Jumping jacks Straddle hops	Jogging Sprinting	Calf and Achilles stretch
Quads	Squats Leg extension machine Leg press machine	Knee bends	Bicycling Hill running Skating Stair climbing	Quad stretch
Hamstring	Leg curls	Back kick	Jogging	Ham stretches
Groin	Abductions and adductions with weight boot Nautilus abduction and adduction machine	Straddle hops Jumping jacks	Skating	Groin stretches Starter's stretch

TRUNK

Muscles	Resistance Exercise	Calisthenics	Endurance	Flexibility
Abdominal	Bent-knee sit-ups on slant board or with weight Various resistance machines	Bent-knee sit-ups	—	Bow
Abdominal oblique	—	Rotational sit-ups	—	Trunk twists
Lower abdominal and anterior thigh	—	Leg-ups	—	Iliopsoas stretch
Lower back*	Good morning exercise Clean and press Various machines	Toe touches	Rowing Swimming Cross-country skiing	William's exercises Cat's back Toe touches Plough*

*Those with back pain or history of back trouble should consult their doctor before doing resistance exercises affecting the back.

---

example, in a basic exercise like the squat (see Figure 6–62), you should pick a weight about 30 percent of your body weight and do a set of eight to twelve repetitions. If you can't do eight repetitions, reduce the weight. If you can do twelve easily, add 5 to 10 pounds more, for your next session. For exercises with smaller amounts of weight, like dumbbell curls, add the next larger weight (usually 2½ to 5 pounds).

This example holds true for most exercises. We will generally indicate an estimated beginning weight in terms of a percentage of your body weight. Another way that some recommend to estimate a beginning weight is to find the maximum you can lift one time and pick a starting weight of about 40 to 60 percent of that. This is prone to problems, especially in beginners or the overly optimistic. In truth, it is hard to find a single, consistent method for estimating starting weight, and we urge you to begin cautiously. For most exercises, we recommend doing a set in the range of eight to twelve each. Of course, for people who have never lifted before, even small amounts of weight are very difficult at first. That is one of the advantages of using weights rather than calisthenics. For example, push-ups, which

exercise your triceps, may be impossible for beginners to do. On the other hand, you can use a 2- to 5-pound dumbbell in a "press" type exercise (see page 133 for an example), which also trains the triceps, and build up from there. Weight training allows you to begin with very small amounts of resistance. (See Chapter 7 for suggested weight training regimens.)

All exercises should follow a warm-up session that combines five to ten minutes of easy aerobics (running, rope jumping, or an exercise bike is frequently used) and careful stretching of the muscles you will be using (see Chapter 7 for regimen details). Your exercises should be arranged to work major muscle groups such as back and legs first, finishing with smaller muscles such as calves and forearms. Good weight training is carried out through a full range of motion, and your training will benefit by good flexibility exercises. Using another period of stretching as a cool-down session is also essential.

The exercises themselves should be done smoothly and slowly both on the lift or concentric phase and the set-down or eccentric phase. Each repetition can take up to six seconds, with about two seconds devoted to lifting and four seconds to lowering. Pause a second or two between repetitions. Technique is even more important than timing. Jerky motion or the noises of weight stacks banging on a Nautilus machine are signs of poor form. And form counts as much here as in all athletics. Weight rooms are usually mirrored to allow you to check your form during a lift. Poor form can mean that you are performing an exercise incorrectly, either using the wrong muscle or lifting too much weight. Poor form as well as too rapid an increase in repetitions or resistance can cause injuries.

And injuries do occur. Most are overuse injuries or are caused by incorrect form. Lifting poorly often calls accessory muscles into play at extreme mechanical disadvantage and leads to strains. A good workout will leave you tired, both peripherally and centrally (see Chapter 2). Your muscles may ache slightly or feel sore and you may have trouble concentrating. But pain, especially in tendons or key areas like your back, is not normal; pain is a warning that injury may occur, and is a signal for caution.

A few final points. Weight lifting is very warm work. You should wear lightweight workout clothes that will absorb sweat, and the room temperature should be between 65 and 70 degrees. Have a towel around to dry your hands between lifts. And you might consider livening up the atmosphere with some music. Finally, many of you will find weight training very enjoyable and want to increase your proficiency and the number of sets you can do. That is the time to find a good coach and learn advanced techniques.

CIRCUIT TRAINING

Circuit training was designed to develop both aerobic and muscular strength and involves a series of weight-training exercises of about twelve to twenty repetitions each, exercising at approximately 50 percent of the maximum you can lift. It generally involves using a series of ten to fifteen stations of resistance equipment. The exerciser moves quickly from one station to the next, with only fifteen to twenty seconds rest between each. The average time per session is about thirty to forty minutes.

This program achieves just about what you would expect. It produces increases in strength comparable to other moderate resistance programs, although less than programs designed to produce maximal strength with high resistance and low repetitions. It also produces some increase in aerobic capacity when measured by maximum oxygen uptake tests. However, these aerobic changes are relatively small when compared with true aerobic training using running, biking, or similar exercises. Similarly, the metabolic benefits of circuit training are disappointing when compared with true aerobic exercise. For example, HDL or "good" cholesterol levels show only slight improvements with circuit training. We feel circuit training is a good exercise program for those who want to concentrate on weight training, but it must be supplemented by a true aerobic training program to achieve balanced fitness.

RESISTANCE EQUIPMENT

Many people are confused about various types of resistance equipment because in recent years there has been a proliferation of exercise machines — and publicity about them. Using these machines has made pumping iron as fashionable as drinking light beer. A review of these types of equipment will help you use them properly.

The Universal Gym was one of the earliest models of resistance equipment and provided a safe means of weight lifting by use of levers, pulleys, and controlled, adjustable stacks of weights. Ten years ago, Nautilus equipment was developed. Nautilus equipment enables you to vary the amounts of resistance at different points in an exercise, enabling you to maintain a truly equal force throughout the complete range of an exercise. It represents true isotonic exercise. This system is designed to extend the active range as much as possible, thereby enhancing flexibility. Real genius has occurred in the promotion of the equipment, so that today it has become a generic term for weight-lifting equipment. The other major manufacturers (for example, Universal Gym, Cybex, and Paramount) have replicated the mechanical advantages of Nautilus, and Cam II has substituted hydraulics for weights, but in the public's mind resistance equipment means Nautilus.

What is the true value of this equipment? Without any doubt, this equipment has led to the popularization of resistance training among athletes — amateur and professional alike. It is relatively safe and relatively easy to learn with a competent instructor, and produces good results in terms of muscular strength and definition.

On the other hand, there are some significant drawbacks. First of all, despite claims, weight lifting with or without the use of these machines produces only a small increase in aerobic capacity. As you know by now from our previous discussions, the routines are primarily high-resistance ones that employ fast-twitch, anaerobic fibers. While "circuit training" does increase your aerobic capacity, it is a very difficult regimen for most amateur athletes to master and its aerobic training benefit can be matched by relatively low-level aerobic exercises.

Second, injuries can occur. The full range of motion against constant resistance that is the advantage of Nautilus can also strain a muscle or dislocate a joint when applied at the extremes of the joint's range. Careful, competent supervision is important. Until you become expert with these machines, you should not use them without a good coach. Too often, resistance machines are made available without any instruction. This is a prescription for trouble — either an acute injury from misuse of the equipment, or, more often, low-back pain from poor technique and straining. If you are going to use this equipment, treat it with respect. There is a lot of leverage at the other end of that bar, and you are still made up of organic material that usually does not win a direct confrontation with iron and steel. Unsupervised exercise equipment in country clubs or racquet centers deserves to be left alone.

Third, one size is supposed to fit all, and if you are shorter or taller than average, you may find that it is difficult to use the equipment without straining.

Finally, training is specific. Exclusive use of Nautilus equipment will build only the muscle groups that are used. It will allow you to develop great skill in Nautilus routines, but this will probably not be translated into a better swing of your tennis racquet or baseball bat. Even more important, athletics demands not only the ability to exert a force, but also subtle elements of balance, coordination, kinesthetic sense, timing, and explosive strength. For these attributes, free weights are a better training method. Lifting a 100-pound barbell requires considerably more skill than lifting the same weight sitting at an exercise machine. But, for the same reason, free weights require considerably more supervision by a knowledgeable coach, and can be riskier.

If your sport demands maximum strength and skill, free weights are preferable. If not, the proliferation of good exercise equipment has provided a real boon for muscular fitness. For most of us, strength training for fitness means using a slightly lower resistance, higher repetition regimen (say eight to twelve repetitions and only one set) than you might want to use for maximum strength and bodybuilding. Most equipment today, regardless of brand, does a good job of providing a full range of motion and isolating the functional muscle groups.

The best resistance-training equipment is found in first-class fitness and health clubs. Since there are more than fifteen hundred such centers in the United States, access to these machines is now relatively easy; a list of fitness centers in your region is available (see the Appendix). But health clubs have disadvantages as well as advantages (for discussion of clubs, see pages 171–173). Many people prefer the convenience and privacy of a "home gym" — which is why sales of home exercise equipment tops half a billion dollars annually. Should you invest in exercise machines for your home?

Stationary bikes and rowing machines for aerobic training at home are excellent. But resistance machines are less successful. You can spend hundreds to thousands of dollars for these machines, but even at the top of the scale, you're asking a lot for one machine to accomplish all the things that ten separate Nautilus machines do. Home resistance machines tend to be bulky, and some are noisy; compact, affordable equipment may not stand up to the demands of frequent use.

But there is an inexpensive, durable, compact, quiet way to get excellent resistance workouts at home: free weights. To get started, all you need are two dumbbells, a 110-pound set of weights, a barbell, and a good bench. With the addition of weight boots for your quads, and using calisthenics to fill in any gaps, you can build muscle strength at home without breaking your budget.

To focus on safe and effective strength training that you can do at home without expensive gear or excessive instruction, we will highlight exercises done with barbells, dumbbells, and calisthenics. They will work well for your wrists, forearms, biceps, triceps, shoulder, chest, upper back, lower back, abdominals, gluteus (buttocks), quads, and calves. A good bench and weight boot will help develop anterior shin, hip adductor, and groin. Hamstrings will need a special leg apparatus or resistance equipment to develop maximum strength.

WEIGHT-TRAINING PROGRAM

Our basic weight-training program requires just eight exercises.

1. Squat (Figure 6–62)
2. Clean and press (Figure 6–58)
3. Hamstring curl (Figure 6–60)
4. Bent-over rowing (Figure 6–37)
5. Bench press (Figure 6–40)
6. Biceps curls (Figure 6–47)
7. Wrist curls (Figure 6–49)
8. Sit-ups (Figure 6–80)

The goal here is general improvement in your most important muscle groups. Each of the exercises can be modified to maintain interest or supplemented if you decide to train for a specific sport. Descriptions of many additional exercises are included so you can progress as you become more proficient. The excercises are grouped according to upper body, trunk, and lower body for anatomic clarity, and to allow you to find the exercise you want for the sport or muscle you are working on. But when doing your program, follow this sequence: always begin with the exercises for your legs, then proceed to your back, chest, shoulders, arms, and stomach in that order. Within each anatomic area, do large groups first, then exercises which isolate or focus on specific muscles. (For example, a bench press — chest, triceps, shoulders — should precede a French press — triceps only.)

UPPER BODY (FIGURES 6–34 THROUGH 6–50)

Figure 6–34: Lateral Raises, Bent Over
(illustrated: can also be done lying on a bench)

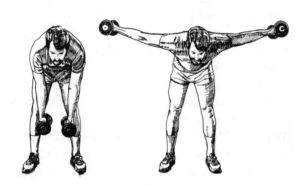

Muscles: Shoulders and upper back; secondarily lower back
Equipment: Dumbbells
Weight/reps: 7½ to 10 percent of body weight per dumbbell; 8 to 12 repetitions
Instructions: Holding a dumbbell in each hand, bend over from the waist until your upper body is parallel to the floor. Let the dumbbells hang straight below your chest and then raise them to your sides, until they are above your torso. Return slowly to starting position.
Comments and cautions: Bend your knees slightly to take the strain off your lower back.

Figure 6–35: Upright Rowing

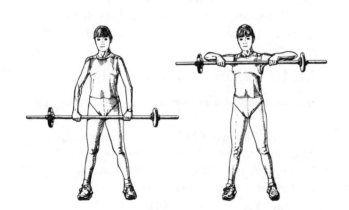

Muscles: Trapezius and deltoids
Equipment: Barbell
Weight/reps: 20 to 30 percent of body weight; 8 to 12 repetitions
Instructions: Hold the barbell with your hands about 6 inches apart, palms facing body. *Slowly* raise the barbell to the level of your neck, keeping your elbows above the bar, and *slowly* lower it down again, moving only your arms and shoulders.

Figure 6–36: Shoulder Shrug

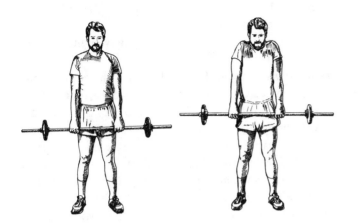

Muscles: Trapezius, neck

Equipment: Barbell

Weight/reps: 40 to 60 percent of body weight; 8 to 12 repetitions.

Instructions: Hold the barbell with your hands about 1½ to 2 feet apart, palms facing inward. Tighten your arms and shoulders, then raise your shoulders as high as possible, trying to touch them to your ears. Slowly lower your shoulders and the bar as far down as possible, moving only your shoulders.

Figure 6–37: Bent-over Rowing

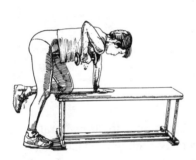

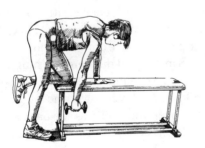

Muscles: Latissimus dorsi, deltoids, and biceps

Equipment: Barbell or dumbbell and bench

Weight/reps: Barbell — 20 to 40 percent of body weight; 10 to 15 repetitions. Dumbbell — 10 to 20 percent of body weight; 10 to 15 repetitions

Instructions: A) Barbell — Hold the barbell with your hands slightly wider than your hips and your palms toward you. Bend over so that your trunk is approximately parallel to the floor, with your knees slightly bent. Let your arms hang down and then slowly pull the weight up to your chest, being careful to move your arms and shoulders only. Then slowly lower the bar back to the beginning position.

B) Dumbbell — Take one step forward and bend your forward knee, keeping your back leg straight. Bend over and pick up the dumbbell, using the opposite arm from your bent knee. Support yourself on the bench with the other hand. Keep your palm turned toward your body and then let your hand hang perpendicular. Slowly bring the dumbbell up to your chest and shoulder area. Then slowly lower it back to the beginning position.

Comment and cautions: This should be done cautiously by anyone with a history of back trouble. Done with one hand, it is safer for your back since you are supporting your weight on your arm and are exercising only your upper body. Thus, we favor the use of a dumbbell for this exercise.

Figure 6–38: Bent-Arm Pull-overs

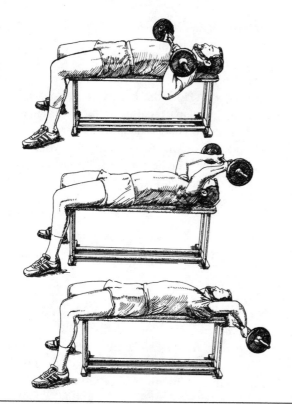

Muscles: Latissimus dorsi, triceps, and deltoids
Equipment: Barbell and bench
Weight/reps: 20 to 30 percent of body weight; 10 to 15 repetitions
Instructions: Lie on the bench with your feet touching the floor and your head hanging over the edge of the bench. Grip the barbell with your palms away from your body and your hands separated by 6 to 8 inches. Let the barbell rest on your chest. Keeping your arms bent, slowly lower the barbell in a semicircle back over your head and then slowly pull the weight back to the starting position.
Comments and cautions: This can cause your back to arch and should be avoided, therefore, by anyone with a history of back trouble.

Figure 6–39: Straight-Arm Pull-overs

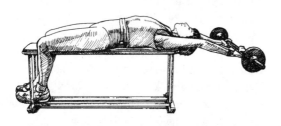

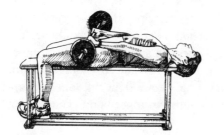

Muscles: Latissimus dorsi, pectorals, deltoids
Equipment: Barbell and bench
Weight/reps: 10 to 20 percent of body weight; 8 to 12 repetitions
Instructions: Lie on the bench with your feet on the floor and your head over the edge. Hold the barbell with your palms away from your body, hands spread about 6 to 8 inches and the weight resting comfortably on your chest. Staighten the barbell out so that your arms are locked. Slowly lower the weight in a semi-circle back over your head as far back as feels comfortable. Then slowly return the weight along the same path until it is directly above your chest with your arms out and extended.
Comments and cautions: This, too, is an exercise that can cause you to hyperextend your back, and therefore should be avoided by people who have a history of back pain. Because you are at a serious mechanical disadvantage when your arms are outstretched and over your head, you should be careful to start with a weight you can easily handle. This exercise is one that is more easily and safely done by various pull-over machines.

Figure 6–40: Bench Press

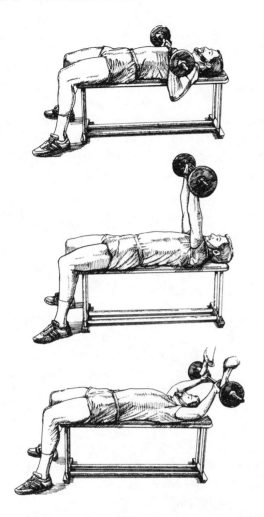

Muscles: Pectorals, triceps, and deltoids

Equipment: Barbell and bench

Weight/reps: 20 to 40 percent of body weight; 8 to 12 repetitions

Instructions: Lie on a bench with your head comfortably situated, your legs straddling the bench and your feet on the floor. Hold a barbell across your chest with your hands slightly wider than your shoulders, palms facing away from you. Push the weight straight up away from your chest until your arms are fully extended, and then slowly lower the weight back down to your chest.

Comments and cautions: This is a classical weight-lifting exercise and primarily builds the triceps and the chest. However, it is easy to arch your back, especially as you get tired, in an effort to get one more repetition going. Thus, it is one of those exercises that you should do carefully to avoid hyperextending the back and potentially getting into trouble, especially if you already have back trouble. In addition, it is easy to build sufficient strength so that you have to use very large weights. Thus, as you get stronger, you will need to have either a rack to support the weight or a "spotter" to help get the weight off your chest if your muscles become exhausted. At this stage, it is useful to switch over to one of the resistance machines, where similar exercises can be done in a safe manner.

Figure 6–41: Lying Lateral Raises, Straight Arm

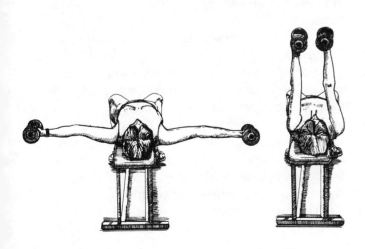

Muscles: Pectorals

Equipment: Dumbbells and bench

Weight/reps: 5 to 15 percent of body weight per dumbbell; 8 to 12 repetitions

Instructions: Lie down on the bench and hold your dumbbells straight above your chest, with your arms fully extended. Keep your arms straight and locked and slowly lower the dumbbells to your sides. Let your arms drop as low as you can comfortably. Then slowly return the dumbbells to the starting position, with your arms still straight out.

Comments and cautions: You may notice pain along the inner aspect of your arm and elbow. If that is the case, you may find it more comfortable to do the following exercise.

Figure 6–42: Lying Lateral Raises, Bent Arm

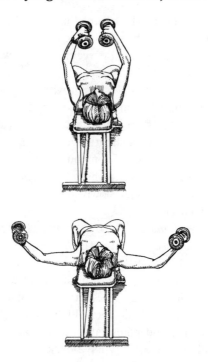

Muscles: Pectorals

Equipment: Dumbbells and bench

Weight/reps: 7½ to 20 percent of body weight per dumbbell; 8 to 12 repetitions.

Instructions: Lying on the bench, hold your arms and the dumbbells extended above your chest. Bend your arms slightly and bring the weights down to your sides as far as you can go beneath the plane of your chest. Return to the starting position.

Figure 6–43: Military Press

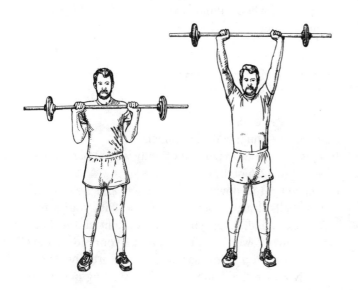

Muscles: Triceps, deltoids, and to some extent trapezius and upper chest

Equipment: Barbell

Weight/reps: 15 to 30 percent of body weight; 6 to 12 repetitions

Instructions: Stand with your feet slightly apart and hold the barbell with hands about shoulder width, palms away from your body. Hold the barbell at about shoulder height, with your hands flexed slightly backward and your elbows down. Slowly push the barbell upward until it is straight above you and then slowly lower it back down to chest level. Try to keep the weight close to the plane of your body.

Comments and cautions: This is the final portion of the most basic lifting exercise, called the "clean and press" (Figure 6–57). It is a basic shoulder and triceps strengthening exercise. Here again, as in all weight lifting, be careful not to arch your back when you lift. This exercise can be done while seated.

Figure 6–44: French Press

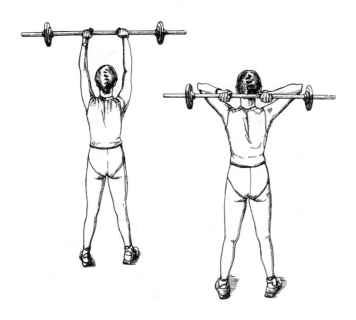

Muscle: Triceps

Equipment: Barbell or dumbbells

Weight/reps: Barbell — 20 to 30 percent of body weight; 10 to 15 repetitions. Dumbbell — 10 to 15 percent of body weight per dumbbell; 8 to 12 repetitions

Instructions: Stand with the barbell held over your head and a narrow grip with only about 6 inches separating your hands, palms facing away from your body. Slowly allow your arms to bend at the elbows, keeping your body and upper arms completely rigid and lowering the barbell in a semicircular fashion until it reaches the back of your neck. At that point, your elbows will be pointed upward. Slowly return to the upright position. You should feel most of the effort in your triceps. This lift can also be done with dumbbells, following the same instructions.

Comments and cautions: This is a very good triceps exercise. It is an excellent conditioning exercise for tennis. It can be done standing or sitting.

Figure 6–45: Side Lateral Raises

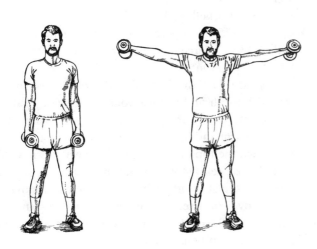

Muscles: Front and lateral aspect of the deltoid muscles

Equipment: Dumbbells

Weight/reps: 7½ to 15 percent of body weight per dumbbell; 10 to 15 repetitions

Instructions: Stand with a dumbbell in each hand at your side. Your arms should not bend during this exercise. Raise the dumbbells in a semicircle out to your sides until your arms are slightly above shoulder level. Slowly return until the dumbbells are at your sides, with your arms straight out. Your palms should be facing down.

Comments and cautions: Be sure to start at the low end of the weight for this exercise, since most of us will find that the deltoid muscles are quite weak when used in this direction. Be careful not to try to advance too quickly either in weight or in repetitions. Rather, continue to stay at the same level for about twice as long as you do with other exercises, giving these relatively small muscles a chance to develop.

Figure 6–46: Front Lateral Raises

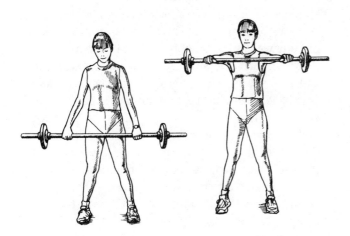

Muscle: Anterior aspect of the deltoids

Equipment: Barbell or dumbbells

Weight/reps: 10 to 20 percent of body weight per barbell, 5 to 10 percent of body weight per dumbbell; 8 to 12 repetitions

Instructions: Stand with a barbell held across your thighs, arms extended and palms facing your body. Your hands should be slightly farther apart than shoulder width. Slowly raise the barbell with your arms outstretched until it is at about eye level, then return to starting position. Follow the same instructions for dumbbells.

Comments and cautions: Use relatively light weights for this exercise and advance both the weight and repetition very slowly to avoid straining these muscles. Give yourself about twice as much time as you would ordinarily before increasing your repetition and your weight load. The deltoids are easily subject to overuse injury by overzealous training.

Figure 6–47: Biceps Curls

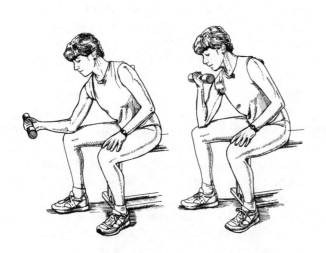

Muscle: Biceps

Equipment: Barbell or dumbbells

Weight/reps: 15 to 30 percent of body weight for barbell, 7½ to 15 percent of body weight per dumbbell; 8 to 12 repetitions

Instructions: Hold the barbell with your arms about shoulder width and against your thighs, your palms facing out. Slowly bring the barbell up, moving only your forearm and hand in a semicircular motion. As you reach the top of the arc, curl your hands inward until the bar nearly touches your neck or chin. Slowly return to the starting position. Try to avoid moving your body. This exercise can be done while standing against a wall to help stabilize your upper body and prevent it from helping out.

Comments and cautions: This is the basic biceps training exercise. It can be done with dumbbells in a similar fashion. The key to a successful exercise is to move your arms only and avoid jerking or getting the weight started by moving your body.

Figure 6–48: Reverse Curls

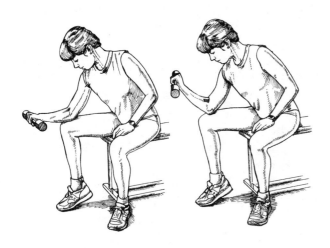

Muscles: Biceps and biceps brachialis muscle and extensor muscles of the forearm

Equipment: Barbell or dumbbells

Weight/reps: 7½ to 15 percent of body weight for barbell, 3 to 7½ percent of body weight per dumbbell; 8 to 12 repetitions

Instructions: Hold the barbell with your arms about shoulder width and your palms facing down. Keep your upper arms still and rotate the bar in a semicircular fashion up to your upper chest. Your elbows should be pointing down at that point. Then continue to rotate the bar closer to your chest by bending your wrists backward. Slowly reverse the motion, returning to the starting position.

Comments and cautions: You will find that you can lift about half the amount of weight with the reverse curl as you can with the regular curl. Here too it is important to keep your body and upper arms still while moving only your forearms, wrists, and hands.

Figure 6–49: Wrist Curls

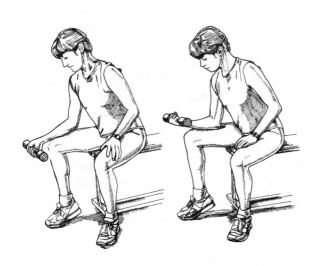

Muscles: Flexor muscles of the forearms and hands

Equipment: Barbell or dumbbells and bench

Weight/reps: 10 to 20 percent of body weight for barbell, 5 to 12 percent of body weight per dumbbell; 10 to 20 repetitions

Instructions: Sit on the bench and rest your forearms on your upper thighs, with your hands spread apart at shoulder width, palms facing upward. Your wrists should extend just over the edge of your knees. Slowly let your fists bend down as far as they can and then curl the bar back as high as it will go, curling it as close as possible to your arm. Return to the starting position.

Comments and cautions: This can be done very well with a dumbbell, with your other hand supporting the elbow of the arm that you are using.

Figure 6–50: Reverse Wrist Curls

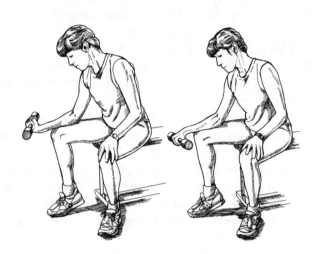

Muscles: Extensor muscles of the forearm

Equipment: Barbell or dumbbells and bench

Weight/reps: 10 to 20 percent of body weight for barbell, 5 to 10 percent of body weight per dumbbell; 10 to 20 repetitions

Instructions: Sit on a bench with your forearms resting on your thighs and your hands over the edge of your knees. Grip the barbell with your arms apart at shoulder width, palms facing down, and slowly allow the barbell to drop down and then bring it back up as far as possible. Slowly return to the starting position.

Comments and cautions: You'll be able to lift approximately half the weight with the reverse curl as you could with the regular curl exercise.

UPPER-BODY RESISTANCE EQUIPMENT (FIGURES 6–51 THROUGH 6–56)

Figure 6–51: Nautilus Pull-over Machine

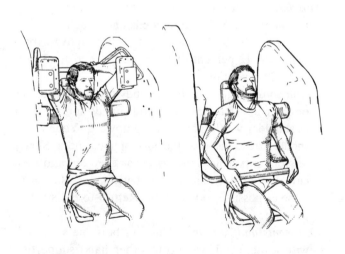

Muscle: Latissimus dorsi

Weight/reps: 40 percent of your single maximum pull-down; 6 to 12 repetitions

Instructions: Press the foot pedal down to bring the bar in the range for you to grasp and place your elbows on the pads. Apply force through your elbows and only rest your hands along the bar. Remove your legs from the foot pedal and slowly let the weight pull your arms back into a stretch position, but do not go so far as to cause discomfort. Slowly, with force applied through your elbows, rotate the bar down to approximately your waist. Hold for one second and then return even more slowly to the original position. When finished with the exercise, use the foot bar to take the weight off your arms before letting go. This is extremely important because at the extreme of motion, the weight can dislocate your shoulder.

Comments and cautions: As with all Nautilus machines, if you are too tall or short, you may have a problem with the conventional pull-over machine. There is a small model for women, but not many clubs have it. Adjust the seat, using a pad for your back if necessary, so that your back is firmly supported.

Figure 6–52: Pull-down Machine

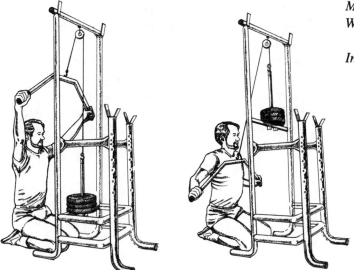

Muscles: Latissimus dorsi and biceps

Weight/reps: 40 percent of your single maximum; 6 to 12 repetitions

Instructions: Sit under the bar of the machine facing the weight pack. Grab the ends of the pulley bar with your palms facing forward. Pull the bar down until it touches your chest, pulling your elbows down and back. Slowly return the bar to the original position.

Figure 6–53: Nautilus Fly — Double Chest Machine

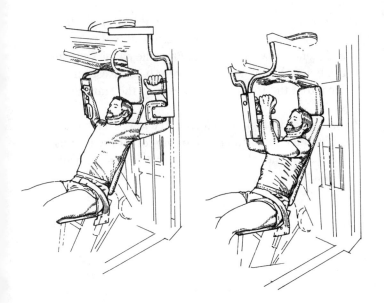

Muscles: Pectorals

Weight/reps: 20 percent of body weight, 8 to 12 repetitions

Instructions: Adjust the seat height so that your arms form a 90-degree angle when positioned against the pads. Ideally, position your shoulders so that they are in the plane of the overhead cams. You may need a back pad to help you sit forward for this. Be sure that your back is flat against the seat back and keep your feet up on the foot rest to lessen the strain on your back. Strap yourself in and, pushing with your forearms against the pad, slowly try to bring your elbows around in a semicircle until they are directly in front of you. Pause for a second and then return to the original position.

Figure 6–54: Nautilus Press — Double Chest Machine

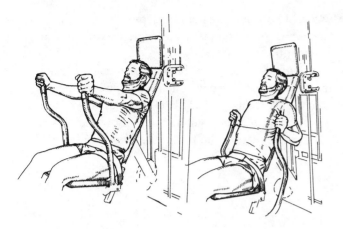

Muscles: Pectorals and triceps

Weight/reps: 20 to 30 percent of body weight: 8 to 12 repetitions

Instructions: Position yourself as in the previous exercise. Push the foot pedal to bring the handles into place in front of you. Grab them with your palms facing forward and push your arms out in front of you slowly, pause, and then come back as far as comfortable.

Figure 6–55: Nautilus Military Press — Double Shoulder Machine

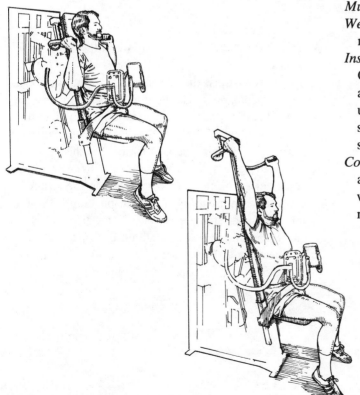

Muscles: Pectorals, deltoids, and triceps

Weight/reps: 15 to 30 percent of body weight; 8 to 12 repetitions

Instructions: Raise your seat to a comfortable position. Grab the handles with a loose grip with your thumbs and palms toward the ceiling. Press the handles straight up, being careful not to arch your back. Rest for one second at the top and then lower to the starting position.

Comment: The higher your seat, the lower the handles are and the fuller the range of motion of the exercise will be. On the other hand, this increases the difficulty markedly.

Figure 6–56: Nautilus Side Lateral Raises — Double Shoulder Machine

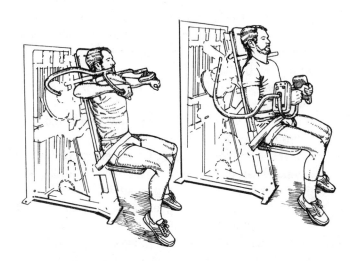

Muscles: Deltoids and trapezius

Weight/reps: 10 to 15 percent of body weight; 8 to 12 repetitions

Instructions: Raise the seat to the point where your shoulders are in the plane of the cams. Put your hands between the handles and the pads, but don't grip the handles. You'll be pushing with the back of your hands, wrists, and forearms. Rotate your elbows upward until they are parallel with the shoulders. Avoid arching your back and keep your head relaxed. Pause for one second and then slowly lower to the starting position.

Caution: As with all deltoid exercises, be careful not to advance too rapidly or to strain.

TRUNK (FIGURES 6–57 THROUGH 6–59)

Figure 6–57: Good Morning Exercise

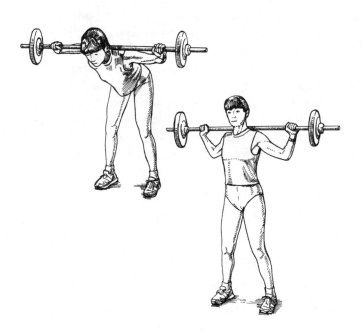

Muscles: Lower back and, to a lesser extent, the hamstrings

Equipment: Barbell (not necessary at first)

Weight/reps: 5 to 15 percent of body weight; 20 to 30 repetitions

Instructions: Stand with your feet at shoulder width. If you use weight, hold a light barbell across the back of your shoulders with your hands slightly wider than your shoulders and your palms facing upward. Bend over to about 90 degrees, bending your knees slightly if you feel any strain on your lower back. Return to the starting position.

Comments: This exercise will develop very good back strength and endurance. Begin without weights, with your knees slightly bent, and with care to avoid tiring your back. This exercise can be very effective in preventing back injuries.

Figure 6–58: Clean and Press

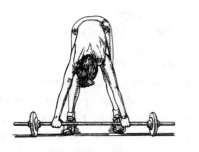

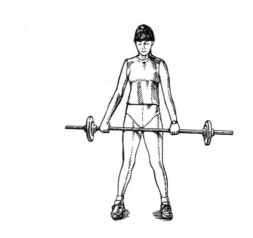

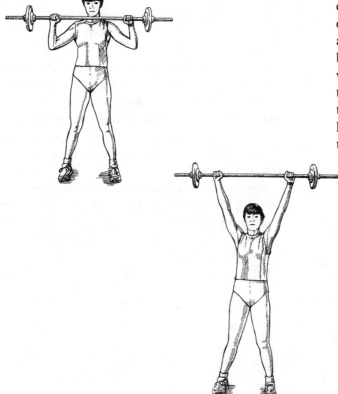

Muscles: This exercise involves your entire body, in particular quads and thighs, lower back, upper back, biceps, triceps, and chest. Your abdomen, calves, and grip muscles come into play as well.

Equipment: Barbell

Weight/reps: 15 to 30 percent of body weight; 8 to 12 repetitions

Instructions: Grab the barbell with a wide grip and your palms facing the floor. Keep your head up, your back straight, your hips low, and your arms completely extended. Straighten your legs, doing the initial portion of the lift entirely with your legs. When your legs and back are straight, your arms should smoothly begin to pull up the weight, with your elbows up and to the sides. As the weight begins to come past your chest, bring your elbows down to finish the motion, raising the weight until it is cradled over your chest at the base of your neck. Then smoothly push the weight upward above your head, fully extending your arms. Lower the weight in a similar fashion, but only bring it to a position just below your knees, not actually putting it on the floor, before beginning another repetition.

Comments and cautions: Form is very important in this exercise, and you should have somebody knowledgeable help you learn how to do it correctly. As in all exercises of this sort, be careful not to arch your back and avoid it if you have back problems. Begin with a very light weight that you can handle easily so that you will first learn the form well before trying to increase the repetitions and the resistance. This lift combines the clean and the military press and is the single most effective weight-lifting exercise.

Figure 6–59: Dead Lift

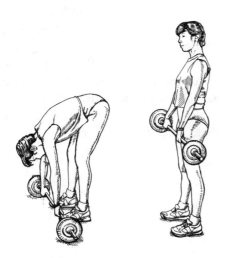

Muscles: Lower back, quads, and hamstrings

Equipment: Barbell

Weight/reps: 30 to 60 percent of body weight; 6 to 10 repetitions

Instructions: In a squatting position, grasp the bar with your arms slightly wider than your shoulders and lying almost against your shins, your palms facing downward. Slowly pull the weight and begin to straighten out your legs, keeping your arms relatively straight. Keep straightening out until you are fully erect and the barbell is held across your thighs. Then slowly lower your body until you have returned the barbell to the floor and are again in a squatting position.

Comments and cautions: This exercise is not for anybody who has back trouble. Very heavy weights can be lifted in this exercise and it is one of the classical competition exercises for weight lifters. If you do get to the point where you are lifting large amounts, be sure to use a special lifting belt to give your back an additional support.

LOWER EXTREMITIES (FIGURES 6–60 THROUGH 6–69)

Figure 6–60: Hamstring Curls

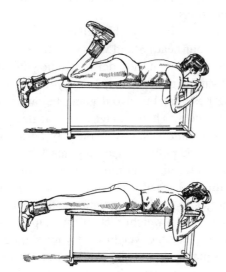

Muscles: Hamstrings

Equipment: Weight boots and a wood block to lift yourself off the floor

Weight/reps: 10 percent of body weight per leg; 10 to 20 repetitions

Instructions: Stand with one foot on the block and, keeping your balance by holding the wall, curl your leg backward until your foot touches your buttocks and then return to the original position. Once you finish the full set of repetitions on that side, shift and do it for the other leg.

Comments: It will be difficult to get enough weight to provide adequate resistance, so increase repetitions. Resistance equipment or leg apparatus on the bench will provide better exercise.

Figure 6–61: Leg Extension

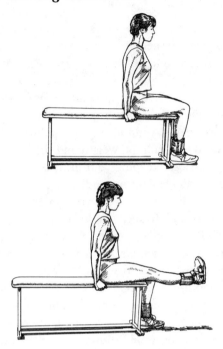

Muscle: Quadriceps

Equipment: High bench and weight boots

Weight/reps: 10 percent of body weight per boot; 10 to 20 repetitions

Instructions: Sit high enough so that your feet clear the floor. Slowly raise your leg until it's straight in front of you and then lower it gently back to the starting position. Perform a full set of repetitions with one leg and then switch to the other.

Comments: See previous exercise.

Figure 6–62: Squat

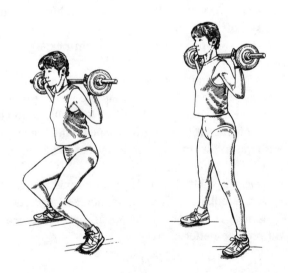

Muscles: All lower-extremity muscles, but in particular, quads, thigh, and hip muscles

Equipment: Barbell

Weight/reps: 20 to 40 percent of body weight; 10 to 15 repetitions

Instructions: Place the barbell over your shoulders behind your head. Stand with your back straight. Your legs should be at shoulder width and your feet pointed outward slightly. Slowly lower yourself into a squatting position, but avoid going below 90 degrees at your knees. Then, straighten up again.

Comments and cautions: You may be more comfortable if you put your heels up on a 1- to 2-inch board. You'll also find that putting a towel or a pad underneath the barbell will make it more comfortable. As you get to a higher weight on this exercise, you'll either need a weight rack or the help of another person to place the weight over your shoulders. Doing full squats below 90 degrees has been blamed for torn cartilage and other knee problems. To avoid that, restrict your exercise to about 90 degrees. The exercise can also be done while straddling a bench and going down only to the point where the buttocks will touch the bench.

Figure 6–63: Lunge

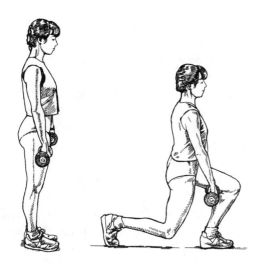

Muscles: Thigh, groin, and hip muscles

Equipment: Dumbbells

Weight/reps: 5 to 10 percent of body weight per dumbbell; 10 to 20 repetitions

Instructions: Hold a dumbbell comfortably in each hand. Step forward with your right foot as far as you feel comfortable. Then lower your body until your left knee almost touches the ground while your left foot comes up on its toes. Keep your upper body straight and look forward. Gradually return to the previous position by straightening up and then bringing your feet together. Alternate feet with each repetition.

Comments and cautions: This exercise can also be done with the barbell. Be careful to do the exercise under control so that you don't come down too hard and fast and suffer a groin pull.

Figure 6–64: Calf Raises

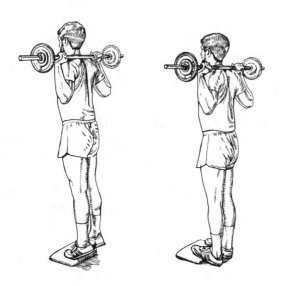

Muscle: Gastrocnemius

Equipment: Barbell or dumbbell, 2-inch-high block

Weight/reps: 40 to 80 percent of body weight; 10 to 15 repetitions

Instructions: Stand straight with the barbell supported across your shoulders and your toes elevated on the block of wood. Slowly raise your body until you are standing on the toes and balls of your feet and then lower your heels back to the floor.

Comments and cautions: Because of the relatively high weights that can be used with this exercise, you may need a weight rack or a spotter to help place the barbell. It can be done somewhat more easily with two dumbbells, hands at your sides. As you become more proficient, problems with balance disappear.

Figure 6–65: Seated Calf Raise

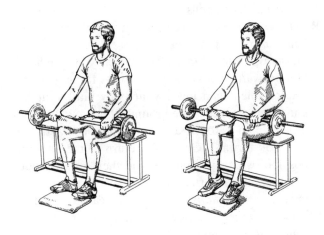

Muscles: Calf and particularly the soleus muscle underneath the gastrocnemius

Equipment: Barbell, bench, 2- to 4-inch-high block, and a towel

Weight/reps 40 to 80 percent of body weight; 10 to 20 repetitions

Instructions: Sit on the bench with the barbell held across your knees and your arms somewhat wider apart than your shoulders. Place your toes on the block in front of you with your heels on the floor. Sit erect and slowly raise both heels up as far as possible and then slowly lower them again. Repeat.

Comments and cautions: Since you'll be using relatively heavy weights, a towel across your knees will make this more comfortable. You'll probably also need a spotter to help you place the weight.

Figure 6–66: Straddle Hop

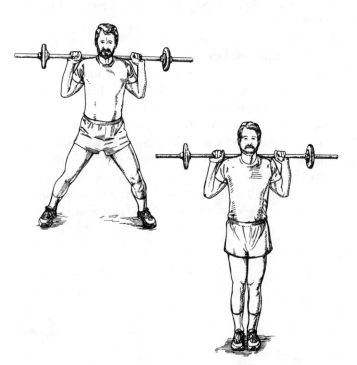

Muscles: Calves, adductors, and abductors

Equipment: Barbell

Weight/reps: 20 to 30 percent of body weight: 10 to 30 repetitions

Instructions: Hold the barbell resting lightly behind your shoulders and your arms as far apart as you can place them comfortably. Hop up and spread your legs about two to three feet apart and then hop and bring them back together again. This constitutes one repetition.

Comments and cautions: You may want to have a pad over your shoulders to help cushion the barbell. Use your arms to keep the barbell itself from bouncing up and down against your shoulders. This exercise is similar to jumping jacks (Figure 6–93) except that you are using the weight to increase the resistance.

Figure 6–67: Lateral Leg Raises

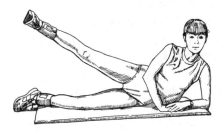

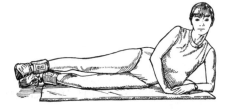

Muscles: Abductor muscles of the thigh, including the gluteus

Equipment: Weight boots and mat

Weight/reps: 10 percent of body weight per leg; 8 to 12 repetitions

Instructions: Lie on the floor on your side. Raise your upper leg as high as you can with your knee straight. Try to get to 75 degrees or more with respect to the floor. Then, slowly lower your foot to the ground. After you have done your repetitions on one side, turn over and repeat for the opposite side.

Comments: This exercise can also be done while standing. Use a small block of wood to elevate you off the floor so that you can freely move your foot with the weight boot.

Figure 6–68: Adductor Exercises

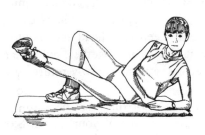

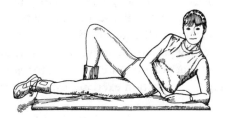

Muscles: Adductor and groin

Equipment: Weight boots and mat

Weight/reps: 10 percent of body weight per leg; 8 to 12 repetitions

Instructions: Lie on your side, but slightly rotate back to about 45 degrees, supporting yourself with your elbows. Place the foot of your upper leg on the mat so that your lower leg can move freely upward. Raise your lower leg about 25 to 35 degrees, keeping your knee straight, and then slowly lower it to the ground. After you have done your repetitions on one side, turn over and exercise the other leg.

Figure 6–69: Leg Spread

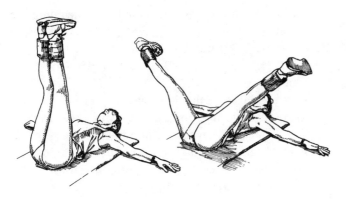

Muscles: Adductors
Equipment: Weight boots and mat
Weight/reps: 10 percent of body weight per leg; 10 to 20 repetitions
Instructions: Lie on your back on a mat. Raise your legs to 90 degrees, holding them together. Support yourself with both of your hands. Spread your legs apart as far as they can go and then slowly bring them back together.

LOWER EXTREMITIES — RESISTANCE EQUIPMENT (FIGURES 6–70 THROUGH 6–73)

Figure 6–70: Nautilus Abductor/Adductor

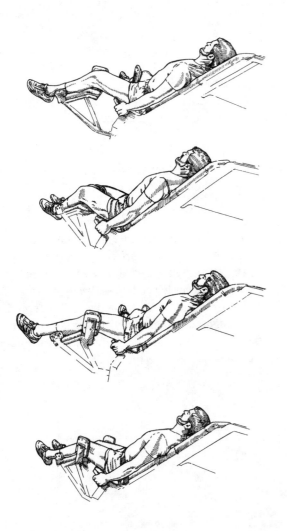

Muscles: Thigh adductors and thigh abductors, including the gluteus and tensor fascia lata
Weight/reps: 30 percent of your maximal single lift; 8 to 12 repetitions
Instructions: Adduction: Adjust the seat so that the inner aspects of the knees and ankles fit against the appropriate pads. You may need a pad behind your back to move yourself forward. Use the adjustment lever to separate your legs as far as is comfortable for you. Slowly contract the adductor muscles, bringing your knees together. Exert all your pressure from your knees. Keep your head and shoulders relaxed. When your knees are together, hold the position for a full second and then slowly return to the original position.

Abduction: Adjust the knee pads so that they are now on the outsides of your knees. Slowly spread your legs as wide as possible until you reach your comfortable limit. Pause for one second and then slowly return to the starting position. The adjustment lever will separate the movement arms, and it's important that you do not begin with too wide an angle during the adduction exercise, especially if you have tight groin muscles.

Figure 6–71: Nautilus Hamstring Curls

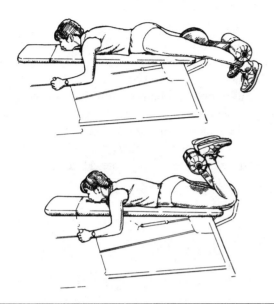

Muscles: Hamstrings

Weight/reps: 40 percent of your maximal single lift; 8 to 12 repetitions

Instructions: Lie face down jon the bench and hook your heels under the rollers with your knees beyond the edge. Grab the handles at the edge of the bench in front of you to provide support. Keep your knees straight. Then bend your knees, exerting force with your hamstrings. Bring your legs as far up as possible. Hold for one second and then slowly lower down to the starting position.

Figure 6–72: Nautilus Leg Extension

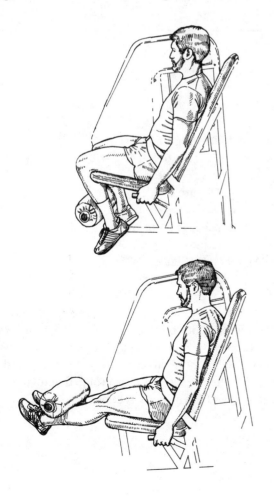

Muscle: Quadriceps

Weight/reps: 40 percent of your maximal lift; 8 to 12 repetitions

Instructions: Adjust the bench so that your knees only extend one inch past the front edge. Hook your feet under the rollers, fasten the lap belt, and grab the handles at the side of the hip to steady your body. Straighten out your legs slowly, concentrating on using your quadriceps until your knees are locked. Stop for one second and then slowly lower to the starting position.

Comments and cautions: There is a natural tendency to arch your back as you get near the end of your set. To prevent back injuries, avoid doing this.

Figure 6–73: Nautilus Calf Raise

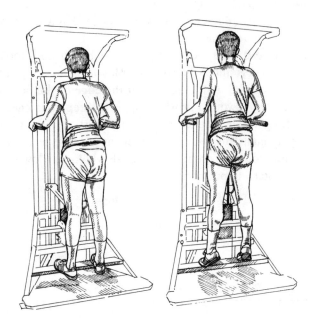

Muscles: Gastrocnemius and soleus

Weight/reps: 40 to 50 percent of your single maximal lift; 8 to 12 repetitions

Instructions: Stand on the first step and put on the padded waist belt. Snap it onto the movement arm. Step back until only the balls of your feet are on the first step. Grab the crossbar to hold yourself steady. Slowly lower your body down until your heels are as low as comfortable, and then elevate yourself on the balls of your feet as high as possible. Hold for one second and then lower yourself to starting position.

CALISTHENICS

Using body weight as the element of resistance, calisthenics are rhythmic, repetitive exercises requiring little or no equipment. Calisthenics develop strength, endurance, and flexibility. They also enhance coordination and balance. Calisthenics can be done holding small weights, thus enhancing muscular endurance and flexibility. Calisthenic exercises allow you to focus attention on the aspects of your body that you need to develop. Because they generally require more strength than athletic activities, they are a good supplementary program for most sports.

Outlined here is a basic calisthenic routine that can be used as part of your FAS(S) program. A basic, balanced program should include:

1. Push-ups (Figure 6–74)
2. Chin-ups (Figure 6–76)
3. Windmills (Figure 6–77)
4. Sit-ups (Figure 6–80)
5. Leg raises (Figure 6–83)
6. Twists (Figure 6–87)
7. Knee bends (Figure 6–94)
8. Toe touches (Figure 6–89)
9. Jumping jacks (Figure 6–93)
10. Side bends (Figure 6–85)
11. Back kicks (Figure 6–95)

As a group, these eleven calisthenics should take at least ten minutes, but they can be extended as you get trained, to allow advanced conditioning. For enthusiasts, a number of more advanced routines are also described. All these exercises are grouped into upper-body, trunk, and lower-body sections.

UPPER BODY (FIGURES 6–74 THROUGH 6–79)

Figure 6–74: Push-ups

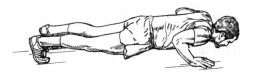
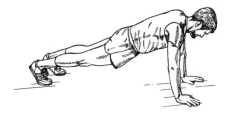

Muscles: Pectorals, deltoids, and triceps

Instructions: Lie on the floor, face down, with your hands placed just to the sides of your shoulders. Lock your body so that your stomach and back do not sag. Push your body up until you arms are straight, with your weight supported on your hands and toes. Then slowly lower yourself down again.

Comment: This is a classic calisthenic exercise and with time everybody should be able to build to 25 or more push-ups. This exercise can be done in the regular position resting on your toes and hands or, in a modified position for beginners, resting on knees and hands. This position reduces the resistance by about half. If you find that you cannot do the regular push-ups, start with the easier ones, build up to about 25, and then move on to the more difficult regular variety.

Figure 6–75: Dips

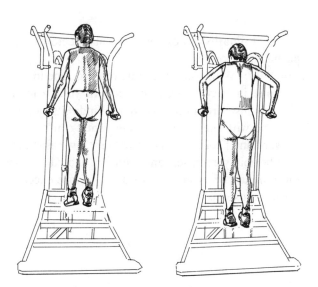

Muscles: The lower pectorals, lats, and triceps

Equipment: Parallel bars

Instructions: Grip the ends of the bars with your palms facing each other. Jump up to the point where you are supporting your full body weight on your outstretched arms and hands. Gradually bend your arms so that your elbows point backward and your body descends to the bar. Then slowly push back up to the starting point. Build up to 25.

Figure 6–76: Chin-ups

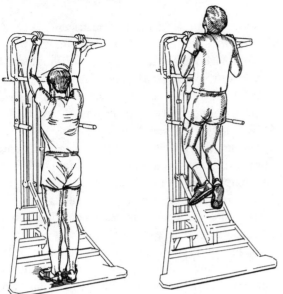

Muscles: Latissimus dorsi and biceps

Equipment: Chinning bar

Instructions: Grab the bar with your hands at shoulder width and your palms facing your body. Hang from the bar and then slowly pull your body up until your chin is just above the bar. Bring your elbows back during the motion. Slowly lower to the starting position. Build up to 15.

Figure 6–77: Windmills

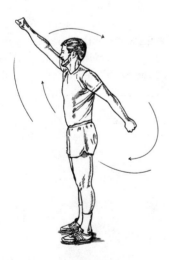

Muscles: Primarily deltoid but also lats, pectorals, trapezius, and rotator cuff

Instructions: With your arms outstretched, one in front and one in back, slowly rotate both your arms simultaneously from the shoulder. Windmills can also be done with one arm at a time. They can be done forward and backward. They are very low-resistance, high-flexibility exercises, and therefore should be done for a minute or two on each side. They are excellent warm-up exercises.

Figure 6–78: Head Rolls

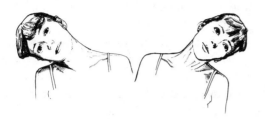

Muscles: Neck and trapezius

Instructions: Bend your chin until it touches your chest and then gradually rotate your head in a circle. Do this slowly, taking a count of four or five to complete one roll. Continue for about 30 seconds.

Comment: This is a good exercise, developing primarily flexibility of the neck. Don't overdo it in the beginning.

Figure 6–79: Wrestler's Neck Bridge

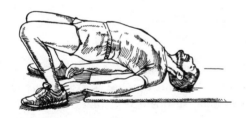

Muscles: Neck and upper-back muscles

Instructions: Lie on your back on an exercise mat. Raise your body so that you are arching your back, with your knees bent and only your feet and the top of your head touching the ground. Rock gently forward, then backward, and then side to side. Gradually build up the number of repetitions and the time that you are in this position.

Comment: This is one of the few exercises to help build your neck strength without the use of very specialized pulleys and techniques. Because most of us start with relatively poor neck strength, begin slowly and build up very gradually.

TRUNK (FIGURES 6–80 THROUGH 6–92)

Figure 6–80: Bent-Knee Sit-ups

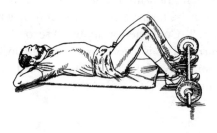

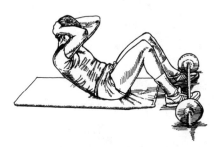

Muscles: Abdominals

Instructions: Ideally this sit-up should be done without your feet hooked under any support, but that is difficult for most people at the beginning. Lie with your knees bent and your arms either at your side, or behind your head depending on how advanced you are. The farther up your arms are, the more weight you have to carry and the more strength you need. Slowly curl up from the head and shoulders first until you are in an upright position, then reverse until you are lying down. Be careful not to arch your back in order to get yourself started and avoid jerky motions. Build up to 50 repetitions.

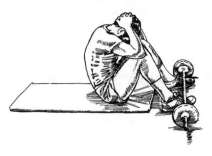

Figure 6–81: Twisting Sit-ups

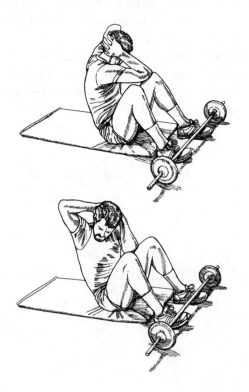

Muscles: Abdominal obliques

Instructions: This exercise is exactly the same as conventional sit-ups except that at the end of your sit-up, you twist your body so that your elbow touches your opposite knee. Build up until you can do 25 to 30 of these.

Figure 6–82: Incline Board Sit-ups

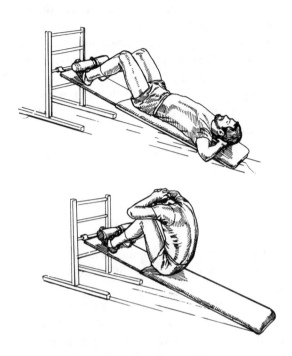

Muscles: Abdominals

Equipment: Incline board

Instructions: Like conventional sit-ups, these are done with your knees bent. However, by using an incline board you are forcing your abdominals to lift you against a greater gravitational pull, which provides much greater resistance. Build up to 20 of these.

Figure 6–83: Leg Raises

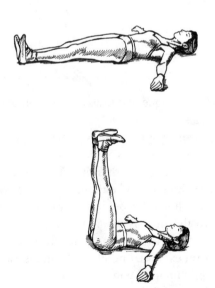

Muscles: Lower abdominal, anterior thigh, and, to some extent, the iliopsoas

Instructions: While lying on you back with your legs outstretched, gradually and smoothly raise your legs as high up as they can go. You can do them one at a time or, for a better effect, raise both at the same time. This exercise is similar to straight-leg sit-ups in that the first 20 to 30 degrees uses the iliopsoas muscle. Therefore, if you have back trouble, you should avoid it. On the other hand, it tends to work the *lower* abdominal muscles better than conventional sit-ups. Build up to 30 of these.

Figure 6–84: Knee-ups

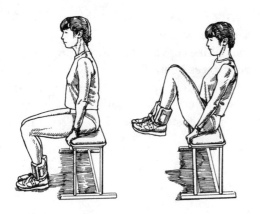

Muscles: Lower abdominals and anterior thigh
Equipment: Bench and possibly weight boots
Instructions: Sit with your hands supporting yourself on a weight bench. Begin by raising your bent knees up to your chest and then slowly returning your feet to the ground. As you get to the point where you can do 20 to 25 of these easily, use weight boots to provide added resistance.

Figure 6–85: Side Bends

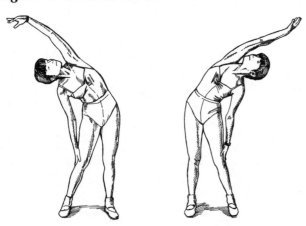

Muscles: The lateral abdominal muscles and muscles along the side of the chest, including to some extent the lats
Instructions: This should be a rhythmic, repetitive exercise. Stand with your feet about shoulder width, hands on hips or linked behind your head, and then tilt laterally first to one side and then to the other. You can also swing your arm above your head to stretch the upper trunk and latissimus dorsi as well. Build up to about 50.

Figure 6–86: Lying Side Bends

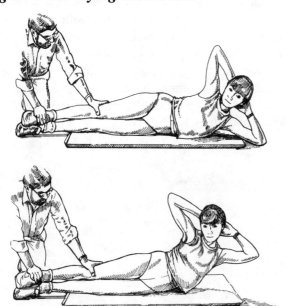

Muscles: Oblique and transverse abdominal muscles and gluteals
Equipment: Support for your feet
Instructions: Lie on your side with your feet held by a friend or underneath a bar. Your arms should be at your sides initially, although later, as you get better, you can link them behind your head. Gradually, bend up to the side as far as you can go and then come back down again. You will find that this is a fairly difficult exercise initially and will take a while for you to build up until you can do it easily and repetitively. Build up to 20.

Figure 6–87: Body Twist

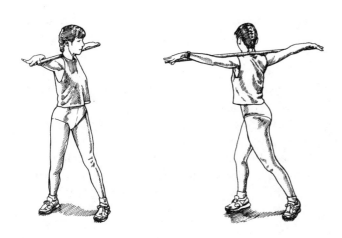

Muscles: Abdominal obliques

Equipment: Unweighted bar

Instructions: This is a low-resistance exercise that will work the abdominal oblique muscles and at the same time increase the flexibility of your back. Put the bar across your shoulder and drape your arms across it. Twist easily from one side to the other, trying to hold your hips still. If your hips tend to rotate, do this exercise while sitting on a bench. Work up to 50 of these.

Figure 6–88: Bent-over Body Twists

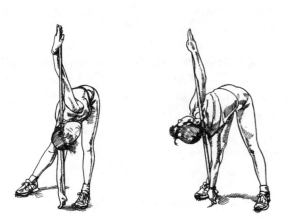

Muscles: Back and abdominal obliques

Equipment: Unweighted bar

Instructions: Put the bar behind your neck and twist your arms over it as in the previous exercise. Bend over at the waist until your torso is approximately parallel to the floor. Then, in a smooth motion, twist to your right, returning only to your starting position with your torso and head facing the floor. Straighten up, then bend over again and repeat, this time twisting to the left. Build up to 25 in each direction.

Figure 6–89: Toe Touches

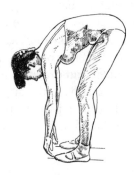

Muscles: Erector spinae of the lower back and hamstrings

Instructions: This exercise should be done smoothly and without strain in order to avoid injury. Stand with your hands above your head. Gradually and smoothly bend over, consciously rounding your spine until you bring your hands as close to the ground as possible. Then let your knees bend slightly and roll back up. Repeat 10 to 25 times. Variations can include alternately touching one foot and the other. Avoid straining or bouncing at the end of the toe touch. Do not do this exercise if you have back trouble.

Figure 6–90: Back Extension

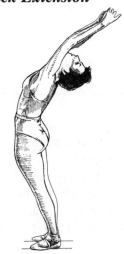

Muscles: Erector spinae

Instructions: This can be done either lying or standing. To do it while standing, assume the same position that you do for toe touches, with your hands above your head, but instead of flexing forward, extend your arms backward and stretch backward, increasing the arch in your back. Do this repetitively. The exercise also can be done at the end of conventional toe touch by just carrying through to this position. Done while lying face down, the exercise involves considerably more resistance. Have someone hold your feet and then raise your chest off the floor just enough so that you are clear. Relax and repeat.

Figure 6–91: Lying Side Leg Raises

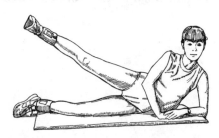

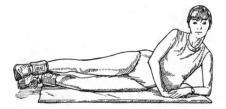

Muscles: Gluteals, abductor of the hips, iliotibial band

Equipment: Mat

Instructions: Lie comfortably on your side with one hand supporting your head, and the other arm at your side. With your knee straight raise your leg up to the side as far as you can go comfortably. Do this repetitively and build up until you can do about 30 on each side.

Figure 6–92: Sit-back

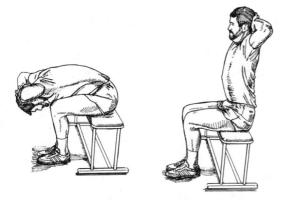

Muscles: Lower back

Equipment: Bench or chair

Instructions: With your hands clasped behind your head, sit up straight and then gradually lower yourself until your chest touches your knees and slowly sit back up again. This is similar to the "good morning" exercise, but with considerably less resistance. Repeat these and build up until you can do about 25 to 30. As with all back exercises, avoid this if it causes back pain.

LOWER EXTREMITIES (FIGURES 6–93 THROUGH 6–95)

Figure 6–93: Jumping Jacks

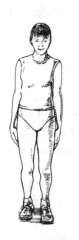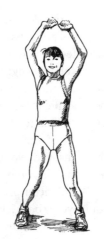

Muscles: Abductor and adductor muscles of the hip and groin

Instructions: Stand with your feet together and your arms by your sides. Simultaneously hop and spread your feet and bring your arms together above your head. Hop again, bringing your feet together, and your arms down to your sides. Build up until you can do 50 to 100 of these. This is a low-resistance, high-endurance exercise. It is also a good warm-up exercise prior to your other exercises.

Figure 6–94: Partial Knee Bends

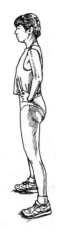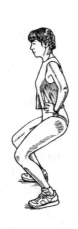

Muscles: Quadriceps

Instructions: Stand with your feet approximately 12 inches apart and your body erect, your hands on your hips. Squat down until your knees are bent no more than 90 degrees and your thighs are parallel to the floor. Straighten up again. Keep your back straight throughout the exercise. Build up until you can do 20 to 30 of these.

Figure 6–95: Back Kick

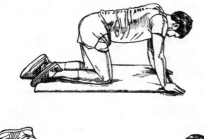
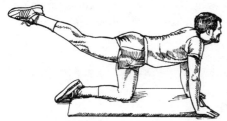

Muscles: Buttock, hamstrings, and lower back

Instructions: Get on your hands and knees in a comfortable position, with your head somewhat upward. Supporting yourself on your right knee, raise your left leg and straighten it out behind you. Simultaneously, raise your head and neck so that you are in a mild extension of your back. Point your toes while doing this. Then smoothly reverse. Repeat this rhythmically, first on one side and then on the other. Build up until you can do 25 to 30 on each side. Avoid this if you have back trouble or if it causes you back pain.

THE IMPORTANCE OF A HEALTHY BACK

Why a special section for your back? First, because proper care of your back needs an integrated set of stretching and strength exercises. Second, how well your back works determines how well the rest of your body works. Third, back injuries are the most common injuries in both daily life and sports (see Chapter 12). Hundreds of books have been written about the human back. By and large, they provide good advice; and by and large, they will be ignored, thus providing good career opportunities for the next generation of orthopedists and physical therapists. We don't expect to put these specialists out of business, but the least we can do is show you what is necessary to prevent back trouble. We recommend this as a separate program that can be done three times a week or more and that will reduce back injuries and pain. If you have back trouble, however, clear these with your doctor.

Our approach combines various exercises and treats the back and its adjacent muscles as an integrated unit. The integrity and function of the relatively weak paravertebral muscles and the ligaments of the lower back depend on the proper function of all the associated structures — namely abdominal muscles, hamstrings, anterior thighs, iliopsoas muscles, and the various ligamentous bands. (See pages 32, 34.)

Whereas the upright posture is a proud achievement of evolution, evolution of the back did not take into account two somewhat contradictory trends: first, the extraordinarily slothful existence of modern man, whose daily physical activity consists of approximately two hundred feet of walking and fourteen hours of semierect posture while sitting; and second, the perverse interest of that same individual in occasional displays of physical prowess, which can result in serious injury. Thus, a program of balanced fitness for the back must take into account all of the adjacent structures and supporting mechanisms, the evolutionary adaptations that have occurred, and the demands of both sedentary time and sport. A balanced program for your back will exercise not only your back, but also its associated groups of muscles and structures. Place particular emphasis on those exercises that correct any weakness or inflexibility that you have. But be careful! If you have back pain or if these exercises produce pain, get clearance from your doctor.

Back Strength and Flexibility Program

1. Begin by doing stretching exercises for your lower back. Lie on the floor and bring up your knees one at a time to your chest and hold the posture for about a count of five. Repeat four to five times. You should gradually be able to bring your knees comfortably to your chest and feel the muscles of the lower back stretch out (Figure 6–12). After these can be done easily, add the cat's back stretch (Figure 6–13).

2. For back flexibility, stretch your hamstrings using the simple hamstring stretch (Figure 6–

3). If they are very tight, do straight-leg raises working with a partner (Figure 6–16).

3. Stretch the anterior thigh muscles by repeating Figure 6–9.

4. Warm up with a series of 15 to 30 back twists done with your arms out (Figure 6–87).

5. Do a set of careful toe touches. Start with about 10 and build up to about 30 (Figure 6–89).

6. The "good morning exercise" can be done standing or sitting. Do about 30 of these without added weight (Figure 6–57).

7. Work on your abdomen, beginning with bent-knee sit-ups (Figures 6–80, 6–81). If you are out of shape, you may have to do only partial ones at first. Be sure to curl your upper body into a sitting position. Build up slowly until you can do 30 to 50 repetitions. Add some variations, including twisting maneuvers where you touch your knee with your opposite elbow. This will build up the oblique muscles of the abdominal wall.

If you have back pain, check with your doctor and wait until the pain and stiffness are gone before you do these exercises. This group of exercises will prevent trouble and, even if you can't do a full FAS(S) program, putting it on your schedule three times a week will pay off.

SPEED TRAINING

Flexibility, aerobics, and strength training are essential for fitness and for sports. Flexibility training will build coordination and improve your reach and range. Strength training will develop power. Aerobic training is crucial to cardiovascular fitness and provides endurance and stamina for sports. But competitive sports require more than just staying power. Once you get to be an athlete, you may start to think about improving your performance. A fourth type of conditioning provides an important complement to the basic three: speed training.

Whereas aerobic conditioning *is* hard work, after you're in shape you will probably find that endurance activities become enjoyable in their own right. Sad to say, the same is not true of speed training; it's work when you first get started and it's every bit as hard even when you reach a competitive plateau. In fact, on a continuum that rates endurance training as work, speed training could fairly be rated as sheer torture. Why do it? The answer is that you *shouldn't* do it if your only goals are fitness and health. But if you want the competitive edge for sports as well, speed training can help.

The idea behind speed training goes back to the distinction between aerobic and anaerobic exercise. Aerobic exercise doesn't build up an oxygen debt because your heart and circulation supply oxygen at the same rate as your muscles need it. Thus, you are limited only by how good a pump your heart is, not how much energy your muscles have. In contrast, anaerobic exercise means your muscles are working so hard that they outstrip their oxygen supply. This has two consequences. First, your muscles have to burn fuel incompletely and inefficiently when they are anaerobic. In fact, muscles get only one-twentieth of the energy from the same amount of fuel when they are anaerobic. Second, waste products such as lactic acid build up and this causes fatigue, cramps, and ultimately pain. If you condition your muscles with anaerobic training, they will be able to function much more efficiently under these adverse circumstances. As a result, you'll have extra speed, which can get you to the finish line and a new personal record, help you beat your opponent on a drive to the basket, or help you charge the net in time to hit a winning drive.

Speed training goes by many names. Physiologists refer to this as anaerobic conditioning. Coaches often speak of it as interval training or repeats. Many athletes call their workouts wind sprints. By any name speed training adds up to just one thing: hard work. The idea is to push your body close to its limits — not once but again and again.

Obviously you run the risk of serious injury if you interpret this to mean nothing more than running full speed until you drop and then scraping yourself off the track to do it over and over again. Proper speed work requires a carefully thought out, tightly controlled plan. It also requires you to be in good shape even before you begin, both in terms of your aerobic capacity and in terms of the flexibility and strength of your muscles and joints. All in all, the most important element in speed training is a delicate mix of the determination to push yourself and the common sense to say "enough is enough."

Sprinting is the best way to build up your speed. You can train by sprinting when you swim, skate, or cross-country ski. You can train for speed on a rowing machine or stationary bike. Most athletes get their speed training through interval drills using their own sport. Running is a good example of the principles of interval training.

To avoid injuries, limit your speed drills to no more than two per week. Needless to say, it is very important always to begin with stretching and jogging so that you are thoroughly warmed up. Only then is it safe to begin speed work. It is very important that you have a carefully thought out plan and a disciplined sense of pace. Your muscles become anaerobic at about 90 percent of their maximum effort, so we suggest that you try to work at 90 percent instead of full throttle. At first you can aim for twenty to forty seconds of sprinting. When you've reached your limit, don't come to an abrupt stop. Instead, walk or jog during the recovery period. As a rule of thumb, allow two to three times as much time for recovery, so that if you sprint for thirty seconds, walk or jog for sixty to ninety seconds. Even this recovery period will not restore you to a daisy-fresh state, but your heart rate will be lower and you will be ready to sprint again. Try to maintain the pace you established in your first interval and go at it for another equal period of time. Cool down once more — and sprint again. Depending upon the kind of shape you are in, you can repeat this cycle three to six times. When you are all through, remember to walk and jog to cool down thoroughly.

As you improve, you can increase the number of sprints, increase your speed, lengthen the distance you sprint, and shorten the recovery period. Remember that this type of speed or interval training is not an end in itself but a means of conditioning for sports. Depending on your ultimate goal in sports and your personal abilities, you may want to hold yourself to one-eighth-mile sprints or build yourself up to a half mile or even more. No matter what your program is, it is vitally important that you listen to your body. If you are stiff or sore, postpone your speed workout. Never combine it with a taxing endurance session, and never do speed work within two or three days of an important competitive event.

Speed training is not for everyone, but if you want to improve your athletic performance, first get in shape aerobically, then give anaerobic training a try. You can use similar sprinting schedules when you swim, bike, skate, row, or cross-country ski to build up your speed for any of these sports. Competitors justify their efforts by saying "no pain, no gain," but if you add common sense to the guidelines we have outlined, you should be able to gain speed without pain or injury. After all, the basic principles of speed training are no different from the fundamental schedule that first got you started: alternate intervals of hard work with intervals of easier exercise so that you will slowly but progressively improve your level of fitness and performance.

Speed training can be a useful adjunct for competitive athletes, but for all of us flexibility, aerobic, and strength training remain the cornerstones for fitness, health, and sports. Assess your goals and abilities so that you can construct a FAS(S) program for your own personal exercise prescription.

7

Putting It All Together: Your Balanced Fitness Program

The FAS(S) program provides you with the building blocks for fitness; now it's time to put these fundamentals together to build a complete fitness program. In the next few pages, you will find a series of training schedules designed to get you started on the road to lifelong fitness. These schedules are written on paper, not etched in stone. They are meant to illustrate training patterns and principles without holding you to a rigid timetable. The schedules are designed to allow for individual modifications and flexibility while still providing a stratified series of goals.

Before you even start your FAS(S) training, you'll need to select your proper entry point. First, be sure you have had an appropriate medical evaluation and that you've been cleared to exercise. Next, review your self-assessment tests from Chapters 1 and 2. Because aerobic conditioning is the key to the entire program, use the results of your cardiovascular fitness test (pages 23–27) to determine your overall starting point. If you are in poor condition, begin with schedule I, week 1 (Figure 7–1). If your score is fair, you may be able to start at the end of schedule 1 or the beginning of the intermediate level (Figure 7–2); week 5 of this chart is a reasonable entry into the system if you are in very good shape, and if your conditioning is excellent, you can start with the more demanding schedule in the advanced conditioning chart (Figure 7–3). Similarly, use the results of your flexibility and strength self-tests to determine the precise training regimen you need at each point.

These training schedules call for a variety of FAS(S) activities at every level. Let's review what each activity entails:

WARM-UP

Plan a warm-up routine that will raise your pulse slowly to get your heart and circulation into gear and will also warm up the specific muscles you'll be using in the following workout. Experiment with various routines until you find the one that's best for you. Review your flexibility self-test and the flexibility section of Chapter 6 to find out what exercises you need most and which are best. Start with static stretches for your arms and upper back, hips, and legs. Next, do dynamic stretching exercises and gentle calisthenics for each area. By now you should be fairly limber, so you can stretch your back muscles. Finally, devote the last two minutes to low-intensity performance of the aerobic work you plan next. For example, if you are on a walk-jog program, conclude your warm-up with two minutes of walking at a leisurely pace. If your schedule calls for a stationary bike or rowing machine, ease into exercise by spending the last two minutes of your warm-up freewheeling or rowing without resistance. We've allotted ten minutes to warm-up but don't skimp; in fact, if you are stiff or if you've been injured, an extra five minutes will be time well spent.

COOL-DOWN

A cool-down will allow your muscles and your heart to make a smooth transition from exercise to rest. Begin with two minutes of low-intensity activity similar to the exercise that concluded your aerobic workout. If you are cooling down from strength training, walking will do nicely. Next, go through a stretching routine similar to your warm-up, adding any exercises you may need for muscles that felt tight or tired during the workout.

Your schedule calls for five minutes of cool-down following most sessions; we've added an extra five minutes following long workouts, but if you have the time, extend your cool-down to the full ten minutes whenever you can.

AEROBICS

The aerobic workout is the key to the entire FAS(S) program. These schedules call for a gradual but pro-

FIGURE 7–1: FAS(S) TRAINING SCHEDULE I: BEGINNING LEVEL

Week	Day 1	Day 2	Day 3	Day 4	Day 5	Day 6	Day 7
1 and 2	10 min. warm-up 15 min. aerobics 5 min. cool-down	Rest	10 min. warm-up 15 min. aerobics 5 min. cool-down	Rest	10 min. warm-up 15 min. aerobics 5 min. cool-down	Rest	20 min. walk
3 and 4	10 min. warm-up 15 min. aerobics 5 min. cool-down	10 min. flexibility exercises	10 min. warm-up 15 min. aerobics 5 min. cool-down	10 min. flexibility exercises	10 min. warm-up 15 min. aerobics 5 min. cool-down	Rest	20 min. walk

(Repeat self-assessment tests for aerobics and flexibility; you should be able to document progress before moving on.)

Week	Day 1	Day 2	Day 3	Day 4	Day 5	Day 6	Day 7
5 and 6	10 min. warm-up 20 min. aerobics 5 min. cool-down	15 min. flexibility exercises	10 min. warm-up 20 min. aerobics 5 min. cool-down	15 min. flexibility exercises	10 min. warm-up 20 min. aerobics 5 min. cool-down	Rest	30 min. walk
7 and 8	10 min. warm-up 25 min. aerobics 5 min. cool-down	15 min. flexibility exercises	10 min. warm-up 25 min. aerobics 5 min. cool-down	15 min. flexibility exercises	10 min. warm-up 25 min. aerobics 5 min. cool-down	Rest	30 min. walk
9 and 10	10 min. warm-up 30 min. aerobics 5 min. cool-down	15 min. flexibility exercises	10 min. warm-up 30 min. aerobics 5 min. cool-down	15 min. flexibility exercises	10 min. warm-up 30 min. aerobics 5 min. cool-down	Rest	30 min. walk

(Repeat self-assessment tests for aerobics and flexibility to see if you are ready to move on; take strength test to plan your progress for schedule II)

NOTE: Individualized modifications of these training schedules may be necessary; see text for details. Additional flexibility exercises and calisthenics for muscular endurance and strength are welcome additions to all three training schedules. If your major workout is the morning, for example, these supplementary exercises can be done at home before bedtime.

FIGURE 7–2: FAS(S) TRAINING SCHEDULE II: INTERMEDIATE LEVEL

Week	Day 1	Day 2	Day 3	Day 4	Day 5	Day 6	Day 7
1 and 2	10 min. warm-up	10 min. warm-up	10 min. warm-up	20 min. flexibility exercises	10 min. warm-up	Rest or walk	20 min. flexibility exercises
	30 min. aerobics	15–25 min. strength exercises	30 min. aerobics		30 min. aerobics		
	5 min. cool-down	5 min. cool-down	5 min. cool-down		5 min. cool-down		
3 and 4	10 min. warm-up	10 min. warm-up	10 min. warm-up	20 min. flexibility exercises	10 min. warm-up	Rest or walk	10 min. warm-up
	30 min. aerobics	10 min. flexibility exercises 20–30 min. strength exercises	30 min. aerobics		40 min. aerobics		20 min. aerobics
	5 min. cool-down	5 min. cool-down	5 min. cool-down	5 min. cool-down	5 min. cool-down		5 min. cool-down

(Repeat self-assessment tests: if you test good or better, you can maintain program at this level)

Week	Day 1	Day 2	Day 3	Day 4	Day 5	Day 6	Day 7
5 and 6	10 min. warm-up	10 min. warm-up	10 min. warm-up	10 min. warm-up	10 min. warm-up	Rest or walk	10 min. warm-up
	30 min. aerobics	15 min. flexibility exercises 30–40 min. strength exercises	30 min. aerobics	10 min. flexibility exercises 20–30 min. strength exercises	40 min. aerobics		20 min. aerobics
	5 min. cool-down	5 min. cool-down	5 min. cool-down	5 min. cool-down	10 min. cool-down		5 min. cool-down
7 and 8	10 min. warm-up	10 min. warm-up	10 min. warm-up	10 min. warm-up	10 min. warm-up	Rest or walk	10 min. warm-up
	30 min. aerobics	15 min. flexibility 30–40 min. strength exercises	30 min. aerobics	15 min. flexibility exercises 25–30 min. strength exercises	45 min. aerobics		30 min. aerobics
	5 min. cool-down	5 min. cool-down	5 min. cool-down	5 min. cool-down	10 min. cool-down		5 min. cool-down

(Most people will achieve excellent fitness at this level; only the competitive athlete will progress to schedule III)

NOTE: The times listed for strength work are approximate only. If you are relying on calisthenics and dumbbells, you should be able to complete your strength work within these guidelines. But if you are using barbells and must pause to set up and change weights, or if you are at a busy health club and have to wait your turn at Nautilus stations, you may require more time. Whereas time is an important variable for aerobic training, it is much less important for strength training; as you improve in strength work, your time may remain constant, but your resistance and repetitions will increase (see Chapters 2 and 6).

gressive increase in the *duration* of the aerobic sessions. But you can and should also individualize the *intensity* of each session according to your own condition. For example, the very first workout calls for fifteen minutes of aerobics — but if you are out of shape, we expect you'll have to intersperse low-intensity exercise in this fifteen-minute period. For example, alternate strolling with walking, walking with jogging, freewheeling with

FIGURE 7–3: FAS(S) TRAINING SCHEDULE III: ADVANCED LEVEL

Week	Day 1	Day 2	Day 3	Day 4	Day 5	Day 6	Day 7
1–3	10 min. warm-up	10 min. warm-up	10 min. warm-up	10 min. warm-up	10 min. warm-up	Rest	10 min. warm-up
	30 min. aerobics	15 min. flexibility exercises 30–40 min. strength exercises	30 min. aerobics	50 min. aerobics	15 min. flexibility exercises 30–40 min. strength exercises		10 min. aerobics 10 min. speed training
	5 min. cool-down	5 min. cool-down	5 min. cool-down	10 min. cool-down	5 min. cool-down		10 min. cool-down
4–6	10 min. warm-up	10 min. warm-up	10 min. warm-up	10 min. warm-up	10 min. warm-up	Rest	10 min. warm-up
	10 min. flexibility exercises 30 min. aerobics	15 min. flexibility exercises 30–40 min. strength exercises	30 min. aerobics	80 min. aerobics	15 min. flexibility exercises 30–40 min. strength exercises		10 min. aerobics 20 min. speed training
	5 min. cool-down	5 min. cool-down	5 min. cool-down	10 min. cool-down	5 min. cool-down		10 min. cool-down
7–9	10 min. warm-up	10 min. warm-up	10 min. warm-up	10 min. warm-up	10 min. warm-up	10 min. warm-up	10 min. warm-up
	10 min. flexibility exercises 30 min. aerobics	10 min. flexibility exercises 10 min. aerobics	30 min. aerobics 30–40 min. strength exercises	80 min. aerobics	15 min. flexibility exercises 30–40 min. strength exercises	15 min. flexibility exercises 30–40 min. strength exercises	10 min. aerobics 20 min. speed training
	5 min. cool-down	5 min. cool-down	5 min. cool-down	10 min. cool-down	5 min. cool-down	5 min. cool-down	10 min. cool-down
10–12	10 min. warm-up	10 min. warm-up	10 min. warm-up	10 min. warm-up	10 min. warm-up	10 min. warm-up	10 min. warm-up
	15 min. flexibility exercises 30 min. aerobics	10 min. flexibility exercises 20 min. aerobics	30 min. aerobics 30–40 min. strength exercises	90 min. aerobics	15 min. flexibility exercises 30–40 min. strength exercises	15 min. flexibility exercises 30–40 min. strength exercises	10 min. aerobics 25 min. speed training
	5 min. cool-down	10 min. cool-down	5 min. cool-down	10 min. cool-down	5 min. cool-down	5 min. cool-down	10 min. cool-down

NOTE: Instruction is very useful at any level, but coaching is particularly valuable at these advanced levels; individualized schedules all depend on your abilities and sports goals. Particular care is needed to avoid injury during periods of intense training. Most athletes will taper off to less intense maintenance programs several times during the year, before building again to their peaks.

pedaling against resistance. As you improve, you'll gradually be able to decrease the low-intensity work until you are spending the entire aerobic period in your training zone, with your heart rate at 70 to 85 percent of maximum.

As the weeks go on, the FAS(S) schedule will gradually take you from three to four weekly aerobic sessions and will extend each session to thirty minutes and beyond. But even if you plateau at thirty minutes, you'll continue to improve because you'll be able to exercise more strenuously week by week without exceeding your maximum aerobic target heart rate. You can mix and match aerobic activities as you wish, and can eventually substitute a variety of lifesports for aerobic training. Chapter 6 details the essentials of aerobic training.

FLEXIBILITY

Don't let the charts fool you — although relatively little time is devoted to pure "flex" training, each warm-up and cool-down also includes stretching exercises, which will improve your flexibility. Review your self-test from Chapter 2 and pick the routine from Chapter 6 that meets your needs best. Many people find a little extra stretching beneficial and enjoyable; try spending the first few minutes in the morning or the last few minutes at night stretching out key muscles and joints.

STRENGTH

Chapter 2 reviews the physiologic basis of strength training and gives you a self-test that will determine your needs. Based on these needs and your own goals, plan a routine from the strength drills in Chapter 6. Remember to include your appearance and injury prevention as well as sports in your goals. For example, if you're bothered by a large stomach, be sure to include several different abdominal exercises in your program. Later, we'll show you some sample programs devised for other people, but remember, only you know your own needs and goals. As with all FAS(S) training, you'll start your strength drills at a basic level and will build up slowly. A typical progression might take you from calisthenics to light dumbbells or "Heavy Hands," with progression to free weights or Nautilus for more advanced conditioning.

REST DAYS

Except at the most advanced weeks, we've built one rest day into each training week. For beginners, this day off is very important to allow your muscles to recover fully. Even after you've improved, you will still benefit from a twenty-four-hour sabbatical. But if you are feeling strong, you can also use the unscheduled day as a swing day, to make up for missed workouts, to do extra work on areas that need improvement, or for the exercises you find most enjoyable. If you eventually work out seven days a week, be sure that you save one or two days for lighter exercise.

WALKING

The first two charts include optional walking days. We are not trying to sneak in extra aerobic sessions. Instead, these are designed to be less-intense, less-formal sessions — just a plain, old-fashioned walk to loosen up your body and clear your mind a bit.

SPEED TRAINING

Speed work is the optional (S) in our training program. You don't need speed training for fitness, but you'll find it very helpful if you go on to competitive sports. Review the precautions and suggestions in Chapter 6 before you get up to speed. And if speed work is not for you, use these days for extra aerobics or strength training.

This series of training schedules should provide the guidelines you'll need to get in shape — and to stay in shape. The essential ingredient in using these charts correctly is to individualize, to write your own exercise prescription for yourself. These ten tips may help:

1. *Use your self-assessment tests.* The cardiovascular tests will determine your entry point, and by repeating the tests you can chart your progress. When you've improved to very good shape, you can maintain your fitness program at that level or you can choose to keep moving up to excellent (and beyond). Use the flexibility tests to select the stretching exercises you need most, and incorporate them into your warm-up, cool-down, and flexibility training. Similarly, the strength tests will tell you which muscle groups need the most work during your strength training.

2. *Let your performance guide your rate of progress.* The charts provide reasonable week-by-week goals — but they are only averages. Some people will go faster, some will need more than two or three weeks at a level before they can move up. Fatigue, aches, and injuries are all signs that you are going too fast. Don't rush — slow, steady, permanent progress should be your goal.

3. *Don't try to make up for missed days*. If travel, illness, or injury interrupts your schedule, don't try to double up to catch up. The rest days, which are built into the schedule, can help compensate for missed workouts. But after a long layoff, drop back one level for each two weeks you've missed, and then resume your progress again, training slowly but steadily.

4. *Set realistic goals*. Health and fitness are the first priority, and the FAS(S) program should give enough balance and variety to achieve this. But if specific sports become important to you as well, modify your program to meet these goals. For example, if long-distance running becomes your thing, add more aerobics, but if you want to improve your swimming, increase upper-body strength work (see Chapter 9). Define what's most important for you, and plan a program that will get you there.

5. *Keep a fitness log*. Figure 7–4 is an example of a useful format. First, note your starting point at the beginning of each week; include your weight, how long you can exercise continuously, and how far you can go.

Next, list your objectives. Be as specific as possible, but pick realistic goals. If you are just starting out, don't set a five-mile race as your first objective — it's better to succeed at a modest goal, like walking and jogging a mile in twelve minutes, rather than to fail at a loftier task that is clearly beyond you. Remember, too, that it's okay to use last week's goals over again if you need to consolidate your progress before moving on. If you have trouble living up to a realistic set of goals, you can even use your goals as a contract that must be honored.

Finally, enter your activities each day, so that you can look back to see if you are meeting the terms of your "contract." Don't forget to include comments about your diet and other fitness goals, ranging from stress management to smoking cessation. Save your log as a permanent record — you may hardly be able to discern progress from one week to the next, but as you look back over the months you'll be proud to see how far you've come, and you'll be motivated to keep working toward total fitness.

6. *Take your life circumstances into account*. You can be a fitness enthusiast without being a fanatic. A limited schedule that you follow faithfully is more beneficial than an ambitious program that is followed only sporadically. Our schedule asks you to commit one hour and fifty minutes per week to get started, and provides maintenance schedules calling for as little as four hours per week. But if this is too much for you, scale down

to a schedule that is realistic and compatible with your other needs. Don't let work or social commitments become an excuse — fitness should be an important priority, and deserves equal time. But other pressures will cause all of us to scale down now and again. Don't feel guilty — do what you can, and build up again when time allows. And if time is the limiting factor, invest your time in the type of exercise that does the most for you: aerobics; use flexibility training in your warm-up, and put strength work aside until you have more time.

7. *Listen to your body*. In the course of exercise and sports it can be surprisingly easy to overlook warning signals from your body. Don't do it. You should be familiar with certain warning symptoms. Chest pain is the most obvious distress signal. Cardiac pain typically causes a dull, heavy pressure in the midchest. The pain may radiate to the neck, arms, or jaw. It is usually brought on by exertion or emotion, but it can come on after a large meal or even without apparent precipitating causes. In general, this type of cardiac pain, which is called angina, is relieved by rest or by certain medications such as nitroglycerin. In some people, however, the pain or angina can be quite atypical, and can be confused with indigestion, gall-bladder attacks, or asthma. The converse is also true, in that noncardiac problems can cause suspicious chest pain. Other worrisome symptoms include undue shortness of breath, disproportionate fatigue, unexpected nausea, sweating, or light-headedness, and a sensation of skipped beats or erratic heart rhythm. Obviously any of these symptoms should lead you to stop exercising at once and get a prompt and competent medical evaluation.

8. *Modify your activity to fit prevailing conditions*. These conditions can be internal or external. By internal conditions we mean the status of your own body. For example, if you have a viral infection, with fever and muscle aches, you should refrain from strenuous exertion. Although you can exercise with a mild case of the sniffles, fever might reflect the spread of a virus in your system. In animal experiments, forced exercise during certain systemic viral infections can lead to myocarditis, or heart inflammation. We don't know if this happens to humans — and we don't want to find out by treating sick athletes. So if you have a fever, confine yourself to gentle stretching exercises. Similarly, if you are injured or even just plain tired, adjust your schedule downward so that your goals for any day match your current abilities. It is just as important to apply this principle to external conditions. Heat in particular can produce a great hazard to your heart and health (see

pages 175–176). Surprisingly, unless you have a tendency toward asthma, extreme cold produces less of a hazard than extreme heat — as long as you dress appropriately and take careful precautions against exposure.

9. *Work yourself back into shape gradually after a layoff*, particularly if it is caused by illness or injury. Any period of inactivity will lead to deconditioning of both your heart and circulation, and of your joints and muscles. This is particularly true in the older age groups, but even young people should try to build themselves back into shape after a layoff. Never thrust yourself into a full workout or highly competitive situation after a layoff until you have tested yourself with less-demanding exercise.

10. *Once you have attained fitness, maintain it.* All the benefits you have achieved will be lost unless you have a maintenance program. In general, you can maintain fitness with a little less time and effort than it took to get you fit in the first place. But you can also use your achievements to move on to more personally challenging forms of exercise and sports (see Part III). Be creative; variety will help keep fitness fun.

How much exercise is enough? Many competitive athletes and "exercise addicts" seem to adhere to a principle expressed first by Mae West: "Too much of a good thing is . . . wonderful." Without commenting on Miss West's favorite form of exercise, we should point out that when exercise and strenuous sports are in question, too much of a good thing can lead to fatigue, impaired performance, and injury (see Part IV). For fitness and health, you should adhere to the "Goldilocks rule": exercise not too much, not too little, but just the right amount.

The right amount for you, however, is a highly individual judgment. From a health point of view, we've suggested a total of 2,000 calories of exercise per week for optimal protection against cardiovascular disease (see page 18). If fitness is your goal, we suggest that you build up to the middle or end of the intermediate FAS(S) chart, requiring four to five hours of training per week. But we hope you'll enjoy fitness as much as we do; our friends and patients generally ask for Goldilocks guidelines at first, but after three or four months of fitness, they are sounding like Mae West.

FIGURE 7–4: SAMPLE FITNESS LOG

Week _____ of fitness program   Dates: Weight at start of week:

Goals for the week: (Record your goals for exercise, diet, and weight)

Day	*Flexibility*	*Aerobics*	*Strength*	*Speed/Sports*	*Comments*
	(Record stretching exercises, including warm-up and cool-down)	(Record type of activity, time spent, distance covered)	(Record calisthenics and weight work)	(Record speed drills, sports and games or other activities)	(Record important data about diet, weather, injuries, medications)
Sunday					
Monday					
Tuesday					
Wednesday					
Thursday					
Friday					
Saturday					
Weekly Totals:					

THE ROAD TO FITNESS: SAMPLE PROFILES AND PROGRAMS

Planning your personalized fitness program may seem complicated and even intimidating at first. But once you get started, the pieces will fit into place. Don't try to plan a lifelong program all at once; instead, divide your goals into small, attainable segments and plan a week at a time. Look over these six case histories; you may find a story that resembles your own, but even if you don't, seeing how others have constructed their fitness programs may help you plan your own.

FITNESS PROFILE: STEPHANIE D.

Stephanie D. is a thirty-four-year-old schoolteacher, married, with one child. She is 5'4" and weighs 134 pounds. She has never participated in competitive sports, but enjoys occasional doubles tennis and backpacking during weekends and vacations. In the past she danced regularly and loved it, but she has found little time for this since her son was born five years ago. She finds her schedule both at work and at home extremely busy and fairly stressful. Stephanie has no medical problems.

Fitness Evaluation

- Cardiovascular — Good.
- Musculoskeletal — Good, except for mild upper body weakness and tight hamstring muscles.
- Psychological — Mild stress.
- Nutritional — Slightly overweight (5 to 10 pounds); diet well balanced.
- Risk factors — None.
- Health life-style — Excellent.

Goals

Stephanie is interested in weight control and appearance, maximizing overall fitness and health, more recreation and enjoyment.

Fitness Prescription

Because Stephanie is starting with excellent health and good baseline fitness, her program has many options. We recommended only modest calorie restriction, relying on increased exercise for gradual, mild weight reduction. She began her FAS(S) training at week three of the intermediate chart. Flexibility training included two hamstring stretches (see pages 104–112), and her strength work concentrated on calisthenics for her upper body and abdominals (see pages 149–155); because of her busy schedule, these could be done in her home without requiring special equipment. For aerobics we advised aerobic dance, rope jumping, or any lifesport of her choice.

Outcome

There was excellent compliance in all areas. After sixteen weeks of aerobic dance, she achieved a six-pound weight loss, excellent strength and flexibility, and excellent cardiovascular fitness. Aerobic dance was enjoyable, but scheduling difficulties added to her stress. For fitness maintenance, she reduced dance classes to one a week, added two fifteen-minute rope-jumping sessions at home, and began weekly singles tennis with her husband; she continued a routine of vigorous calisthenics and stretching exercises daily.

FITNESS PROFILE: ERNEST S.

Ernest S. is a forty-three-year-old accountant, married, with three children. He is 5'10" and weighs 210 pounds. He has never participated in sports and has no medical problems.

Fitness Evaluation

- Cardiovascular — Poor.
- Musculoskeletal — Poor flexibility, good lower-body strength, fair to good upper-body strength.
- Psychological — No difficulties.
- Nutritional — 40 to 50 pounds overweight; high-fat diet.
- Risk factors — One-pack-per-day smoker, cholesterol borderline-high, family history of heart disease (father had heart attack, uncle had stroke).
- Health life-style — No routine medical care.

Goals

Ernest is aiming for weight loss, risk-factor reduction, and recreational sports with his children.

Fitness Prescription

Although healthy at present, Ernest has multiple risk factors for heart disease, and is starting from a very low level of fitness. Hence he needs a comprehensive program, including medical screening, behavioral modification, and an exercise program which starts slowly and progresses gradually. His plan:

1. Smoking cessation.
2. Low-fat, low-calorie diet.
3. Daily walking, beginning with fifteen minutes at a modest pace until a medical evaluation is completed and an exercise prescription is prepared.
4. Comprehensive medical examination. Because of obesity, smoking, family history, and poor fitness, a stress test should be done before serious training. Ernest's test showed poor fitness but no evidence of heart disease.
5. Exercise prescription: Begin FAS(S) training at chart one, week one. Stationary biking for aerobics initially, then gradually shift to a progressive swimming program, starting with weekly lessons and building to thirty-minute swims three or four times weekly. Swimming and bike riding with children, hikes with family when repeat self-testing reveals improvement to average cardiovascular fitness.

Outcome

Ernest lost twenty-eight pounds, his smoking decreased to one pack per week, and his cardiovascular fitness level was above average after six months. Ernest chose swimming for maintenance fitness and began playing soccer with his children. Additional lower-body flexibility exercises (see pages 104–109) were prescribed to avoid injury.

FITNESS PROFILE: JAMES McW.

James McW. is a twenty-eight-year-old unmarried software engineer. He is 5'11" and weighs 162 pounds. Jim ran cross-country in high school, but did not run regularly again until one year ago. He is now averaging forty miles per week, and enters races at least once a month. However, frequent leg injuries have interrupted his training repeatedly. Jim has no medical problems.

Fitness Evaluation

· Cardiovascular — Excellent.
· Musculoskeletal — Excellent strength, poor lower-body flexibility.
· Psychological — No difficulties.
· Nutritional — Weight ideal; high-fat, high-salt diet.
· Risk factors — Family history of heart disease (father had heart attack at age fifty-nine).
· Health life-style — Excellent.

Goals

Jim's objectives are injury prevention and improved racing times.

Fitness Prescription

Jim's overall fitness is already excellent. Rather than prescribe a formal FAS(S) schedule, we concentrated on correcting his one weakness (inflexibility) and meeting his goals (improved racing).

1. Twenty minutes of stretching exercises daily, emphasizing back and legs (see pages 104–113).
2. Warm-up and cool-down programs before and after each run.
3. Reduce running to twenty-five to thirty miles per week and omit racing until injury-free. Add swimming and biking to supplement running. When injury-free, build running mileage to forty to forty-five miles per week, and add speed training twice weekly.
4. Reduce dietary fat and salt without caloric restrictions. Check blood cholesterol profile.

Outcome

Jim's compliance with the program was excellent. He continued competitive running, but without injuries, and his personal record for the 10-kilometer (6.2-mile) road race was reduced from 47 minutes 12 seconds to 41 minutes 45 seconds. Jim is lifting weights at home to maintain balanced strength and is considering training for a triathlon.

FITNESS PROFILE: RUTH S.

Ruth S. is a fifty-year-old married housewife with three daughters, the youngest of whom is college age. She is 5'3" and weighs 117 pounds. When her children were young, she biked with them and played tennis frequently, but she has not exercised regularly for eight years. She has no medical problems, but she complains of fatigue and poor sleep.

Fitness Evaluation

· Cardiovascular — Fair.
· Musculoskeletal — Flexibility and strength, fair to good.
· Psychological — Mild stress and moderate depression.
· Nutritional — Well-balanced diet.
· Risk factors — Blood pressure, borderline-high.
· Health life-style — Last saw doctor six years ago.

Goals

Ruth wants to "feel better" and improve her overall health and fitness.

Fitness Prescription

Ruth is healthy, but does not feel well. She needs both a medical evaluation and a comprehensive fitness program.

1. Comprehensive medical checkup to be sure that her fatigue is not caused by illness. Annual checkups thereafter.
2. Dietary salt restriction because of borderline-high blood pressure. Periodic blood pressure checks.
3. Begin FAS(S) at chart one, week five. For motivation and companionship, aerobic dance is recommended.
4. Refresher tennis lessons and a return to tennis suggested.
5. Psychological evaluation and counseling if energy and mood do not improve in two to three months.

Outcome

Ruth attained very good fitness in four months, with a greatly improved energy level. Ruth is now continuing in advanced aerobics and she's joined a health club to do Nautilus exercises to improve muscle tone, strength, and her appearance. She participated in short-term counseling, and has started a part-time job at a design firm.

FITNESS PROFILE: EDWARD E.

Edward E. is a fifty-four-year-old divorced attorney. Although at 5'9" he weighed 230 pounds and smoked one pack of cigarettes per day, he considered himself perfectly healthy until he had a heart attack two years ago. He had been a high-school football player and college wrestler who stayed "in shape" with weight lifting or Nautilus one to three times weekly. Other medical problems discovered at the time of his heart attack include high blood pressure and gout.

Fitness Evaluation

· Cardiovascular — Poor.
· Musculoskeletal — Strength, good to excellent; flexibility, poor to fair.
· Psychological — High stress, moderate depression after heart attack.
· Nutrition — 60 to 70 pounds overweight, high-fat diet.
· Risk factors — Family history of heart disease (older brother died of heart attack at age fifty-one, sister has high blood pressure), high cholesterol, high blood pressure, smoking, stress.
· Health life-style — Last medical routine examination two years before heart attack.

Goals

Edward wants to prevent additional heart damage, lose weight, and "enjoy life."

Fitness Prescription

Edward E. already had serious medical problems by the time he sought help. His fitness program required careful medical supervision. Two months after his heart attack, he enrolled in the Harvard Cardiovascular Health Center. He had a comprehensive medical examination, including stress testing and a blood cholesterol profile. He was started on an extremely low-fat, low-salt, calorie-restricted diet, under the close supervision of a nutritionist. Ed was also enrolled in smoking-cessation classes; initially unable to stop smoking, he succeeded after a second session. He was instructed to give up weight lifting because this isometric form of exercise raises blood pressure substantially. Instead, he was enrolled in a closely monitored, medically supervised aerobic exercise program at the Health Center.

Outcome

Over a period of six months, Ed lost sixty-five pounds and lowered his blood cholesterol from 280 to 210 (high-normal). His blood pressure returned to normal, and he was able to discontinue high blood pressure medications. His exercise program consisted initially of low-level biking at the Center and a home walking program. After two months, repeat testing showed that his cardiovascular fitness had improved from "poor" to "good," and he was enrolled at our track for supervised jogging. After four months he was able to jog five miles in fifty-five minutes with ease, and he was "graduated" to unsupervised jogging, checking his heart rate by himself.

Over the past year and a half, Ed has returned to the Center one to three times weekly to jog under loose medical supervision with fellow "alumni" of the cardiac rehabilitation program. He has regained fifteen pounds, but he does not smoke, and gets regular medical care. Psychiatric counseling was suggested but refused. However, Ed's post-heart-attack depression has entirely resolved and he has changed to a less stressful job.

FITNESS PROFILE: SHARON Z.

Sharon Z. was an avid downhill skier until eighteen months ago, when she developed asthma at age thirty-six. Wheezing prevented her from skiing, and her weight increased from 122 pounds to 137 on her 5′6″ frame. Sharon was a good all-around athlete as a girl, but as a magazine editor she felt that she did not want to devote time to competitive sports. She had no other medical problems, but was taking medications for her asthma.

Fitness Evaluation

- Cardiovascular — Good.
- Musculoskeletal — Lower-body strength and flexibility, good; upper-body strength, fair.
- Psychological — Mild stress.
- Nutritional — 5 to 10 pounds overweight; well-balanced diet.
- Risk factors — None.
- Health life-style — Excellent.

Goals

Sharon sought overall fitness and an "athletic" look.

Fitness Prescription

Sharon demonstrates how a single medical problem — in this case, asthma — can interfere with an active life-style. But in most cases, appropriate adjustments in medical treatment or exercise programs can allow exercise for fitness and recreation.

We suggested regular exercise training, beginning with week seven of the beginning chart. For aerobics, swimming was recommended because it does not usually exacerbate asthma. After four weeks, Sharon began a light weight-lifting program to increase upper-body strength for swimming (see pages 128–136).

Outcome

Sharon became an avid swimmer and now averages five to six miles per week. She participates in regional masters swim meets. She joined a health club and uses Nautilus equipment at least twice a week for strength and muscle tone. Her asthma medications remain the same, and she has not lost weight, but she is pleased with her trimmer look.

Fitness did not come easily for these six people, and it may not come easily for you. But with planning, patience, and persistence, you'll get there. And once you do, you'll discover something remarkable: fitness is fun. You'll discover that you are an athlete in your own right, and that exercise fulfills a basic human need, the need to play. A healthful life-style will become automatic, and fitness will be woven into the fabric of your daily life. You'll have to maintain your good diet, health habits, and exercise program to retain these benefits. But even if attaining fitness is work, maintaining it will be fun. You are, after all, an athlete.

HEALTH CLUBS: ARE THEY RIGHT FOR YOU?

Along with increased participation, the American exercise boom has produced a change in style: people no longer work out in the gym — instead, they engage in exercise training at the fitness center. This chapter has been devoted to a comprehensive fitness program that you can accomplish right at home, and the next three chapters will outline sports that will keep you fit without a fitness club. Health clubs are not necessary for fitness — yet they can be a great asset for some people. Is a health club right for you?

There are three reasons to join a health club: motivation and companionship, instruction and supervision, and equipment and facilities.

Perhaps the most important contribution a club can

make to your fitness program is motivation. Most people find that fitness itself is all the motivation they need — when they see how much better they feel and look, they are forever hooked on exercise. But getting started is another matter. The first two to four months can be hard going. If you enjoy group activities, a health club can really help you get started on your fitness program. Many clubs offer weight-control programs, which can also help with motivation. Even if you prefer to work out alone, a club can help motivate you by giving you a special time and place to exercise. And for some people, the membership fee itself can be a helpful commitment — the only way to get your money's worth is to use the club.

A good health club can also provide instruction and supervision. Most people can attain fitness by using the FAS(S) program without further instruction. But if you need extra help, consider a club. In general, the people who benefit most from a supervised fitness program are those at the extremes of the fitness spectrum. If you are very out of shape and have never exercised, good instruction can help teach you how to exercise effectively and safely. At the other extreme, coaching can be very helpful for people who are in excellent shape and who are training to "go for it" in sports and competition. In particular, coaching can be extremely helpful in designing and monitoring a strength-training program, using either free weights or resistance equipment.

The third reason to consider a health club is the equipment you can use there. You can save money by purchasing your own stationary bike or rowing machine for home use — but if you want to use both, to say nothing of a treadmill, ski simulator, weight room, or Nautilus apparatus, a health club makes sense. Many clubs have whirlpools, which can help with minor injuries; swimming pools can be a major reason to join a club, but most clubs lack pools. Finally, some clubs have tracks, racquetball or squash courts, or tennis facilities, which are a real inducement to people interested in sports as well as fitness.

Among the most heavily promoted facilities at some clubs are saunas, steambaths, and hot tubs. Whirlpools can help with the rehabilitation from injury (see Chapter 11), but saunas and steambaths should be viewed as devices for enjoyment or relaxation rather than as fitness aids. Your muscles may feel good after a sauna or steambath, but they won't be any stronger or more flexible. Don't be taken in by claims of weight loss

resulting from these treatments — if you lose weight, it will be because you are dehydrated; this type of weight loss is only temporary, and can impair your performance or even damage your health. Always be sure to drink enough to replace the sweat you lose in a sauna or steambath.

Both saunas and steambaths can also produce overheating; never enter one right after you exercise, because the cumulative heat loads of exercise and the hot room can raise your body temperature to dangerous levels. Instead, after you exercise go through your cooldown routine before you use the sauna. Don't use a sauna or steam room that is too hot, don't stay too long, and don't take a cold-water plunge immediately afterward, because this practice can stress your heart. In fact, people with heart problems are best advised to avoid these treatments altogether.

All in all, if fitness is your goal don't expect help from a sauna or steam room. Use them with care for relaxation, but don't join a fitness club for its sauna.

If you decide to join a club, which one should you choose? First, consider your local Y. Often overshadowed by sleek and sexy new clubs, the Y's have a long tradition of high-quality instruction and excellent classes, which may give you everything you need at a bargain price. Other places to look for bargains are your local schools and colleges. Although hours are generally limited, some schools do allow the public to share their facilities for a modest fee.

Even among the new generation of health clubs there are important differences. Clubs range in type from health spas and salons to centers offering very specialized workouts. Membership costs also vary widely. At the lower end are the franchised spas, which cater chiefly to women. Group classes and weight-control programs are the main advantages of the typical women's health club. Many have added exercise equipment such as treadmills and bikes, but they are often underutilized. If you join this type of club, you'll have to be sure that your program includes enough aerobic exercise, a shortcoming of many spas.

The next group of clubs, considerably more technical, are those that specialize in weight training. These days, most offer Nautilus equipment, but many have free weights and exercycles as well. The best of these have very knowledgeable lifting coaches, who can be very helpful with your strength training. Some of these clubs are rather oriented to competition, and many stress strength as an end in itself, rather than promoting balanced fitness. So if you join this sort of club, you'll have to review the program to be sure you're getting enough aerobic exercise.

Among the best clubs are the multipurpose facilities. Here, too, there are differences. All will provide space, equipment, and instruction in aerobic exercise, weight training, and flexibility. Some combine this with educational classes, aerobic dance, running programs, or swimming pools, and many add a social dimension. Others, so-called scientific clubs, emphasize very careful pre-exercise evaluations and often focus on one aspect, such as cardiovascular training or sports fitness and rehabilitation for amateur athletes.

If you decide to join a club, investigate the competing facilities in your area with care. Beware of "front-end loading," where fees for the first three to six months are much greater than for the rest of the term, or where life memberships are sold for a discount. If all your money is up front, they don't expect you to be around for very long. Ask for the credentials of the people "on the floor," the coaches. Some clubs have "fitness specialists" whose training is only in sales power — they are adept at lifting your money from you. A reputable fitness club hires people with at least undergraduate degrees in fitness who are supervised by someone with advanced training and degrees. Access to an athletic trainer, physical therapist, dietician, or physician are other important features.

Look at the people at the club, and especially at the ones who will be the coaches. By and large, they should fit your image of what you want to become. If they are out of shape, it is not likely they can help you get into shape. If they are all "muscle heads" (i.e., bodybuilders) and you want a balanced program, find another place. If they are all men, ask about programs for women and vice versa. Most good clubs provide facilities and programs for both men and women.

Ask about the initial evaluation, planning, and instruction. If you are looking for a full program at the beginning level, you should get a full evaluation of your needs and goals leading to an exercise prescription — your individual program.

Look at the equipment. Begin with the locker room. Showers are a must. If they don't have showers, they don't expect you to sweat, and if you don't sweat, you can't get into shape. Saunas and Jacuzzis are nice, but extras. There should be a wide range of exercise equipment. Despite claims, most of us cannot achieve complete training on any one set of equipment. There should

be a full selection of aerobic equipment (good stationary bikes, treadmills, rowing machines, and perhaps extras such as cross-country skiing devices) as well as free weights and resistance equipment. An attractive ambience and an upbeat mood will also help keep you coming to your club.

Finally, a good club should have convenient hours and realistic membership limits, so that even at peak time you can hope to get a good workout without too much waiting. Pick a club located near your home or office so that travel time doesn't become a hassle or, even worse, an excuse to "postpone" your workout.

THE TRANSITION TO SPORTS: TIPS FOR THE EMERGING ATHLETE

You can work your way to fitness without playing any sports: you can exercise for flexibility, aerobics, and strength at home or at a health club without entering a race, joining a team, or putting your name on a tennis ladder. But sports can add to your fitness program by providing variety, challenge, camaraderie, and competition. Sports help make fitness fun.

You can use lifesports (see Chapters 8 and 9) to provide the A in FAS(S) right from week one, or you can train on exercise equipment to get into shape for sports, which can in turn maintain and extend your fitness level. At any level, a few tips may help smooth the way as you become an athlete:

· *Keep a fitness log.* This is just as important for the emerging athlete as it is for beginning FAS(S) training. Hopefully, you have your original log and can continue it. If not, turn back to page 167 to review the principles of the fitness log.

· *Be flexible.* Although you should set goals and do your best to meet them, it's important not to become overly rigid. You will have to back off if you are injured or ill — instead of feeling guilty, do what you can safely and comfortably, and then gradually return to your schedule. Don't try to make up for missed days or lost miles — you are asking for trouble if you overcompensate and do too much too soon. Best of all, design a schedule with enough "give" to accommodate the unexpected events that will cause temporary detours on the road to fitness.

· *Build in variety*. Nobody ever said that variety is the spice of fitness — but a varied routine will add fun and enjoyment to your program. There are many ways to do this. You can alternate sports — run one day, bike the next, play tennis two days later, and so forth. You can also alternate weight-lifting exercises to keep from getting stale. In this book alone there are plenty of exercises to choose from for each of your major muscle groups. Or even if your only fitness activity is jogging, vary your routes. No matter what your sport, remember to vary the intensity of your workouts, so that your muscles will have an easy day or two to recover from a hard workout.

· *Plan a balanced fitness program*. All athletes require a balanced program, but masters (above age forty) and seniors (above age fifty) just cannot get away with cutting corners the way younger people can. You really have to pay attention to details in planning your program. Don't abandon the basics in favor of one sport only. Remember to get your quota of flexibility, aerobics, and strength training even when you make the transition to sports.

· *Proceed at a slow but steady pace*. Getting into shape can be a slow and even a painful process; the transition to sports is less difficult for people who are already fit, but it still takes time. Your goal is a lifetime of fitness — there's no need to set any records for getting fit fast. Obviously it will take you longer to get fit at fifty than it would at twenty-five, but it's *never* too late to start. Once you've achieved fitness, you should find it both easy and extremely enjoyable to maintain your peak condition at any age.

· *Stay lean*. In general slim athletes have more speed, more stamina, and fewer injuries. As you grow older, your body uses fewer calories. Regular exercise will help you burn excess calories, but you may have to trim your appetite as well. Avoid excessive intake of salt and fat. Eat a balanced diet that includes complex carbohydrates as the main calorie source. Fiber and roughage are good for you — but not before you exercise.

· *Exercise regularly*. Weekend athletes are the most vulnerable to injuries, and this is doubly true in the masters and seniors categories. It's harder and harder to come back from a layoff each year.

Plan to exercise three to five times a week so that you can avoid losing ground during a layoff. Clearly, as the seasons change you may have to change from outdoor to indoor activities. If you have an injury, switch to a form of exercise that will not stress your injured tissues. This approach will enable you to keep your heart and lungs in shape even if you have to rest an injured arm or leg for a period of time.

· *Take lessons*. Many people have the mistaken idea that coaching and lessons are exclusively designed for kids or beginners. This is not true. As you grow older, you may want to take up new sports either for the fun and challenge of it, or so that you can stay active as your capacities and personal interests and desires change. Good technique will also help prevent injuries. Tennis elbow is a case in point, for this common ailment strikes mostly middle-aged weekend players who can swing hard enough to damage their tissues but who "lead with the elbow" during the backhand stroke. "Old" players can and should learn new tricks. You can learn a twist serve at thirty or a two-handed backhand at forty. But as you get older, lessons from a pro are increasingly important for you to learn new techniques the right way. Leave some extra time to acquire these skills. Coaching, experience, strategy, and, of course, training will enable you to stay surprisingly competitive with much younger individuals.

· *Exercise with companions*. It's very helpful to trade tips and share experiences with other emerging athletes. You can learn to avoid problems before they occur, and you will also get help with your motivation if a buddy is checking up on you. In addition, you may find it much easier to work out with a companion than to do it alone — you will pick each other up and establish a smooth rhythm that will enable both of you to work harder and go farther. If you can't find a friend who is at your level, join a club or group that has members at all levels, including yours.

· *Enter competition*. There is no substitute for athletic competition to keep you inspired and motivated. Needless to say, the great majority of us will be competing for fun rather than for victory. In the older age groups particularly, it is vitally important to pace yourself realistically even during a race or tournament. Given these provisos, "competitive" events can be great fun at any age. The AAU holds age-grouped swimming meets throughout the country. Similarly, the Athletic Congress sponsors races and track events in which entrants are classified according to age. The Super Seniors are tennis players who stage regional and national tournaments for players in their sixties, seventies, and eighties. If you are not up to regional standards, you can still organize age-grouped tourneys or ladders at your athletic club. In addition to competing yourself, watching other athletes can also be inspiring and instructive. Don't restrict yourself to your own age group only. You'll get a boost from playing well against younger individuals also.

· *Pay extra attention to little things.* As you grow older, your body will have less tolerance to stress. Try to protect it by choosing appropriate footwear and clothing. Similarly, beginning athletes and older athletes have less ability to compensate for fluid losses, so be sure to maintain good hydration and avoid extreme heat. Even sunlight is a factor, because it accelerates skin aging and can cause skin cancer — so use a sunscreen lotion and wear appropriate clothing including a hat or visor if necessary. If your vision changes so that you need eyeglasses, be sure to pick safety lenses for sports. In fact, even if you don't need glasses, you should consider eye protectors for all racquet sports.

· *Listen to your body.* Despite your best efforts to prevent injuries with a balanced fitness program, problems may still arise from time to time. Don't stubbornly ignore injuries. You should also know the warning signs of heart trouble, including chest pain and/or shortness of breath, light-headedness, weakness, pallor, and excessive sweating. But you must know your body and how exercise affects it in order to interpret its messages appropriately. For example, even with a diligent warm-up, you may experience some shortness of breath when you begin exercising. Many people make the error of throwing in the towel at this point. Don't give up too soon. Remember that this early breathlessness is perfectly normal, and that if you keep going at a modest level you will soon become comfortable once again. You'll get your "second wind." Know

what your body can do, use it to its safe maximum, and listen to its messages — with time, you'll find that you have the body of an athlete with surprising potentials and capabilities.

COPING WITH THE ENVIRONMENT

Unless you restrict your exercise to the temperature-controlled confines of your home or health club, you will have to cope with a variety of environmental conditions in all forms of exercise and sports. Let's outline the key techniques that will allow you to cope successfully.

The most obvious advice we can give you is to use common sense. Speaking as doctors, we would hardly think it necessary to have to advise people to stay cool in the heat and warm in the cold — but as athletes, we understand that it can be difficult to apply reason and restraint when you have programmed yourself for a long run or arranged court time for a tough tennis match. So at the risk of belaboring the obvious, we will remind you that it is most important to use plain old common sense in planning your exercise schedule when the weather is adverse. This does not mean that you should head for an air-conditioned movie every time the thermometer hits 90 degrees, or for a roaring fire every time it snows. You can continue to exercise in virtually any weather as long as you prepare yourself appropriately, dress properly, listen to the messages of your body, and pick an appropriate sport. Swimming, for example, is ideal during extreme heat, and a whole variety of indoor sports and exercises can keep you fit during the worst winter weather. But with some careful planning, you can even enjoy land sports in summer and outdoor sports in winter; let's look at some specific ways in which you can adjust to climatic extremes so that you can exercise safely all year round.

HEAT

How hot is hot? Summertime temperatures of 80 degrees are delightful for a cool drink on the patio, but even this modestly warm weather can be troublesome if you exercise strenuously. In fact, the American College of Sports Medicine recommends that long-distance races should be canceled when the environmental temperature exceeds 83 degrees. The reason that temperatures above 80 degrees are potentially hazardous is that your body generates a tremendous amount of heat when you exercise strenuously. Your body is only about 25 percent efficient in translating the energy generated by your muscles into work; the remaining 75 percent is converted into heat. The amount of heat you produce is directly proportional to the intensity with which you exercise. Elite marathoners, for example, can generate nearly twenty times more heat when they run all-out than they do at rest. These athletes often have temperatures of 103 or 104 degrees at the end of a summertime race. This elevation of body temperature is not itself harmful, but if the body's mechanisms for dissipating excess heat are swamped, body temperature can rise even higher — with potentially disastrous results.

Body heat can be lost directly to the environment by radiational cooling, but as ambient temperatures approach body temperature, this mechanism for heat transfer becomes very inefficient. During summertime exercise, the major way in which your body cools itself is by the evaporation of sweat. During all-out effort, you can produce up to two quarts of sweat in an hour. At least 20 percent will drip from your body, but if the remaining 80 percent were entirely evaporated, you could shed as much heat energy as it takes to bring an ice cube to a boil. Obviously when the humidity is very high, the air is saturated with water, so sweat will not evaporate efficiently. Because of this, high humidity is a major risk factor for heat injury. Direct sunlight also adds heat to your body, adding to your troubles. On the other hand, a summer breeze will help dissipate heat by convection.

Finally, the state of your own body is another important consideration. Elderly people or young children are much less tolerant to thermal extremes than are healthy young adults. Similarly, if there is an abrupt transition from cool weather to oppressive heat, you are much more likely to have trouble than you would if your body has had a chance to acclimatize gradually over a period of three to seven days.

There are three distinct patterns of heat illness in athletes: heat cramps, heat exhaustion, and heat stroke (see Chapter 12). Cramps are very painful, heat exhaustion is debilitating, and heat stroke can be lethal. Obviously the best treatment of all is prevention. A few simple guidelines should keep you out of trouble:

1. Do not exercise in extreme heat or humidity. During a summer heat wave, switch to swimming; if you must run or play tennis, choose early-morning or late-evening hours and do your best to avoid direct sunlight. Cut down on the intensity and duration of your exercise. Give yourself at least a few days to acclimate if you are confronted with a sudden heat wave. Above all, listen to your body: don't exercise at all if you're feeling ill, and be sure to rest immediately if you feel poorly during summertime sports.
2. Dress appropriately. All participants in warm-weather sports should wear light-colored, loose-fitting, brief garments. Joan Benoit Samuelson won the first Olympic women's marathon wearing a cap in the Los Angeles summer heat. Emulate her fitness, but not her haberdashery: if you wish to shade your face, wear a visor instead of a hat so that you will not interfere with normal heat loss from your head. A headband can prevent sweat from running into your eyes, and wristbands will keep your hands dry.
3. Drink.
4. Drink.
5. Drink.

Hopefully you'll get the message without even more repetition — fluid replacement is critical to avoid heat injury during summertime sports. Water can also be very helpful if it's splashed onto your skin. Your body will get rid of lots of heat as the water evaporates. This will help keep your body temperature down; as a result, you'll sweat less, and will therefore get less dehydrated.

COLD

Wintertime can also be hazardous to the athlete. Those at greatest risk are hikers, runners, skiers, and skaters, but a few guidelines are worth emphasizing for all winter athletes.

Cold weather can produce three injury patterns: frostbite, exposure, and hypothermia (see Chapter 12). Cold temperatures are the greatest risk factor, but wind, dehydration, lack of proper protective equipment, and especially skin moisture add to the risk. Fatigue, injury, or anything else that forces you to slow down or stop exercising before you're safely back to a warm lodge can be particularly dangerous.

Quite obviously, prevention is the best policy. Avoid prolonged exposure to extreme cold especially if wind is present. In severe cold, stay close to civilization and always go out with a buddy. Never go out at all unless you are in top shape; even if you are healthy, cut back on your schedule in very bitter conditions. Above all, stay dry — your clothing will lose its insulating properties when it's wet, so frostbite, exposure, and hypothermia are much more likely.

Appropriate clothing is critical for winter sports. Each sport has its particular clothing requirements. The basic principle, however, is to wear multiple layers of thin, flexible clothing. We are particularly fond of a new synthetic fabric, polypropylene, for the inner layer because it's very flexible, comfortable, and lightweight; at the same time polypropylene is very warm and has a marvelous ability to wick moisture away from your body. Wool is also a good insulator, but is itchy and less comfortable. Cotton longjohns tend to get soggy with perspiration and are therefore much less comfortable and much less effective. Silk longjohns are coming back into fashion for some skiers; elegance notwithstanding, silk does retain a moderate amount of moisture and is therefore less desirable than polypropylene for active winter sports.

For an outer layer, wool has been traditional, but here, too, synthetics are gaining favor. Fabrics coated with Gore-tex are particularly desirable because they are water-repellent, lightweight, wind-resistant, and flexible. In addition to these excellent properties Gore-tex has many pores, which will allow your body to "breathe" so that sweat will evaporate and you will stay drier and warmer. Gore-tex has long been the favored outer shell for runners, but is now also gaining favor among skiers, who also prefer down as an ideal insulator for outer garments.

Be particularly careful to keep your hands, feet, and head warm and dry. A face mask can help protect the skin of your face during very cold weather, or you can try a thin layer of Vaseline to protect your skin and exposed areas.

You may be surprised to learn that hydration is also extremely important for winter sports. You can sweat amazingly heavily during strenuous winter sports. Drinking almost any fluid will do the trick, ranging from water to a wide variety of more appealing warm beverages.

Winter sports can be uniquely challenging and exhilarating, but they do require special precautions. Prepare yourself appropriately and listen to the messages from your body. If environmental conditions are very extreme, or if there is any question at all about your fitness or health, switch to indoor exercise until conditions improve. If you have asthma, you may have to

be particularly careful, because cold weather and exercise can combine to produce attacks of wheezing. People with disorders of the heart and circulation must also be particularly careful. But with these provisos in mind, you should be able to exercise happily and safely in all but the most extreme of winter conditions.

POLLUTION

It's no secret that air pollution is becoming an increasingly serious problem in industrialized societies. Pollution is a particularly serious concern in urban areas, in manufacturing regions, and in places where automobile traffic is dense. And pollution is particularly troublesome when thermal inversions produce heavy, still air, which causes industrial and automotive fumes to accumulate.

In the United States, there are two major types of atmospheric contaminants. Photochemical pollution, or smog, arises chiefly from motor vehicle emissions. Automotive exhaust also contains carbon monoxide, but atmospheric concentrations are not high enough to impair seriously oxygen delivery in the body. Photochemical pollution is most troublesome in urban centers, especially in the western states. The second major type of pollution is sulfur oxide and various particulates. These contaminants arise from the combustion of fossil fuels and are most prominent in the industrial centers in the eastern and central parts of the country.

Pollution and smog can produce coughing, chest discomfort, breathlessness, and eye irritation in healthy people; patients with heart and lung ailments can develop even more serious problems. Although the long-term effects of repeated exposure to atmospheric pollutants has not been clarified, it seems likely that such exposure constitutes a significant health hazard.

Naturally, the urban athlete suffers because of pollution. Doctors John Nicholson and David Case studied the effects of pollution on sixteen runners in New York City. Their subjects were all healthy volunteers who were asked to jog for thirty minutes in Central Park or along FDR Drive during peak rush-hour traffic. All of the subjects showed a substantial rise in blood carbon monoxide levels; for the entire group, carbon monoxide levels were increased approximately threefold at the end of just thirty minutes of strenuous exercise.

Of course, runners are not alone in their susceptibility to auto fumes. The same study showed that simply standing quietly near New York City traffic increased carbon monoxide blood levels more than twofold. The runners' levels were somewhat higher because their breathing volumes were greatly increased by exercise; however, even nonrunners showed the effects of pollution.

What does this mean for those of us who run, bike, or walk in urban areas? The brilliant success of the 1984 summer Olympics in smoggy Los Angeles is reassuring, and at this point there is certainly nothing to be alarmed about. We don't know if the changes in blood carbon monoxide levels have any long-term ill effects, but common sense suggests that you'd be wise to avoid traffic as much as possible by exercising far away from busy roadways and by avoiding peak rush-hour times. These precautions are particularly pertinent during summertime, when air quality is often only fair or poor. Finally, if you experience unusual respiratory symptoms, shortness of breath, fatigue, or just plain lack of energy during exercise in urban areas, ask yourself if pollution might not be playing some role. If the answer is yes, don't give up exercise, but do try to find a sport or a location that will keep you away from industrial and automotive fumes.

HIGH ALTITUDE

Thin clear mountain air can produce problems for athletes (and tourists) who attempt to get away from it all by traveling to high altitudes. Mountain climbers obviously are at the greatest risk for high-altitude illness, but in our mobile society it is not unusual for skiers, hikers, trekkers, and other travelers to find themselves at high elevations. Whereas mountain climbers are generally knowledgeable and well prepared to deal with high altitudes, skiers and others may not have given the matter sufficient thought.

Even modest altitudes can affect athletic performance. The percentage of oxygen in the air decreases progressively as you ascend from sea level. Since your body's demand for oxygen is greatly increased when you exercise, the higher you go, the less energy and endurance you will have. Some competitive runners and skiers purposely train at modest altitudes of four to five thousand feet, hoping that the additional work will give them extra endurance when they return to sea level. Most authorities feel that a well-conditioned athlete can exercise quite normally at elevations up to about five thousand feet. But at higher altitudes, performance is bound to suffer. Maximum oxygen uptake decreases by at least 3 percent for each thousand feet of elevation above five thousand feet. It's not surprising, then, that running times have been consistently slower than expected when the Pan-American Games and Olympics were held in Mexico City at an elevation of about seven thousand feet; this is particularly true of medium- and long-distance events, which place a premium on endurance.

You can help counteract the effects of altitude by getting yourself into optimal shape, and above all by giving your body time to acclimatize gradually at high altitudes before you begin any strenuous exercise. Once you are acclimatized, a carefully planned progressive training program will help you do your best. But if you have any chronic medical problems or if you are in the older age group, you must proceed with particular caution before you do any strenuous exercise at high altitudes.

Impaired athletic performance is one thing, but illness is quite another — and high altitude can produce illnesses that range in severity from mild to catastrophic. In general, high-altitude illness is not a significant risk at elevations below eight to ten thousand feet, but at these levels important problems can occur, including mountain sickness and accumulations of fluid in the lungs or brain (see Chapter 12).

Don't make the mistake of dismissing mountain sickness as an exotic problem restricted to trekkers and mountain climbers. Many ski resorts and lodges in the American West, in Canada, and in Europe are situated at eight thousand feet or higher. The avid skier with a short vacation is understandably tempted to hop out of the airplane and onto the slopes as rapidly as possible. Fortunately, serious problems at these resorts have been rare, but we would certainly urge you to stage your ascent if at all possible, and to give yourself some time to acclimate before you exercise strenuously once you've arrived at your destination. If you have underlying medical problems, these precautions are all the more important. And if you experience any symptoms, be sure to stop exercising and get medical attention; often medical attention is available only at lower altitudes. A crucial element in the treatment of high-altitude illness is, in fact, a descent to lower elevations.

FLUID AND FOOD REQUIREMENTS

It is surprising indeed that the body's fluid balance (see Chapter 4) is so poorly understood by athletes, coaches, and even trainers. Athletes are often cautioned against drinking water because fluids are rumored to cause bloating, excess weight, or sluggishness. Cramps and fatigue are erroneously attributed to drinking before or during competition. And in extreme cases, dehydration is actually encouraged to "build character" or "toughness." In fact, all of these common dicta are entirely wrong — appropriate fluid intake *prevents* fatigue, cramps, and weakness, while dehydration impairs performance and can even lead to life-threatening illness.

Nor is the athlete alone in these misconceptions. Dehydration, or "sweating it out," is a common way for wrestlers, boxers, and lightweight crew members to "make weight." In most cases they are smart enough (and thirsty enough) to spend a long while at the drinking fountain en route from the scale to the ring or shell. But the idea that dehydration is helpful for weight control has unfortunately extended beyond athletics. Fluid restriction is recommended in various crash diets, and some physicians even prescribe diuretic medications for weight reduction. These practices are to be deplored — dehydration is safe for "making weight" *only* if it is modest in degree and is substantially corrected before exercise. And dehydration has no place — and no effect — in long-term weight control.

Surprisingly, as we've said before, heavy exercise can produce a significant loss of fluid in cold weather also, both through perspiration and as a result of the dry atmosphere.

What are the hazards of falling behind in your fluid replacement? The first effect is impaired athletic performance; you will tire more easily and have less strength and endurance if you become dehydrated. If dehydration is allowed to become pronounced, some very serious conditions can result, such as a fall in blood pressure or damage to kidney function. And, in warm weather, heat exhaustion and even heat stroke can be triggered by dehydration during exercise.

Dehydration can also have troublesome effects after your workout is completed. Fatigue and irritability can persist for hours if fluids are not replaced. Our patient John M. illustrates this point. He began exercising for fitness and health and made very nice progress, so that by six months he had lost nineteen pounds and was running five miles per day. We were delighted, and we assumed that he was, too. But he returned to the office complaining of fatigue and conflicts with his wife. At first, John had done his jogging in the morning before work. But when he reached four miles a day, he found himself too tired to function at work, so he switched his jogging to the evenings. His wife complained, not so much because of the one-hour delay in dinner but because John was now tired and grumpy every night, and was a "lost cause" after his six-mile Sunday run. The solution was simple: water. John was just dehydrated. He felt "washed-out" because he was *dried* out. Now he drinks at least sixteen ounces after each run and has plenty of energy and high spirits after jogging each morning.

As John discovered, you cannot rely on your body's automatic fluid regulation system to tell you how much to drink during and after exercise. The fluid shifts that accompany exertion begin very early, and thirst lags quite far behind. And even when you begin to feel thirsty, the other physical and mental sensations of sports competition may well distract you from thirst and cause you to underestimate your fluid needs seriously.

All of this leads up to a simple but very important message: drink early and drink often. Fluid replacement should be part of your game plan before you start competition. You should begin drinking before you even begin exercising. Don't worry about slowing down because of a few ounces of water — scientific studies have shown that even a bellyful of water (one pint or more) just before exercise does not impede performance. Plan to drink during your event as well. The changeovers between games in tennis, time-outs in basketball and soccer, and the breather between shifts in hockey all give you plenty of time to keep up with your fluid needs. Most road races provide water stations so that long-distance runners can keep drinking as they go. It can be hazardous to drink while running, however, so you will have to stop for a few seconds. Don't let the lost time deter you — Bill Rodgers stopped for water six times en route to his 1975 Boston Marathon victory. If you are running or biking on your own without a race, you should plan routes that will allow you to stop for water.

How much should you drink? Obviously this depends on how much water you lose — fluid requirements increase as the intensity and duration of exercise increase, and as the heat and humidity rise. You can quantitate your fluid needs very precisely by checking your weight; since a pint of water weighs about a pound, you need to drink a pint for each pound you lose during exercise. Weigh yourself before and after you exercise, but be sure to strip down both times so that sweat-laden clothing won't give you false readings. You'll be surprised by how much sweat you lose during a workout. You don't have to be a champion athlete to learn from

Alberto Salazar's experience during the 1984 Olympic Marathon. Salazar lost twelve pounds — 8 percent of his body weight — during the race. This amounts to one pint every eleven minutes — no wonder he failed to win a medal. Weighing yourself is not as silly as it sounds: competitors in Hawaii's grueling Iron Man Triathlon (2.4 miles of white-water swimming followed by a 112-mile bike race and a 26.2-mile marathon) are weighed regularly and are forced to drop out for medical reasons if they lose more than 10 percent of their body weight. For most of us, however, weighing in during sports is neither practical nor necessary. Common sense, experience, and thirst will enable you to estimate your needs quite nicely. As a rule of thumb, we suggest drinking six to eight ounces within ten minutes before you start out. During exercise, four to six ounces for each ten to fifteen minutes should keep you in the ball park. You will need much more water in the summer. And it's always a good idea to drink liberally as you cool down after exercising.

Should your fluids be cool? This is largely a matter of personal preference. Since one reason for fluids is to keep your body temperature normal, cool fluids may be helpful. Even ice-cold water will not cause cramps or other problems. But if you are more comfortable with the idea of tepid fluids, go ahead with them — the only critical thing about fluids is that they be wet.

What fluid is best? Here, too, personal preference is an important determinant. Just look at what runners drink during a marathon — the variety is staggering, ranging from cola drinks to orange juice to beer. We too have a preference: plain water. Others advocate various commercially available sugar-electrolyte solutions (ERG, Gatorade, etc.). Our reservations about these beverages are based on several factors. First, sugar is not necessary unless you are exercising for more than three or four hours, and it can delay the absorption of fluids from your stomach. Second, the salt and potassium are not needed during exercise, when the blood concentrations of these electrolytes may actually rise. But although we favor water itself, we are happy to see athletes drinking whatever is their own personal cup of tea.

If the fluid requirements of athletes are usually underestimated, the food requirements are typically overestimated. Your "pre-game" meal should be nothing more than a light snack of low-roughage, low-fat, high-carbohydrate food such as yogurt, toast and jam, or custard. And even this light meal should be eaten at least two hours before you exercise strenuously. Candy bars or other concentrated sweets will *not* provide "extra energy" for sports, and may actually give you less energy by impairing your body's ability to mobilize its own energy reserves. You will not need calories during exercise unless you are participating in extreme endurance events such as ultramarathons or triathlons, in which case calories are crucial to keep you going *beyond* four or five hours of strenuous exercise. All of this may sound a bit spartan — but after you cool down, drink up, and shower, you will be able to indulge your appetite without worrying about your athletic performance. But don't forget tomorrow; if you run five miles but eat for six miles, you will gain weight despite all your exercise.

There you have it. In Part II, we've taken you from your doctor's office, to a balanced "FAS(S)" fitness training program in your home or club, to your pre-game fluids. For fitness, you can simply maintain this program indefinitely. But we hope you'll choose to come with us the rest of the way — to Part III, covering sports for fitness and fun.

III

SPORTS FOR FITNESS AND FUN

A Selection of Activities for Recreation and Health

8

Lifesports I: Walking, Jogging, and Running

Although the terms are often used interchangeably, exercise and sports are not synonymous. You can use the FAS(S) program to get into excellent shape without playing sports at all. On the other hand, you can go bowling three times a week and play golf and softball every weekend without being at all fit. Exercise is necessary for fitness. Sports are an added attraction — a form of recreation and socialization that can bring variety and stimulation to your fitness program. To play well, and to avoid injuries, you should get into shape for sports. And if you choose your sports well, you can use them to stay in shape and to develop new degrees of fitness.

Which sports are best for you? As you look over Figure 8–1, you'll see that many different sports can be used for aerobic training. You will note that some very popular sports, such as doubles tennis, golf, bowling, and softball, are very low on the list. This is because all of these sports include prolonged periods of inactivity. We are not trying to discourage you from playing golf or baseball; if you enjoy them, continue playing for recreation, but add more intense exercise for aerobic conditioning and health. Figure 8–1 also compares the aerobic value of these sports by showing you the maximum oxygen uptake of high-quality competitors in these sports. We are not saying that an elite runner is a better athlete than a champion golfer — but he is in better aerobic shape.

Although aerobic conditioning is the most important health benefit of exercise, total fitness has other dimensions as well. Figure 8–1 compares representative sports in terms of their contributions to strength, flexibility, and coordination.

As an athlete, you can choose whatever sports suit you best. As doctors, we'll try to point out the fitness benefits and also the possible drawbacks in the major sports. Let's start with the sports that can do the most for you, the lifesports.

WHAT ARE LIFESPORTS?

What do walking, running, swimming, rowing, biking, cross-country skiing, skating, and aerobic dance have in common? Although these sports may seem quite different at first glance, the bottom line for each is that they are excellent aerobic conditioning activities. Each of these sports can be good for your health; in trying them for yourself, we hope you'll discover not only the fitness benefits but also the fun and pleasure that you can get from them.

We call these activities lifesports because they are quite literally just that: sports that can be carried out through a long lifetime. In turn, they can help enrich and even prolong life as part of a balanced fitness and health program. From a medical point of view, all of these sports share an important physiological characteristic: they are all endurance or dynamic or aerobic activities. In all of these sports you'll be using large muscle groups in a rhythmic, repetitive fashion for pro-longed periods of time. You can — and should — raise your heart rate to 75 to 85 percent of its maximum; you'll be working hard but not all out, and when you attain fitness, you'll be able to sustain this intensity for thirty minutes or longer. Regular aerobic or endurance training is the best way to get your heart and circulation into shape, and is the best way to attain the metabolic benefits of exercise. And, if you're like the rest of us, you'll feel more energetic, less tense, and a good deal happier about yourself and your life.

We've already explained the fundamental aspects of fitness. Now let's get down to some practical "how to" issues for sports. Each of these lifesports offers the opportunity to train alone or with other people, either in a noncompetitive fashion for fitness and recreation, or at the competitive level. And many of these activities can be extended to extreme levels of endurance, such as marathon running, swimming, biking, or cross-country skiing.

Finally, although these lifesports can be entirely ful-filling and rewarding in their own right, they can also serve as the basis of stamina training for the competitive or team sports we'll discuss in Chapter 10. This is par-ticularly true of running, the common denominator of endurance training for all sports.

All aerobic sports are excellent conditioning activities (see Figure 8–1). They all burn calories very efficiently and can be sustained for prolonged periods of time once you get into shape. These sports differ in terms of the specific muscle groups they utilize and in the strength, flexibility, coordination, and skill that they require. You can choose your sport based on these criteria, but most of us will also be heavily influenced by practical con-siderations such as climate, facilities available, the time required, costs, and so forth. In fact, a mixture of life-sports is probably better than an exclusive diet of any one.

Of all these sports, running is our favorite, but our reasons for stressing it are not parochial: running takes little skill, training, and equipment, is inexpensive, and is very efficient in terms of the exercise value you get for each hour you invest. It can be carried out in vir-tually any climate, and is universally used as a condi-tioning activity for other sports. Let's begin then with a look at walking, jogging, and running for fitness, rec-reation, and competition.

FIGURE 8–1: A COMPARISON OF SELECTED SPORTS: REQUIREMENTS AND BENEFITS

Activity	Requirements for Equipment and Facilities	Skill and Coordination	Flexibility	Aerobic Power (Endurance)	Strength	Fat Loss
Brisk walking	low	low	low	moderate	low	moderate
Jogging	low	low	low	high	low	moderate
Running	low	moderate	low	high	moderate	high
Swimming	high	moderate	high	high	moderate	moderate
Rowing	high	moderate	moderate	high	high	high
Aerobic dance	moderate	moderate	high	high	moderate	high
Biking	moderate	moderate	low	high	moderate	high
Skating	high	moderate	moderate	high	moderate	moderate
Skiing						
Cross-country	moderate	moderate	moderate	high	moderate	high
Downhill	high	high	low	low	moderate	low
Tennis						
Singles	high	high	moderate	moderate	low	moderate
Doubles	high	high	moderate	low	low	low
Basketball	high	high	moderate	high	moderate	moderate
Soccer	high	high	moderate	high	moderate	moderate
Baseball	high	high	low	low	low	low
Golf	high	high	moderate	low	low	low
Bowling	high	moderate	low	low	moderate	low

WALKING

Human beings are the only primates with an upright posture, and there is a lesson in this observation. We are not engineered to lie down, sit down, or even stand around; instead, man is ideally engineered for walking and running. Sadly, industrialized Western society seems to have forgotten this. Walking was once the basis for human transportation, and was an integral part of daily life. Now, walking is what you do to get from your car to an elevator or easy chair. We are surrounded by a bewildering variety of motorized, mechanized, labor-saving conveniences. We save labor all right, but with a price in mental stress and physical sloth. It is no coincidence that modern engineering miracles include cardiac monitors and heart-lung machines for bypass operations. We certainly don't want to denigrate the tremendous importance of these devices, nor do we advocate a return to the nineteenth century. But we do strongly urge adding exercise back to modern living. Walking is a great place to start, if not for transportation, then for health and even sport.

Even the most slothful and inert of us walks. Can this commonplace, humble activity be part of your fitness program? Yes. In some ways walking is an ideal form of exercise. Universally available and convenient, it requires little equipment and costs next to nothing. It does not require specialized techniques, instruction, or skill. Whereas jogging and running share all of these advantages, walking has the additional advantage of being less traumatic, particularly for the legs and back. When you walk, one foot is on the ground at all times, so your weight does not come pounding down. When you jog, both feet are off the ground at the same time — at least briefly. The faster you go, the longer you are airborne; competitive runners may have a "flight time" approaching 45 percent. Runners may pay a price for this speed, grace, and intensity, however, in terms of the shock that must be absorbed each time they come back to earth.

Walking is an ideal form of exercise for many people who are elderly or ailing. Walking is also an excellent starting point for people of any age who are very deconditioned, and can be the basis for a logical progression to jogging, running, and other conditioning activities and sports. A reliable and inexpensive form of transportation, walking is also an excellent recreational activity. You can walk alone for peace and solitude, or with companions for socialization. You can explore new sights, both rural and urban. You can clear your head and get away from it all with a good long walk.

The major drawback to walking is its relative lack of intensity. If you weigh 150 pounds you will consume about 100 calories per mile of walking, jogging, or running. However, if you are strolling at one to two miles per hour, you'll get very little conditioning benefit. If you walk briskly at three and a half to four and a half miles per hour, you can raise your heart rate to its target level, consume 350 to 450 calories per hour, and get yourself into shape. But once you do get into shape, you will need more intense exercise to progress further. Jogging and running are logical ways to do this, as we'll see shortly. Or you may choose to expand your horizons into one of the other lifesports in Chapter 9. But if walking remains your passion, you can learn race walking, which can be an intense competitive sport and is a demanding and excellent conditioning activity.

EQUIPMENT AND CLOTHING

Whether you're walking simply as part of your daily life or for fitness, good shoes should always be a part of your attire. As physicians, we always advocate function over fashion, and this is particularly true when it comes to women's footwear. Walking gear is basically identical to running gear, as detailed on pages 190–192; comfortable, loose-fitting clothing and well-fitted jogging shoes are all you'll need to get started.

SETTING YOUR GOALS AND GETTING STARTED

Even before you establish a formal fitness program, you can and should start walking. Assuming that you are properly shod, try to build as much walking as possible into your daily routine. If you are driving, try to find a parking spot *farther* away from your destination so that you can get in a little walking. On public transportation, get off the bus one stop early and walk. Whenever possible, use the stairs, particularly when going up. Those of you who work on upper floors may groan, and although we walk to the thirteenth floor of the hospital several times daily while making rounds, we can understand your point. But there is nothing to stop you from getting off the elevator at the ninth or tenth floor and walking the rest of the way. Walk every chance you get for recreation, sightseeing, shopping, and transportation. Take a walk during your lunch hour. Even a "mini-walk" during a coffee break can help clear your mind and invigorate your body.

Walking for transportation will help, but if you make walking the foundation of your fitness program you'll have to do more. As with so many things in this life, the first step in your fitness program is likely to be the hardest. Even before you take that first step walking, however, you should formulate a plan of attack. Start by reviewing your self-evaluation tests from Part I and your personal goals and FAS(S) fitness plan from Chapter 7 (Figure 7–4). You should also be sure your fitness log is all set so that you can begin charting your progress from day one. If you are in good shape, you may want to begin at a higher level, either with brisk walking or with jogging. But if you are in average to poor condition, a more modest walking program is an ideal way to work yourself into better shape so you can move up safely and smoothly.

You should give yourself the best possible conditions when you get started. Pick a time of day when you feel alert, unhurried, and relaxed. Try not to eat for two hours preceding your exercise session. Although you can walk in virtually any weather, you'll get off to a better start if the temperature is moderate and the air dry. Similarly, although you can walk over any terrain, you'll be best served by selecting a smooth, flat route at first.

As with any endurance training, the next step is a warm-up. Although slow walking can be used to warm you up for brisk walking, we suggest gentle calisthenics and stretching exercises so that your muscles will be loose and flexible and therefore less prone to injury. A warm-up period will also give your heart and circulation a chance to get into gear gradually. Stretching exercises, particularly those which will loosen up your Achilles, calves, hamstrings, and hips (see pages 104–113), are an ideal routine before walking. These same exercises can and should be used in a cool-down period once you finish your exercise session.

The benefits of exercise depend on three factors: intensity, duration, and frequency. If your goal is to attain true fitness through walking, you'll have to walk long, hard, and often, because even brisk walking is only moderately intense exercise. Initially, you should plan perhaps fifteen minutes a day or twenty minutes every other day. Your pace will depend upon how well you feel. Use either the "talking pace" concept or your target heart rate to judge the intensity of your effort (see pages 114–115). Most people start at a pace of two and a half to three miles per hour. As you improve, try to bring your pace up to three and a half to four miles per hour, assuming that you don't get winded or exceed your target heart rate. Once you can sustain this brisk walking for fifteen minutes daily or twenty minutes every other day, you should increase the duration of each exercise session. But move up gradually, adding perhaps five minutes to each session every week. This may not seem like much, but over a month or two your progress will really add up; you'll find yourself walking three to four miles in forty-five to sixty minutes, and your fitness log will document your progress. You can also get some additional benefit by walking briskly during daily activities, but don't push to your fitness pace if you've just had a big meal, if you are in street shoes, or if you're burdened by heavy clothing or bundles.

If you can continue at this level at least four times per week, you'll do yourself a lot of good. But you will probably find yourself wanting an even harder workout, and we encourage you to move on. One way to do this would be simply to extend the duration of your walk. Another good trick is to add hills, which will get different muscles into shape (such as the quadriceps muscles on the front of your thighs) and also give more of a workout to your heart and circulation. Walking up stairs will have similar benefits; you use three times more energy going up stairs than down, and you build up your quads in the process. You can also increase the training benefit of walking by wearing a backpack. Even a modest load of five to ten pounds will increase the benefits of your walk. We prefer a backpack to hand-held weights because of a better distribution of the load on your body, but some people feel awkward about wearing a pack and prefer to carry the extra weight in their hands. You can do this with specially designed weights such as "Heavy Hands" or weighted gloves or wristbands. If you choose to carry weights in your hands, they should be comfortable, and your right and left hands should be balanced so that your stride remains smooth.

The English romantic poet Shelley tells us "if winter comes, can spring be far behind?" Even in the idyllic world of fitness, however, spring and summer will be inevitably succeeded by fall and then winter. How can you continue walking during the inclement weather? Except in deep snow or on icy surfaces, you can keep walking even in very cold weather (see pages 196–197 on winter jogging). And you can always take your walking program indoors. Shopping malls are ideal for this, as are treadmills, either at a health club or at home. Whatever tactic you choose, keep walking year round, so you can keep fit year round.

Walking is a basic activity of all humanity. Put walking back into your life. Walk for fitness, walk for transportation, walk for recreation. With each step, you'll be taking a stride toward fitness, health, and fun.

TECHNIQUE

Because walking is so universal, you may not give style and technique any thought. Indeed, walking is so natural that formal coaching and training are not necessary except for competitive walkers. But a few tips may help. Try to keep your posture upright and erect. Hold your head high with your gaze fixed on the road ahead instead of on the pavement at your feet. It's very helpful to let your upper body do some of the work. Hold your hands at your sides, with your fingers in a relaxed position, and swing your arms rhythmically front and back. Bring your right arm forward at the same time that you swing your left leg forward; obviously, your left arm will swing forward with your right leg on the next stride. I think you'll be surprised at how much power and speed you can get from swinging your arms, particularly when you pick up speed. It may actually be easier for you to concentrate on your arm motions and let them establish your pace, but pay at least a little attention to your feet and legs. You should land on your heels and roll forward onto your toes so that you can push off from behind your body.

Perhaps the most important thing is to establish a comfortable rhythm. The training benefits of your walking depend principally on your velocity, or speed. Velocity in turn will be determined by the length and frequency of your strides. For most people, stride length adjusts itself quite automatically, so you can concentrate on the frequency of your strides to establish your pace. Try to build up a good cadence or rhythm. You may even want to count strides per minute to be sure you are on target, or you may choose to purchase a jogger's watch, which can beep out a predetermined cadence to pace you the way a metronome guides a musician.

The final element in technique is your breathing. Again, the goal is to establish a rhythmic, smooth breathing pattern; when you build up to a brisk pace, you will probably find yourself breathing mostly through your mouth.

All this may sound like a lot to remember, but a little thought about technique can be helpful. You may even want to ask a friend to have a look at your stride with these guidelines in mind to make some suggestions. But for most of us, walking really does come very naturally and the odds are good that you'll find yourself moving right along with no more thought than a "heel-toe and away we go."

SAFETY TIPS AND PRECAUTIONS TO AVOID INJURY

One of the things you'll appreciate most about walking is its freedom from injuries. As you begin to extend your range and advance your speed, you may be subject to some of the foot and leg problems experienced more often by runners (see pages 197–199 and Part IV). And like runners, you'll have to learn to deal with dogs, cars, and environmental extremes (see pages 196–197). Finally, if you take your walking on the trails to do some serious hiking, you should give some thought to the effects of high altitude on your heart and lungs (see Chapter 7).

ADVANCED WALKING FOR COMPETITION

Most of us think of walking as transportation, recreation, or fitness training, but walking can also be an excellent competitive sport. In fact, race walking was one of the most popular competitive sports in the eighteenth and nineteenth centuries. Race walking was accepted into modern international competition in the 1908 Olympics, and was quite the rage in America in the twenties. Although the popularity of race walking declined subsequently, it is now on the rise again, sometimes under the synonyms power walking, aerobic walking, or even health walking.

Race walkers are those funny-looking men and women striding along, looking like penguins with their tails on fire. The stride may look funny but is actually very effective. The only rules of competitive race walking are that one foot must be on the ground at all times, and that the knee be extended so that the leg is straight when the foot is striking the ground. The rest of the gait can vary, but in order to be competitive, race walkers adopt a relatively stereotyped stride. This involves a great deal of swiveling at the hip and also a great deal of arm pumping and swinging to gain power and speed. This stride helps develop the upper extremities a lot more than even jogging does; all the upper-body motion also means that you can burn more calories (110) walking a mile in twelve minutes than you can jogging a twelve-minute mile (96 calories).

Because one foot is always in contact with the ground, race walking is less traumatic to the feet and legs than is jogging. Good race-walking technique involves an erect posture, rhythmic coordination of arms, legs, and breathing, and an efficient stride that includes a firm heel stride, balanced forward roll, and strong push-off. A good walking technique can even make you a more efficient runner.

The race-walking technique, however, does require training, and is in fact harder to learn than jogging and running techniques. If you are interested, you should begin by seeking out a race and watching the competitors. Then contact a race-walking club in your area. Most race-walking groups are very interested in recruiting new members, and offer clinics and instructional sessions to that purpose. There are also national race-walk organizations and publications that can be helpful (see the Appendix).

Are race walkers "real athletes"? Yes, indeed. Ray Sharpe set a new world's record for the mile walk at the 1983 Melrose games. His time was a blistering (no pun intended) 5 minutes 46.21 seconds, so that Ray was walking faster than most of us can run. And the longest Olympic event is not the marathon (42 kilometers) but the 50-kilometer race walk, won in 1984 by Mexico's Raul Gonzalez (3 hours, 47 minutes, 26 seconds).

Not surprisingly, race walkers are among the most fit athletes. In one study, race walkers had a maximum oxygen uptake of 63 ml/kg/min (see page 12 for an explanation of this test). Race walkers are right up there with the best athletes, achieving oxygen-uptake levels that are exceeded only by elite long-distance runners, cyclists, swimmers, cross-country skiers, national-class racquetball players, and rowers. This means that top-flight race walkers are as a group more fit than tennis and soccer players, football players, basketball stars, and bodybuilders. Clearly, we should all have renewed respect for walkers.

HIKING AND ORIENTEERING

One nice feature about walking is that you can take it off the road and into the countryside. Hiking and backpacking are excellent ways to maintain your fitness while enjoying the beauties of nature. You'll want to leave your jogging shoes behind and get good hiking boots as well as appropriate clothing and, if your hike is a long one, appropriate food and beverages to bring with you. Obviously you'll need to find a good trail, and in most cases you'll probably want to hike with one or more companions. You'll do best if you get yourself into shape before you begin serious hiking; backpacking and hiking can then be used as excellent ways to stay in shape. You can get information about hiking from organizations listed in the Appendix.

If you are really serious about nature and fitness, you may want to look into orienteering. Orienteering began as a Scandinavian sport in 1898 but was not taken seriously in this country until the early 1950s. Even today orienteering is still a relatively unknown sport. Perhaps that's because it's so demanding, requiring not only physical fitness but a lot of mental agility. Orienteers call their sport "cunning running."

The strategy of orienteering is to follow a map to get from point A to point B as quickly as possible. That may sound easy — until you realize that points A and B are not separated by a smooth track or a well-traveled path, but by woods, hills, and streams. All you have to aid you is a map, a compass, and your wits. You'll have to be able to move rapidly on the flat parts of the course and to climb and scamper over rocks and hills. Orienteers are tough and they must dress tough. They wear special shoes, which are rigid with very little padding because of the soft ground in the woods. Shin guards are usually used to protect the legs and are worn over knickers; long-sleeved shirts are important to protect the arms from branches, and goggles should be worn to protect the eyes.

Championship orienteers are among the most fit of endurance athletes. U.S. champion Eric Weyman, for example, does not consider himself a competitive runner, but he has turned in a 2:38 marathon. But the sport also has room for beginners. Orienteering meets generally offer a variety of courses, ranging from relatively easy one-and-a-half-mile routes for beginners, to demanding five- to eight-mile courses for advanced competitors.

Clearly, orienteering isn't for everybody. But if it appeals to you, you can get more information from sources listed in the Appendix.

Walking for fitness has many virtues. It does not take special skills or athletic abilities, it requires only inexpensive equipment, and it is completely convenient. Walking has great versatility, being well suited for someone just getting into fitness, while also retaining its place as a competitive sport for world-class athletes. Walking is as enjoyable for people who prefer solitude as it is for people who want companionship on the road to fitness. And walking is nearly injury-free.

Walking's major drawback is the time it requires. After you've walked your way to fitness by building up from fifteen minutes a day, you'll need at least forty-five minutes four times a week or one hour three times a week to maintain high-level fitness with walking alone. You can maintain fitness by running for half that time. But if you enjoy walking, it's well worth the investment of time. And walking is also an excellent complement to swimming or rowing, which develops the upper body, as part of a total fitness program.

JOGGING AND RUNNING

If walking is such a good fitness activity, you may ask, why run? Indeed, many people can attain and maintain fitness through walking alone, but jogging and running give you the additional intensity factor. For example, suppose you are capable of walking a mile in sixteen minutes or jogging a mile in eight minutes. In either case, you've consumed about 100 calories in traveling that mile, but the jogger has another eight minutes left over, and if he is able to extend his jogging for another mile he will have achieved more than twice the benefit as the walker in exactly the same amount of time.

But this increased intensity of effort carries with it an increased risk of injury. Jogging and running can place a lot of strain on your hips, legs, and feet, but with appropriate equipment, stretching, warm-ups, and proper technique, you should be able to avoid serious problems. Once you are able to do this, you'll have all the benefits of walking (convenience, low expense, adaptability to all seasons, etc.) with the additional benefits of the intensity factor. As with walking, you can choose to jog or run alone, but if you prefer competition, running will give you many more opportunities for such group activities than will walking.

We've been using the terms jogging and running interchangeably, yet there are differences. The differences, however, are ones of degree. Jogging differs from walking in that the jogger will have both feet off the ground at some point during his stride. Running differs from jogging only in that it is faster, so that the runner is airborne for more time than is the jogger. Because of this, there is no formal definition separating jogging from running. Some may adopt the egoistic definition that they run, but anybody who is slower jogs; most people going at a pace of nine or ten minutes per mile or faster consider themselves runners, whereas people in the ten-plus-minutes-per-mile range generally think of themselves as joggers.

Does speed make any difference in terms of the benefits? Not much. If you weigh 150 pounds and cover one mile in eight minutes you'll consume approximately 98 calories. If you quicken your pace to a rather snappy six-minute mile, you'll add no more than 4 calories per mile; similarly if you cut back to a comfortable ten-minute-per-mile pace you will not lose more than 4 calories. All in all, the distance you cover and the regularity of your running are more important than speed alone in determining the benefits you can derive from jogging. In terms of caloric consumption, body weight is a much more important variable than is speed: the heavier you are, the more calories it will take to move you one mile (see Figure 8–2).

FIGURE 8–2: CALORIES USED PER MILE OF RUNNING

Weight	Pace per Mile		
(lbs.)	6 min.	8 min.	10 min.
120	83	79	76
130	89	85	82
140	95	92	88
150	102	98	94
160	109	104	100
170	115	111	106
180	121	117	112
190	128	123	118
200	135	129	124
210	141	136	130
220	148	142	136

EQUIPMENT AND CLOTHING

Although running is an inexpensive sport that requires relatively little equipment, some attention to your gear can make a big difference is terms of enjoyment, safety, and injuries.

The only really crucial piece of equipment will be your running shoes. As a result of the running boom in America, running shoes have become a multimillion-dollar industry. This means that you'll have many excellent shoes from which to choose. It also means that you'll be subjected to a tremendous barrage of conflicting claims and slogans. Don't be confused by all this hype. Remember that flashy colors and stripes won't help you at all when you move from the showroom to the roads. Nor will endorsements by Rodgers, Benoit, Salazar, or even Simon and Levisohn help you out; after all, *you* are the one who will be wearing the shoes — so take your time and pick a pair that will give you comfort, support, and durability at a price you can afford. Prices vary tremendously, ranging from under forty to over one hundred dollars for a pair of good running shoes. In general, you can expect to spend fifty to seventy dollars. Don't be dismayed by this outlay: good shoes should last you for 750 miles or more, and they do represent the single greatest expense you'll face. Although many different makes and models are suitable, we'd suggest that you stick with a "name" brand with good quality control rather than trying to save a few dollars by picking an off brand.

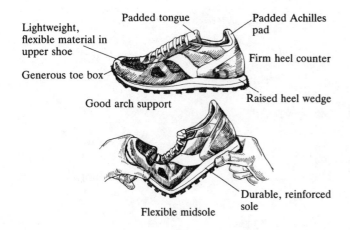

Lightweight, flexible material in upper shoe

Padded tongue

Padded Achilles pad

Firm heel counter

Generous toe box

Good arch support

Raised heel wedge

Flexible midsole

Durable, reinforced sole

FIGURE 8–3: *What to Look for in a Running Shoe*

Running shoes come is two varieties: training shoes and racing flats. First you'll need training shoes (see Figure 8–3). Find a shoe that is comfortable for you. It should feel supportive without being snug or constricting. Both the tongue and the Achilles pad should be well padded to prevent irritation and tendinitis. The "uppers" should be light and flexible; most manufacturers have abandoned leather in favor of nylon mesh, polyester, or other synthetics. Suede is often used for reinforcement and strength. The shoe lining should be comfortable and moisture-absorbent. Most insoles are made of a firm foam rubber. Some insoles provide built-in arch supports, which can be helpful but are not truly necessary for runners. (In fact, if you have structural or biomechanical abnormalities of your foot, you should consider a specially molded-to-measure insole called an orthotic to provide support and gait correction.) The heel counter should be firm, to provide hind foot stability. The heel itself should be raised on a heel wedge so that the height of the sole and wedge in the back of the shoe is two to three times greater than the sole beneath the ball of the foot. Since you'll be landing on your heel, this will give you greater shock absorption and will also take pressure off your Achilles tendon.

The midsole of the shoe should be flexible, and the toe box should be rounded and at least one and a half inches high. Flexibility is important so that you can push off properly, and a large toe box is important to avoid injuring your toes and nails by excessive pressure during push-off. Many sole materials and designs are available. Try to find one that is rated high for durability. Look for reinforcement in the heel, particularly along the outer side. This is where most runners strike first, and hence is the area that will wear down first. A studded sole is particularly useful for running on slippery or wet surfaces.

Despite all these factors, shoe selection is really pretty easy. We suggest that you shop at a store that specializes in running gear so that you'll have a wide selection and also a salesperson who knows about both running and shoes. Be sure to wear your athletic socks so that you can get a realistic fit. Take your time: try on several brands, and always lace up both the right and the left shoes, since your feet are bound to be at least a little different. Jog around in the store to see if the shoe is really comfortable. And when you've found the right shoes, inspect them carefully for manufacturing defects.

Runners often spend hours selecting shoes only to destroy them through neglect. Shoe maintenance hardly requires an engineering degree. Untie your shoes *before* you take them off so that you don't stretch out the uppers. When your shoes are wet, allow them to dry out slowly at room temperature; even the heat of a radiator can cause buckling, because the soles and uppers dry at different rates. Above all, inspect your shoes for signs of wear. Abnormal wear patterns may be the first clue to a problem in your stride that might lead to injury. Even normal wear can lead to injuries if your shoes lose their bounce and cushioning. You can make minor repairs yourself with "Shoe-Goo" or you can have your shoes resoled at low cost. But if you've run enough to wear down a pair of shoes, we'd suggest that you splurge and reward yourself with a new pair. In fact, most serious runners have several pairs in use, so that they can be broken in gradually and allowed to dry out between runs in wet conditions.

One of the nice things about jogging is that except for good running shoes, you can decide on the rest of your clothing and equipment needs as you go along, based strictly on your own comfort. Running togs have also become a big industry, and you can spend many hundreds of dollars to outfit yourself. In fact, some of the new synthetic fabrics can be comfortable and advantageous — but if your idea of style and comfort includes a pair of old gym shorts or a much-used sweatsuit, these will serve your purposes fine.

A few guidelines about clothing may be helpful. In warm weather your running outfit should be as brief as possible. A pair of shorts and a singlet will generally do the trick; men may even choose to run shirtless. Your clothing should fit you loosely and should be porous or absorbent. Cottons are fine, but the newer nylon synthetics have gained favor with most serious runners. Light colors will help reflect sun and heat away from you, which is very important in the summer; bright colors are also a safety feature. A sweatband can help absorb perspiration and prevent it from dripping down into your eyes, and wristbands can be useful to keep your hands dry and also to dry off your face as you run along. Many women find a firm, supportive bra to be desirable, but underwear selection for men and women is strictly a question of comfort; an extra pair of shorts can help protect men in very cold weather.

Cooler fall and spring weather is ideal for running. Temperatures above 75 degrees can be hazardous for intense exercise, but your shorts and singlet should keep you fairly comfortable when it's between 60 and 70 degrees. Temperatures in the 50s generally call for a T-shirt and shorts, which is why so many runners like to collect T-shirts from races and fun runs. When it cools

off to the upper 40s, you can respond by switching to a long-sleeve T-shirt or a three-quarter-sleeve baseball shirt. High-topped socks may add to your comfort in the mid-40s. Because a lot of your body heat is lost through your head and hands, you will probably want to add a pair of cotton gardening gloves and a hat or earband when it's about 45 degrees.

Temperatures in the low 40s generally bring out the sweatsuits. As we said earlier, any comfortable pair of sweats will do the trick. A sweatshirt that zippers up the front is useful, because you may find yourself getting quite warm when you run, especially when the sun is out or the wind is at your back. When this occurs, you can roll up your sleeves and unzip without having to stop and undress. Similarly, a hood will give you additional flexibility, because it will enable you to stay warm if you turn into the wind or if your pace slows so that you cool off.

Temperatures below the freezing point generally call for even warmer clothing. A woolen or acrylic ski cap will keep your head and even your body much warmer than will the baseball or biking caps that many of us wear in warmer temperatures. Similarly, you should switch from light cotton gloves to warmer fabrics such as woolens. In fact, mittens are much better in cold weather because they retain heat better. Multiple layers of light, flexible clothing are also the best way to keep your body warm at lower temperatures. The cheapest way to achieve this is simply to throw on a pair of cotton long johns under your sweatsuit. As the temperature declines to the 20s or teens, you can add additional layers in the form of a jersey or turtleneck, extra shorts, extra socks, and extra gloves. It's quite amazing how warm you can stay with multiple layers of light clothing. Layers will enable your body to retain a tremendous amount of the heat that is generated when you run, and will also allow you to unzip and cool off if you start to overheat during exercise.

Although these inexpensive, traditional athletic outfits of long johns, shirts, and sweatsuits will do the trick, we should point out that many runners find the newer synthetics to be very advantageous, in comfort if not in price. Long underwear or turtlenecks made of polypropylene are much better than old-fashioned cotton long johns. These fabrics are very lightweight and flexible; they fit much like a dancer's leotard, allowing you maximum flexibility and comfort. They are also very warm, but most importantly, they have an amazing ability to wick perspiration away from your body. Because your skin and the polypropylene layer next to it stay dry, they will also tend to stay much warmer. You'll have less chafing and skin irritation, and you won't be weighed down by heavy, water-saturated clothing. Polypropylene is more expensive than cotton long johns, usually costing thirty to forty dollars for a set. But if you do a fair amount of winter running, it's well worth the investment.

Many runners favor nylon or polyester synthetic running suits over traditional cotton sweats. Again, cost is a major disadvantage, since these synthetic running suits may cost from fifty to one hundred dollars, but they are lightweight, flexible, and comfortable. They also help break the wind, which is a big plus for winter running. Their bright colors are a nice safety feature, and some even have reflectorized strips, which are mandatory for safety after dark. For an even more streamlined look, consider running in Lycra tights, which will cling to your legs without constricting your stride.

Perhaps the most remarkable synthetic available to runners is Gore-tex. Gore-tex was originally developed for medical use; in fact, it's the standard fabric for arterial grafts that are surgically implanted to repair or replace damaged blood vessels. We are not encouraging you to wear your aorta on your sleeve, but Gore-tex turns out to be an ideal fabric for running suits. It is light, warm, and wind resistant. Most importantly, it is waterproof, but has one-way pores so that it breathes well and perspiration can leave the body. Gore-tex is also washable and very durable. It sounds too good to be true, but like all good things there is a price associated with it. You can expect to pay $125 to $225 for a good Gore-tex running suit. Clearly, it's not an appropriate investment for beginners, but the hard-core runner who expects to run right through the winter will find Gore-tex extremely helpful in severe cold, and especially in cold rain. Gore-tex is now available in running suits, hats, mittens, and even shoes.

There are very few other things you'll need for running. If you plan to walk or run at night you should wear a reflectorized vest at all times. If you find jogging by yourself boring, a headset-type radio or tape player can provide great companionship. Remember, however, to keep the volume low enough so you can hear traffic noises, and don't let the music distract you from listening to messages of discomfort or warning from your body. Another equally optional item that you may find useful is a moisture-resistant watch. Unless you are training seriously, you don't really need the precision of a digital stopwatch, but even beginners will find them

helpful to keep track of how long they spend jogging and walking.

All of this gear can fill a closet and empty a wallet. Still, running is simple and inexpensive when compared to most other sports. But with the exception of a good pair of shoes, we'd suggest that you start out with a minimal investment in clothing, using any old pair of shorts and sweats that you have on hand at first. As you get fit, you can reward yourself with new items of clothing. Let your own experience and taste be your guide; quite literally, you can suit yourself.

SETTING YOUR GOALS AND GETTING STARTED

The first steps you should take as a jogger should not involve your feet, but your mind. Plan ahead. First review your fitness self-assessment profiles (Part I) and set up your exercise log (see Chapter 7). In planning your first month's schedule, decide if jogging will be your major fitness activity. If you want a mix of activities, biking is an excellent supplement to running for building leg strength, whereas swimming, rowing, and weight training are excellent complementary activities, because they build up your upper body, which is not likely to benefit from running alone.

Your actual starting schedule will depend on just how fit you are. If you are out of shape, if you are in the older age groups, or if you have medical problems, you should start by walking. And no matter what shape you are in, you should review Chapters 1 and 6 to understand the principles of aerobics, your target heart rate, and especially medical screening tests, precautions, and warning signals. For the time being, let's assume that you have gotten yourself into good shape with a progressive walking program, so that you can comfortably walk one mile in fifteen minutes or two miles in thirty to thirty-five minutes. Now let's get you started jogging.

Even if you are in good shape as a walker, you should plan to make the transition to jogging a gradual one. Although brisk walking for prolonged periods is good conditioning for your heart and circulation, you'll be using different muscles when you jog. You'll have to give these new muscle groups a chance to get into shape gradually.

You will find it easiest to get started in spring or fall, but if the spirit moves you in less hospitable seasons, you should get going then and there. If you dress appropriately, you can jog at any time of the year. Try to find a level route so that you don't face the extra challenge of hills at first. As with any form of exercise, you should plan to jog on an empty stomach at a time of day when you are alert, relaxed, and unhurried. As with any exercise program, it's very important to begin with a warm-up and conclude with a cool-down period. Stretching exercise and gentle calisthentics are ideal for this purpose. We'd suggest a ten- to fifteen-minute routine encompassing Figures 6–1 through 6–11 (pages 104–107).

Now let's finally get out on the road.

Beginners just getting into shape for jogging can plan to exercise aerobically for about fifteen minutes every other day, plus five to ten minutes each for warm-up and cool-down. You'll be using your target heart rate or the "talking pace" to guide the intensity of your exercise (see pages 114–115). But for most of us it would be difficult to jog for a full fifteen minutes at this pace when first getting started. Instead, you should plan to alternate walking and jogging. If you are on a track or can measure distances fairly accurately, you can start with 100 yards of brisk walking followed by 100 yards of jogging, continuing these cycles in an alternate fashion. You can then gradually increase the distances you jog to 200 and then 400 yards, which is about a quarter of a mile. Over a period of a few weeks, you can decrease the amount of walking and increase the amount of jogging. Hopefully, by the end of a month or so, you'll be able to jog continuously for ten to twelve minutes and cover a mile or more in this period of time.

You can be justifiably proud of yourself when you are able to jog a mile, but you should not rest on your laurels. Instead, we'd suggest that you continue this slow, steady progression until you are able to jog for three to four miles. It may take you three months to get there, but at this point you will have attained good levels of cardiopulmonary fitness. If health is the principle goal of your exercise program, you can simply maintain this level of three to five miles of jogging per day, three to five times per week. Not only is this optimal for health, but it will be an excellent conditioning program for your legs that will help you in many other sports, ranging from tennis to basketball. But many joggers will have gotten the bug by then, and will want to move on to more serious long-distance running and even road racing. We'll discuss advanced training techniques for the enthusiast in just a moment.

First, let's go back briefly to the starting line. We talked about using distance as a guide for your train-ing, but if you don't have accurate yard and mile markers you can do the very same thing by looking at your watch and using time to guide you. Start out by walking briskly for a minute, then jog for a minute; alternate these cycles for your fifteen-minute exercise period. Gradually increase the amount of time you jog while keeping your one minute of walking constant. When you can jog comfortably for five minutes, cut down on the periods of walking, so that over a period of four to five weeks you can jog continuously for ten to fifteen minutes, covering perhaps one to one and a half miles without stopping. Then gradually increase your distance as discussed earlier.

This alternate walking/jogging scheme may seem a bit tame, particularly when you look at all the fit people running by. But remember they all started at the beginning just like you. Moreover, your training schedule utilizes the exact same principles that guide the veteran racer. You, too, are doing interval training. In the case of the racer, his intervals are sprinting and his recovery periods are jogging. In the case of the beginner, of course, the intervals are jogging and the recovery periods are walking, but the underlying theory is the same, and the practice will enable you to improve and progress at a gradual, measured pace. It may seem slow and even boring at first, but give it three months before you quit. Aerobic exercise is hard work initially, but when you get to the stage where you can exercise comfortably at high intensity for twenty to thirty minutes, you'll probably find it quite rewarding and enjoyable in its own right. You'll also see and feel the health benefits of endurance training. You'll be healthier, and you will have established an excellent base for many other athletic activities, if sports are your goal.

Perhaps the most important advice we can give you is to be patient and persistent without being rigid or fanatical. Balance enthusiasm with restraint and excitement with common sense. We want you to make progress at a steady pace, but don't succumb to the temptation to overdo it. You should alternate hard exercise days with easier days, particularly at first. You may even want to work out every other day so that your muscles will have plenty of time to recover. But if you choose to exercise daily, try to cut back on your pace or distance on alternate days until you get into shape. Listen to your body. If you are injured or ill, take some time off until you recover. You can use these days off to do extra strength or flexibility exercises, which will serve you well. If you have aches, pains, or other discomforts while you are jogging, remember that it's okay to stop and walk or stretch until you fell better. It's important to have an overall fitness plan, but you should reevaluate that plan depending upon your progress and the way you feel. If you are doing well, it's fine to move up more quickly — but don't take shortcuts such as cutting down on your warm-ups and stretching. If, on the other hand, your progress is a bit slower, don't give up. All of us can get into shape with enough time and patience.

For many emerging athletes, getting started is the hardest thing of all. Shyness or self-consciousness can be the first barrier. A well-known running authority, Hal Higdon, suggests that you can overcome this by starting out as a "closet jogger," by which he means jogging in place at home until you feel more confident. While this can help some people, we'd generally recommend an outdoor walking program to get you started. Mental confidence can also be built up by thinking about all the successful runners who started out in worse shape than you are in, and who built up slowly but steadily to very good levels. If you don't know anyone personally who did so, just watch the back of the pack at a local road race. You'll see people of both sexes in all sizes, shapes, and ages who can and do enjoy jogging.

If you don't know anyone who has made the transition from sloth and obesity to running and fitness, feel free to think of me (HBS). In Chapter 1, I told you how I went from a 200-pounder who couldn't jog a half-mile to a 160-pounder who actually enjoys running fifty miles. The moral is simple: if I can do it, so can you. Or think of Patti Catalano. Patti was a 148-pound smoker who began to jog to lose weight. And lose she did: at her racing best, Patti weighed in at a sleek 104 — a staggering reduction of almost a third of her body weight. This didn't come easily — Patti built up to 120 miles per week plus calisthenics, Nautilus, and stretching. She also became a world-class runner who has set many records; her 2:29:34 in the 1980 New York City Marathon was a new record for American women. Obviously it's rare to achieve these heights, but the same message applies: you'll never know if a top athlete is lurking within you unless you try.

A few other tips may help motivate you. Try to make exercise part of your daily routine. While some people enjoy the solitude of running alone, many are greatly helped by finding friends to share their daily runs. Try to find a partner of similar abilities so that you can progress together. Health clubs and running clubs are ready sources of companionship, and when you get into

shape, fun runs or races can be enjoyable. Races will also help build variety into your schedule, and can go a long way to relieve monotony and provide motivation. If you feel good on a particular day, let yourself go and run a little farther or faster. Vary your routes. Perhaps the greatest help of all can come from other people who have made the transition from sedentary living to jogging to running. Many beginning joggers find a guru to provide encouragement and advice. Experience is a great teacher, and fellow runners can give you many little tips that we have not included here.

A final bit of advice: use your exercise log. Record your daily activity, your resting and exercise heart rate, your weight, and also the way you feel before and after each run. If you find yourself a little discouraged after a month or so, just look through your diary. Your progress may be difficult to appreciate on a daily basis, but when you look back over the weeks you'll be amazed at how far you've come. But don't let filling in the diary become an end in itself. It's okay to skip days, and it's especially important to back off if you are ill or injured. If you have to take some time off, don't try to make it up by starting back at even higher levels. Instead, you should put yourself back a few notches and ease yourself into shape.

What should be your ultimate goals as a runner? This is a highly individual question and the answer depends on how you are using running. If you are jogging for health, every little bit helps. Dr. Peter Wood and his co-workers at the Stanford Heart Disease Prevention Program found that as little as 8.6 miles per week produced measurable health benefits in terms of improved blood fat profiles, body fat measurements, and exercise capacity. Dr. Ralph Paffenbarger's study of seventeen thousand Harvard graduates showed that the equivalent in about twenty miles per week provided optimal protection from heart disease, so we'd suggest this as an excellent goal for the average person who is jogging for health.

This general range is also ideal for those of you who want to use running as conditioning for other sports. Running is the best way to build "legs" or endurance for a whole variety of athletic pursuits. Many professional athletes have discovered this; one example is Baltimore Oriole pitching great Jim Palmer, who ran five miles every day in the off-season, and found that his endurance on the mound remained remarkably good over the years.

All in all, fifteen to twenty-five miles per week seems a good target range if you are running for health, for the physiological benefits of the training effect, or for endurance training for other sports. But if you are like so many of us, once you get to this level you'll find that running has become enjoyable and challenging in and of itself. You might be a candidate for long-distance running.

TECHNIQUE

Jogging and running, like walking, are very natural activities and should not require special coaching or instruction. Whereas elite runners do have a characteristic grace and smoothness, there is really no right way to run. All of us have had the humbling experience of being left in the dust by someone with an awkward gait or clumsy stride.

Your goal should be to run in a relaxed, rhythmic fashion. Don't worry about speed; instead, concentrate on consistency and smoothness. At first, resist the temptation to time yourself and don't try to alter your stride for speed. Use total distance or total time as your goals and concentrate on smoothness, comfort, and rhythm.

In general, an upright posture is best, with your back straight and your gaze fixed on the road ahead instead of at your feet (Figure 8–4). Carry your arms at about waist level, with your elbows at close to 90 degrees, so that your forearms are parallel to the ground. Your

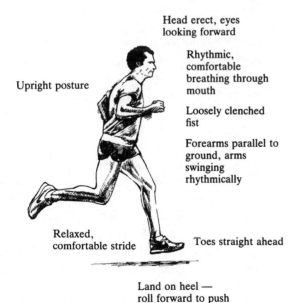

Head erect, eyes
looking forward

Rhythmic,
comfortable
breathing through
mouth

Upright posture

Loosely clenched
fist

Forearms parallel to
ground, arms
swinging
rhythmically

Relaxed,
comfortable stride

Toes straight ahead

Land on heel —
roll forward to push
off onto toes

FIGURE 8–4: *Good Running Form*

fingers should be curled loosely instead of clenched into a tight fist, which tenses up all of your muscles. Swing your arms rhythmically backward and forward, so that your left arm is moving forward at the same time as your right leg advances, and conversely. Once you have mastered this rhythm, you can actually use your arms to adjust the stride of your legs. When you pump your arms more, you will get extra power for hills or for speed. Similarly, when you start to tire, you'll find yourself slouching forward and shuffling your legs. Concentrating on a smooth, rhythmic arm thrust can often help correct these problems. Your breathing should also be rhythmic and comfortable; most runners find that they automatically breathe through the mouth.

Leg motion varies greatly among runners. In general, elite runners have a fairly high knee lift and long stride, but many very good runners find that they can save energy with lower knee lifts and somewhat shorter strides. There really is no fundamental distinction between runners who lope along with a high kick and those who tend to shuffle with less knee lift. In fact, some wonderful long-distance runners, such as Rod Dixon, tend to run with something of a "shuffle."

Footwork is important. You should concentrate on landing on your heel and then rolling forward to push off with the ball of your foot and great toe. Sprinters tend to land on their toes, but joggers and distance runners should land on their heels, roll forward, and push off all in one flowing, rhythmic motion. Your toes should be straight ahead. If you find that you roll your foot outward or toe-in excessively, you may tend to develop injuries. A friend may be able to spot this in your stride, or you may be able to diagnose it yourself by noting an abnormal wear pattern on the soles of your shoes. If you are pain-free, efficient, and comfortable, it's not important to make major corrections, but if you start getting aches and pains, you should consider asking a coach to evaluate your stride. In some cases, a visit to a sports podiatrist may be needed so that you can be fitted for special shoe inserts, or orthotics.

SAFETY TIPS AND PRECAUTIONS TO AVOID INJURY

Safety is of utmost importance. Try to find a golf course, park, or path where you can run; a soft surface will help cut down on injuries caused by pounding the pavement, and you won't have to worry about traffic. If you are lucky enough to get off the pavement, be sure that the surface is smooth and regular so that you don't turn an ankle or trip and fall. Many high schools and colleges have outdoor tracks with a forgiving cinder surface, which can be ideal both for beginning joggers and for serious runners who want speed training. Unfortunately for many of us, these idyllic conditions are hard to come by. If you have to share the roads with vehicular traffic, try to minimize problems by running when traffic flow is light. Always use the sidewalk when it's available, and try to avoid heavily traveled streets and roads. You should always run facing the flow of cars, and you should be particularly careful at intersections. Above all, run defensively. You cannot count on drivers to be careful and considerate; instead, make it your business to get out of their way. Light-colored clothing can be helpful, and reflectorized vests are a must after dark.

While four-wheeled vehicles are your greatest worry, four-legged animals can also cause concern. Dogs are best avoided by means of an impromptu detour, but if necessary, they can generally be controlled by a firm command of "go home." When confronted with dogs, some runners reach for a nearby stick or stone, while others may actually carry aerosol sprays, squirt guns filled with dilute ammonia, or horns. In general, however, we have found it best to respect the canine territorial instinct by simply turning tail and avoiding encounters altogether.

For women joggers, two-legged animals can also cause concern. Considering the number of women runners, assaults are really quite uncommon, but they are by no means rare. These problems can generally be avoided with a little advance planning. Your best protection is to run with a companion. Avoid isolated areas, and try not to run after dark. Be aware of conditions in your neighborhood and do a little asking around before you plan a new route, either at home or when you are traveling to new cities.

Many of the other safety precautions for runners are no different from the safety tips for other athletes (see Chapter 7). Runners should be particularly careful about the following:

- Avoid rush-hour traffic and cut down on mileage during smoggy summer days to minimize your exposure to air pollutants.
- Don't eat for two hours before your run; make your last meal a light snack featuring food high in complex carbohydrates and low in fat and roughage.
- Protect your skin. Heavy sweating can produce skin chafing and blisters during running. A thin layer of Vaseline applied to the groin or under arms can help prevent these problems. Men who wear shirts or braless women joggers can experience painful irritation of the nipples. "Jogger's nipples" can be prevented by applying Vaseline or circular plastic Band-Aids before you run.
- Drink plenty of water before, during, and after your run, especially in warm or humid weather. You may want to carry a plastic squeeze bottle with you to provide some of this water. You should also plan your routes so that you can stop and drink at fountains. Firehouses and police stations generally have bubblers and are usually accommodating to thirsty runners; gas stations and luncheonettes also have water, but tend to be less hospitable.
- Avoid extreme heat. Even in moderately warm weather, cut down your mileage, run at dawn or dusk, dress lightly, and drink, drink, drink. The 1976 Boston Marathon was run in record 95-degree heat. Salvation that day took the shape of a garden hose. Surburban runners can also run for the hoses during the summer by running through lawn sprinklers whenever possible; in addition, you can douse yourself at drinking fountains. And remember that a cool shower is the fastest way to cool off at home.

Not even world-class athletes are immune to heat problems. One example was the collapse of Alberto Salazar following his strong finish at the Falmouth Road Race in August 1978. Salazar's temperature was nearly 106 degrees, and he required emergency medical aid to avoid life-threatening illness. During the summer it would be best for you to run with a partner, or at least to stay near populated areas where you can get help. Above all, listen to your body. Warning signs include weakness, lightheadedness, nausea, and confusion. If these occur, you must cease running. Rest in the coolest place you can find, and drink cool fluids. Emersion in cool water is extremely effective. If confusion or collapse occurs, heat stroke is a threat and emergency medical care is mandatory. While awaiting help, first aid should include administration of cool fluids if the victim is alert, and application of ice or cold water to the skin.

- In extreme cold, you should plan shorter runs and try whenever possible to run with a companion. Midday is the best time for winter running so that you can take full advantage of whatever warmth is available from the sun. Be particularly conscious of the wind. With the wind at your back you will probably feel quite warm if you are dressed appropriately (see pages 191–192), but when you turn into the wind you'll start to cool down fast, and you'll rapidly become a believer in the wind-chill factor. It's best to head into the wind when you start your run, so that you can have the wind at your back when you're on the way home and may be tiring. Vaseline can be used to protect your face from the wind, but some runners prefer wearing a ski mask. Obviously it's best to avoid bitter cold conditions, with wind-chill factors lowering temperatures below zero. But unless you have asthma or other medical problems, you can run safely and comfortably in amazingly cold weather with appropriate clothing and precautions.

· Moisture is actually a greater hazard during the winter than is the cold. Running in the rain can be great fun at 60 degrees and only mildly uncomfortable at 45, but at 32 degrees it can be life-threatening, because your clothing will lose its insulating properties when it's wet, and your body will lose heat very rapidly. An overlooked puddle that soaks your socks can lead to serious frostbite, so be sure to stay dry during winter by wearing waterproof gear and, even better, avoiding moisture.

· Winter also brings special problems with the road surface. Most runners would agree with Renoir that "snow is one of nature's illnesses." Hard-packed snow is a reasonable surface, but you should wear running shoes with waffled or studded soles for best traction. You'll also have to slow down and run very, very carefully. Ice, however, is extremely hazardous, and should be avoided altogether by runners. Even when road crews have begun to clear streets, winter running can be hazardous because you'll have to compete with automobiles for scarce passable roadway. The secret is not to win the confrontation with automobiles, but to avoid it. Even with the best motivation in the world, cars maneuver poorly, stop slowly, and skid easily on winter streets. Once again, our advice is to run defensively. If snow and traffic combine to produce hazardous conditions, take a few days off, find an indoor track, or take up cross-country skiing.

· Above all, use common sense and caution during the winter. Plan shorter runs. Choose routes where you can easily get to warmth and transportation if you become tired or have an injury. Let someone know your route and approximate timetable, and don't deviate from your plans. Run with a friend if possible. Carry money and an I.D. and possibly some candy. Stay well hydrated, and be particularly careful to warm up adequately before you even get out your front door.

RUNNING INJURIES

We've been accentuating the positive aspects of running for health, recreation, or competition, but we do want to give you a balanced account; hence, it's time to talk about running injuries.

It has been estimated that twenty million Americans jog or run. If that is the case, then we would guess that twenty million Americans have had running injuries at one time or another. But don't let this figure frighten you; whereas virtually all runners are liable to have problems at some time, the great majority of these are quite mild. Sixty percent of runners will have to miss at least some running because of injury, but only 15 percent will have injuries severe enough to warrant medical attention. Although all runners are vulnerable to injury, some of us are more injury prone than others. In general, the most significant injuries tend to occur during transitional stages, when you're progressing from being sedentary to being a jogger, when moving from jogging to long-distance running, or when making the final transition from long-distance running to competitive racing.

Many running injuries can be prevented by wearing good shoes, choosing a good running surface, doing exercises for strength and (especially) flexibility, and, above all, by selecting an appropriate distance and pace. Even if you can't prevent injury altogether with these measures, you can limit the damage to mild problems that you can often treat yourself.

Why do running injuries occur? A little arithmetic will give us the answer. Let's assume you jog with an average stride length of three feet. That means that every mile will involve 1,760 strides. Once you've built up to twenty miles per week, you'll be subjecting your body to the repetitive impact of foot upon ground 35,200 times weekly. On a yearly basis this translates to a truly impressive 1,830,400 strides. With each stride your feet will absorb a force up to eight times greater than your body weight; in just one mile, each foot will have to absorb more than 100 tons of impact force. Running is great for your heart, lungs, and circulation, for your body's metabolism, and for your psychological makeup, but it certainly subjects your feet and legs to a considerable degree of trauma. You can minimize that trauma with good footwear that absorbs shock and by running over a forgiving surface, which will further dissipate impact. Even so, there's just no way of avoiding stress on your lower extremities.

The specific causes of running injuries are varied and complex, but they pare down to the same pitfalls that can affect any athlete: overuse, overstress, impact, biomechanical defects, improper equipment or technique, and structural abnormalities in your body itself. Chapter 11 explains these problems — and tells you how to overcome them.

The final major causes of injuries are inflexibility and muscle imbalance. Dr. George Sheehan has a nice way of classifying the major muscles involved in running into opposing pairs (see Figure 8–5). At the level of the abdomen and hip, the abdominal muscles in front are counterbalanced and opposed by the iliopsoas muscles at your back. At the hip and thigh, the large quadriceps muscles of the thigh are counterbalanced by the hamstrings at the rear. At the knee and calf, the pretibial shin muscles in front are counterbalanced by the gastrocs or calf muscles behind. At each level, the front member of each muscle pair is weaker and is overpowered by the much stronger rear member. The muscles on the front can therefore become excessively fatigued and hence injured; to prevent this, do exercises to strengthen these weaker muscles. In contrast, the rear member of each pairing is naturally stronger, and is further built up by running. With strength, unfortunately, come tightness and shortening, which can also lead to injuries. To prevent this, it is very important to stretch these muscle groups. Chapter 6 shows you how to strengthen the weaker muscles and stretch the stronger ones.

Not surprisingly, running injuries are almost entirely confined to the lower body (see Figure 8–6). Although runners may be more vulnerable to these problems, once "running" injuries occur they are virtually identical to similar injuries sustained by other athletes. Chapter 12 explains in detail how you can manage these ailments. Except for the knee, which is the most commonly injured part of the runner's body, these injuries are most common at the foot and ankle, and grow progressively less common as you move up the body to the hip and back. Figure 8–6 illustrates the most common running problems.

One special problem facing runners is instability of the foot — excessive pronation or, less often, excessive supination. Pronation is not a conspiracy thought up by

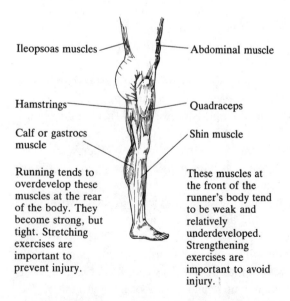

Ileopsoas muscles

Abdominal muscle

Hamstrings

Quadraceps

Calf or gastrocs muscle

Shin muscle

Running tends to overdevelop these muscles at the rear of the body. They become strong, but tight. Stretching exercises are important to prevent injury.

These muscles at the front of the runner's body tend to be weak and relatively underdeveloped. Strengthening exercises are important to avoid injury.

FIGURE 8–5: *Inflexibility and Muscle Imbalance — Major Causes of Running Injuries*

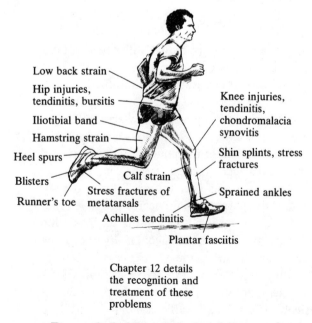

Low back strain

Hip injuries, tendinitis, bursitis

Iliotibial band

Hamstring strain

Heel spurs

Blisters

Runner's toe

Stress fractures of metatarsals

Achilles tendinitis

Calf strain

Plantar fasciitis

Knee injuries, tendinitis, chondromalacia synovitis

Shin splints, stress fractures

Sprained ankles

Chapter 12 details the recognition and treatment of these problems

FIGURE 8–6: *Major Running Injuries*

shoe manufacturers and sports podiatrists to sell special shoes and orthotics. Pronation is simply part of any normal stride. When you land on your heel and shift your weight forward to push off with your toes, your foot will naturally tend to roll inward. This inward rolling is pronation — but if it becomes excessive, pronation will flatten the natural arch of your foot, causing inflammation and pain in your foot or heel as the stress accumulates mile after mile (see Figure 8–7). Ankle, knee, and even hip pain can result if you do not correct

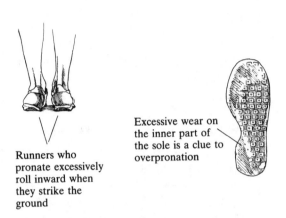

Runners who pronate excessively roll inward when they strike the ground

Excessive wear on the inner part of the sole is a clue to overpronation

FIGURE 8–7: *Excessive Pronation*

this problem. Excessive supination, or outward rolling of the foot, is less common but can also cause injury. You can tell if your gait is abnormal by having a friend watch you run or by checking your shoes for abnormal wear (see Figure 8–8). If you are an overpronator, look for special shoes designed to limit pronation or get orthotic inserts, which will stabilize your gait in normal shoes. A straight stride will help prevent many running injuries.

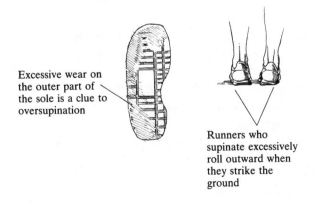

Excessive wear on the outer part of the sole is a clue to oversupination

Runners who supinate excessively roll outward when they strike the ground

FIGURE 8–8: *Excessive Supination*

ADVANCED LONG-DISTANCE RUNNING AND RACING

In general, *joggers* are motivated by considerations of health, whereas *runners* have come to enjoy the sport in and of itself. And, in this scheme of things, *racers* are those who have turned to the roads for competition. Racers are runners who have become goal oriented, not necessarily in terms of winning, but in terms of achieving ever better times and establishing personal records at various distances.

We encourage everyone to exercise, and everyone whose health permits to consider jogging and running as part of his or her exercise program. We do not, however, encourage everyone to race. Competitive running places unique stresses on your body and can lead to injuries. But if competition is your thing, there are certainly ways to train effectively and avoid injuries as well.

Suppose you find yourself jogging or running up to twenty miles a week without pain or strain. Now you want to run faster, harder, and longer. You can achieve some of these goals simply by plugging along and progressively doing more of what has worked so well for you thus far. But some changes in your training schedule will accelerate your progress, and some changes in your routine can help prevent injuries. A few tips:

· Increase your stretching and strength work. The more you train, the more your muscles may become tight and/or imbalanced. Counteract this problem before it occurs. If exercises are not your thing, you can bike or run stairs to build your quadriceps, and swim to build your upper body.

· Increase your caloric intake to fuel your additional mileage. Now that you are fit enough to train for racing, you should be at ideal body weight. Reward yourself: eat to maintain that weight. You don't have to be gaunt to be a serious runner.

· Don't abandon the running shoes that have gotten you this far. If you decide to buy a pair of racing flats, break them in carefully and then reserve them for races of ten miles or less. For your daily workouts you need the comfort and support of good training shoes, especially as your mileage increases.

· Keep a runner's log. Your training log helped you get fit, and it can help you train properly for advanced running as well. Record your weight, diet, mileage, road conditions, and race times and note how your body feels. Review your entries each month and plan ahead according to your findings.

· Listen to your body. Don't push yourself too hard to attain arbitrary speed or distance goals. Don't try to "run through" injuries or fatigue — rest up, and readjust your schedule to fit your body's needs. Don't attempt to overcompensate for missed workouts or injuries; instead, work your way back to full training gradually after a lay-off or injury. And don't attempt to maintain a competitive peak all year long; build up to an important race and then allow your training to ebb a bit until it's time to peak for the next race.

· Increase your mileage slowly, adding no more than 10 percent per week. Your mileage will depend on your goals. For health, fifteen to twenty-five miles per week is ideal. For road races of five to ten miles, a base of thirty-five to forty miles per week is reasonable. For marathon running, fifty to sixty miles per week is necessary, and competitive marathoners may do twice that much.

· Vary your distances, alternating longer and shorter runs. As a rule of thumb, your "collapse point" will be about three times your daily average. For example, if you are averaging five miles per day, don't try to extend your longest run beyond twelve to fifteen miles.

· Vary your pace. About 90 percent of your training mileage should be at a pace that is substantially slower than your race pace. But the other 10 percent should be speed work.

Your speed work can take several forms: (1) Interval running on a track or on the road — after warming up, sprint at 90 percent of your maximum for 100 yards, jog 200 yards to recover, repeat the cycle four to eight times, and then cool down and stretch. As you improve, increase the distance you sprint to 220 or even 440 yards (one-quarter mile) — but always give yourself twice your sprint distance to recover. Intervals are exhausting and require lots of discipline. (2) A less taxing way of getting speed work is to intersperse your training pace with "surges" or "pickups" of faster running. This technique is called "fartlek" running — a Scandinavian term that translates as speed play. (3)

Tempo drills — after warming up, run for a predetermined distance at your ideal race pace, then cool down with slower jogging. If your goal is a five-mile race at a seven-minute-per-mile pace, you might start with one mile of tempo running; but as you improve you can extend your distance until you approach your target.

Whatever form your speed work takes, always remember to warm up and cool down thoroughly. Stretching is particularly important. Postpone your speed work if you are ill, injured, or overly tired. Don't plan more than two speed workouts per week. Try to do your hard runs with a friend of similar abilities.

· Run hills. Like speed running, hills will give you high-intensity training. If you maintain your normal pace while running uphill, you'll push toward your anaerobic threshold. Hills will also build your quads. Be careful not to overextend yourself on the way *down* — downhill running is easy on your breathing but hard on your legs. Serious runners know that "uphills train, downhills strain"; don't learn this lesson the hard way.

· Consider running twice a day as your mileage increases. Doublets are less taxing physically and mentally.

· Enter races. Don't race to win or even to run your hardest every time. Racing is a good form of speed work, and it also offers motivation, companionship, and fun. Always remember the first commandment of racing: Pace thyself.

· Join a running club so that you can get individual training tips and coaching.

Does all this hard work and meticulous attention to training pay off? Indeed it does, and the effects of training can be measured in the exercise laboratory as well as on the track. During the five-year period when he reigned as America's premier miler, Jim Ryun's VO_2 max varied between an excellent 65 ml/kg/min and an astounding 81 ml/kg/min. Clearly, the major variable was neither heredity nor age, but training and conditioning. Ryun's results varied with his level of fitness, but success on the road depends on more than success in the lab. Training builds speed, endurance, efficiency, and strength. Hard work also builds will and determination. But that extra bit of desire, confidence, and tactical skill comes from racing itself. All in all, you must train hard to race, and race often to win.

THE MARATHON — AND BEYOND

As doctors we are not encouraging you to train for a marathon, but as runners we are unashamedly enthusiastic. Legend has it that the first marathoner was a messenger named Pheidippides, who collapsed and died after a run from Marathon to Athens in 490 B.C. Tradition notwithstanding, the marathon is not a sadomasochistic event. Quite the reverse is true: marathon running should be both safe and enjoyable — if you train for it properly. Again, a few tips may help:

· Unless you are an extraordinary athlete, don't attempt a marathon until you've been running regularly for one to two years and have a well-established base of thirty to forty miles per week.

· Give yourself a full three months of intensive training prior to your first marathon. Gradually build to fifty to sixty miles per week and maintain that base. Include some hills and speed work. Include at least one long run (thirteen to eighteen miles) per week, and run at least one twenty-miler three or four weeks before the race. Taper your mileage down for two weeks before the marathon.

· Pick your first marathon according to the four C's: course (flat), climate (45 to 55 degrees), crowd (supportive and friendly), and companionship (run with a friend, ideally one who has completed a marathon previously).

· Run intelligently. Your goal should be to finish feeling good, so you shouldn't even think about your time during your first marathon. Start slowly; listen to "coach" William Shakespeare: "Too swift arrives as tardy as too slow" (Romeo and Juliet). Aim for a steady pace — the marathon is really two races, the first twenty miles and the last 6.2, so you'll need to keep something in reserve. Drink plenty of water. Enjoy the race, interact with the crowd, observe the scenery, and do your best to relax. Needless to say, you should also listen to your body; if cramps, injuries, or excessive fatigue occurs, you should walk, stretch, rest, or even drop out altogether. Remember that in every marathon at least one elite competitor will drop out; Bill Rodgers has dropped out of five marathons, including his first attempt at Boston in 1973. There will be other races on other days, if you stay healthy, so don't push yourself to the point of injury, utter exhaustion, or collapse.

Running as a mass-participation sport in America is relatively new, dating back perhaps fifteen years. Despite this, no fewer than fifty thousand Americans have completed at least one twenty-six-mile, 385-yard marathon, and at least five thousand have completed this estimable achievement in a truly excellent time of three hours. Fifty thousand Americans can't be wrong, nor have they invested months of training and countless hours of effort for health alone. Marathon running can be fun. Although motives for marathoning range from competition to overcoming personal handicaps to achieving what once seemed unachievable, the bottom line should be enjoyment and satisfaction. Perhaps all those gaunt marathoners are just doing what comes naturally, living up to the ancient biblical prediction that "many shall run to and fro" (Daniel 12:4).

For the veteran marathoner, what comes next? Again, if we were to speak as physicians only, we would not encourage you to think beyond the marathon any more than we would have encouraged you to train for marathoning in the first place. Only a minority of joggers and runners will choose to become marathoners, and only a minority of marathoners choose to go beyond. But you may be interested to know that for the true fanatic, marathoning can be just the *beginning*. *The Wide World of Sports* has acquainted all of us with the Ironman Triathlon, which serves up 2.4 miles of ocean swimming and 112 miles of biking as appetizers for a standard 26.2-mile marathon. Although triathlons are just now becoming popular, there are increasing numbers of these events, and many involve much shorter distances that are within the reach of dedicated human beings who are not necessarily superstars.

Or if running is your thing, you can look into ultramarathoning. If marathoning requires unusual physical and/or mental traits, ultramarathoning may be considered as a fringe activity. But for some of us, an ultramarathon is the logical extension of an enjoyable activity. An ultramarathon is any race of thirty-one miles or more; the most common distances are thirty-one miles, fifty miles, or sixty-two and a half miles (one hundred kilometers). And if that's not enough for you, you can look for hundred-mile races, twenty-four-hour races, or even six-day races. Even these awesome events seem like sprints to the likes of Don Choi, whose ultramarathon began May 1, 1985, and finished fifteen days, six hours, fourteen minutes, and seventeen seconds later, when he became the second man in history to complete a thousand-mile race.

In a very real sense, ultramarathons are throwbacks to the early days of road racing precisely because they are fringe events. You won't find sixteen thousand participants in an ultramarathon — in fact, the first one I (HBS) ran had only sixteen entrants. In many of these events there are no T-shirts, no bottled spring water, and no yogurt — just dedicated runners and officials doing their thing. But the numbers are increasing: in 1969, only seventy Americans ran ultramarathons; but in 1981, 3,967 completed at least one ultra.

Although the runners themselves do not complain about the loneliness of ultra-long-distance running, many splendid athletes such as Ray Scannell, Stu Mittleman, and Marcy Schwann have never received the recognition they deserve. Barney Klecker is hardly a household name — and yet Klecker set the world record for fifty miles in 1980, running a phenomenal 4:51:25. This translates to two *consecutive* 2:26 marathons. Klecker did this with a VO$_2$ max of "only" 62 ml/kg/min, well below that of many elite marathoners. But when he leaves the lab and gets on the road, he is clearly as good as any endurance athlete in the world. Although ultra-marathoners are obscure in the U.S., they have achieved national prominence in other countries. The annual fifty-four-and-a-half-mile run between London and Brighton, England, is one example. Even more famous is the yearly Comrades Marathon in South Africa. This race is run from Durban to Pietermaritzburg one year and in the opposite direction the next. The difference is substantial, since the two cities are separated not only by fifty-four miles but also by 2,100 feet in altitude. 1983 was an uphill year — and 5,867 runners (including 177 women) made the trip through the "Valley of a Thousand Hills." A 117-pound South African archae-

ologist named Bruce Fordyce won in 5:30:12, setting a new record for the uphill direction. You'll never find a Bruce Fordyce running suit — but his abilities and accomplishments surely deserve as much respect as Frank Shorter's or Bill Rodgers's.

Whereas some elite ultramarathoners run "only" 100 to 120 miles per week in training, Stu Mittleman and others often put in more than 200 miles per week. What are the health consequences of all this running? Only time will tell. But we can get some reassurance from the story of Earle Dilks, who participated in the 1928 Transcontinental Foot Race, set the 100-mile record in 1928 and ran 117 miles in twenty-four hours in 1931. Ultimately, Dilks cut down to six miles a day — at age eighty.

How do ultrarunners do it? You do not have to have the genes of a world-class athlete to be a successful ultramarathoner. Ask Joe Michaels, who has run twelve ultramarathons since he began running in 1980 — after his recovery from coronary bypass surgery at age thirty-nine. The equation is the same as for any human achievement in or out of sports: talent plus work equals success. Ultramarathons are relatively uncommon in America, but in other cultures ultralong-distance running is part of daily life; the fabled Tarahumaras Indians of Mexico have been running hundreds of miles per week for generations. Perhaps it all goes back to the biblical wisdom of Isaiah: "They shall run and not grow weary" (40:31).

Please remember that we are not trying to tempt our readers to join us in these admittedly extreme events. But we are eager to point out that the limits of human endurance are truly extraordinary. With good health, a little innate ability, and a lot of training and determination, even ordinary mortals can achieve extraordinary feats with their feet.

9

Lifesports II: Swimming, Rowing, Aerobic Dance, Biking, Cross-Country Skiing, and Skating

By now, our enthusiasm for walking, jogging, and running should be quite obvious. We emphasized these activities in Chapter 8 because they take little equipment and no skill, they are available to people at all levels of fitness, and they are also adaptable to a wide range of climatic conditions, so you can do them virtually year round. Finally, most other sports incorporate running into their training regimens and use many of the same training techniques. Therefore, if you understand running, you will have a good foundation for understanding other sports. In fact, the aerobic benefits of other lifesports can be readily compared using running as a standard; Figure 9–1 shows you the "running equivalents" of these sports so that you can easily figure out the relative effort required for each.

Of course, running is not a perfect form of exercise: running will not develop your upper body and may overstress your feet and legs, leading to injuries. Moreover, some people are just not built for running; if you are overweight or if you have problems with your legs or feet, running may even do more harm than good. And, though we hate to admit it, some people just don't like to run. But don't give up on fitness just because running is not your thing. Happily, there are many other lifesports, and in this chapter we'll detail the way each can contribute to your fitness program. Each of these sports has its own unique attributes. Not all of them may be right for you, but this chapter will present the pros and cons of each lifesport so that you'll know which ones you'd like to try for yourself.

The best fitness programs depend on a *mixture* of sports rather than on a slavish devotion to one form of exercise alone. It may take some trial and error to find out which sports you like best, but even the process of trying them out can be great fun. Ultimately, you can develop confidence in several areas so that you can have variety in your exercise program, which will keep you mentally fresh and also give your muscles a balanced and varied workout.

SWIMMING

Life on earth evolved from the water. Although man has been a terrestrial animal for eons, it is perhaps

---

FIGURE 9–1: "RUNNING EQUIVALENTS" OF OTHER LIFESPORTS

To get the same benefits of jogging 1 mile, you should:

Swim	¼ mile
Row	¾ mile
Cross-country ski	1 mile
Bike	5 miles
Jump rope	6 minutes
Aerobic dance	8 minutes
Skate	10 minutes

---

appropriate that we return to an aquatic environment for fitness and for fun. In fact, surveys of recreational habits in America consistently show that swimming is our nation's favorite sport. We suspect that the majority of Americans who classify themselves as swimmers enjoy paddling around as a form of recreation instead of carrying out serious lap swimming for fitness. We hope we can stimulate you to add lap swimming (which can be quite enjoyable in its own right) to other forms of recreational swimming and diving. And once you get into shape, you can use swimming to explore all sorts of new horizons, ranging from snorkeling to long-distance lap swimming to competitive swimming.

In many ways, swimming is *the* ideal form of exercise. Swimming is excellent training for *cardiopulmonary endurance;* you'll get all the benefits of aerobic fitness, including increased work capacity, a slower heart rate with a stronger cardiac pumping capacity, a lower blood pressure, and an improvement in your blood fat profile.

Each of the lifesports can help you attain cardiac fitness, but swimming has some unique advantages for your muscles and joints. First of all, swimming requires you to use virtually all of your major muscle groups, so you'll be able to develop *balanced muscular strength*, particularly if you vary your strokes. Because the major propulsive force in swimming is pulling by the arms rather than pushing by the legs, you will tend to develop your arms, shoulders, and trunk somewhat more than your hips and legs. Hence swimming can be an ideal way to complement running, biking, or skiing to obtain truly balanced muscle strength.

Swimming is also an excellent way to develop *flexibility* of your muscles, ligaments, and joints. As you swim, you'll be moving all of your major joints through a large range of motion against the resistance of the water. As a result, swimming is one of the few sports that does not require a lot of supplementary stretching or strength work, although these forms of land exercise can be useful, especially for competitive swimmers. Since swimming will require you to use all parts of your body in smooth, rhythmic fashion, it is also a good way to improve your *coordination*.

Perhaps the most important advantage of swimming, however, is its relative freedom from injury. You can thank the buoyant force of water for the protection that your muscles, ligaments, and joints enjoy. In the water, your body weighs only 10 percent of what it does on land; while you swim, your weight is evenly distributed and supported by the water, so you can get a very good workout without the pounding that your legs take during running and other land sports. Also, it is very hard to overdo it during swimming, since the aquatic environment tends to restrain you from pushing yourself harder or longer than you should.

Swimming is the ideal exercise for people who are overweight. The buoyancy of water will protect you from the injuries that plague so many heavy people who take up running or other land sports. And body fat in turn makes it easier to float and provides insulation against cold water. But don't get the wrong idea: if you swim seriously, it's better to be lean, as you can see from even a quick look at the sleek shape of champion swimmers. Mary T. Meager will testify to this. At 135 pounds she set world records in the 100- and 200-meter butterfly, but at 146 pounds she fell way off her own record pace and was finishing out of the money. Mary gave up ice cream and candy — and won the Olympic gold in the 100-meter butterfly in Los Angeles. If you are overweight, swimming will help you burn off extra calories and reduce your body's fat content, but a little restraint in the kitchen will help as well.

Swimming is very efficient: you can burn a large number of calories in a reasonably short period of time. As with any sport, the number of calories you burn depends on your body size, how fast you go, and how long you keep at it. You can estimate the work load of swimming by comparing it with jogging and running (see Figure 9–1). Because of the resistance and drag of water, swimming is approximately four times more work than is running. If, for example, you burn 100 calories in jogging a mile, you can get the same metabolic benefit from swimming just one-quarter mile. Of course, swimmers travel a good deal slower than runners, so a person who is able to run a mile in ten minutes would probably require the same ten minutes to swim his quarter mile. As you get into shape and improve the efficiency of your stroke, both your speed and endurance will pick up. If you become a good swimmer, you can expect to consume up to 800 calories in one hour of freestyle or crawl stroke swimming; the breaststroke and backstroke are somewhat less demanding, and would therefore average 600 calories per hour for a good swimmer. These energy levels are quite comparable to running, and are clearly superior to many other recreational sports such as tennis.

Swimming is adaptable to all age groups and fitness levels. Because of the protective aspects of the water itself, aquatic exercise can be an excellent way to start a fitness program for people who are very out of shape or who are recovering from illness or injury. Joe Namath, for example, swam one and one-half miles per day to keep in shape while recovering from knee problems. Many aquadynamic exercises can even be performed by nonswimmers! Swimming can also be an excellent form of exercise for people with various handicaps. It's no accident that Franklin Delano Roosevelt installed a pool in the White House during his presidency. Incidentally, swimming has been one of the favorite presidential sports ever since. President Kennedy enjoyed and benefited from swimming because of his bad back, and President Johnson was also a regular swimmer. President Nixon closed the White House pool (instead of avoiding water, perhaps he should have avoided Watergate). President Ford reopened it and swam twice daily while he was in the White House. President Reagan includes swimming in his comprehensive fitness program, drawing on the skills he developed in youth during six summers as a lifeguard.

Quite obviously, swimming is also ideal for summertime sports. Whereas land sports are exhausting — and even dangerous — in hot, humid weather, the cool water will keep you fresh and energetic even if you swim on the hottest August day. And since your body won't overheat while it's in cool water, you won't have to worry about drinking lots of fluids to prevent dehydration.

To critics, a disadvantage of swimming is the solitude factor. You can't socialize while you swim, so lap swimming is fundamentally a lonely activity. Many people find the solitude beneficial, but for others lap swimming is boring; if you want to socialize, you will have to do so at poolside or elsewhere in your swim club. Solitude notwithstanding, swimming does have important *psychological* benefits. Swimming shares the exhilaration and relaxation of other aerobic and endurance sports, but some swimming advocates claim that the rhythmicity and coordinated breathing of swimming provide additional mental relaxation. And enthusiasts further point out that the buoyancy of water and the way in which swimmers are insulated from noise and external stimuli produce additional relaxation. We are not aware of any good scientific comparisons of the psychological benefits of swimming and other sports, but we do know that once you become a confident, competent swimmer, you'll find it both extremely relaxing and pleasantly invigorating.

Swimming is an ideal form of exercise, but alas, it's not perfect. The major drawbacks in swimming are logistical: you need water. For most of us this means a swimming pool. And unless you live in the Sunbelt, you'll have to rely on an indoor pool for much of the year. It takes time and effort to get to the pool, which takes time away from exercise itself. In most cases, there is at least a modest membership fee involved. These are, however, rather minor inconveniences, and once you get in the swim of things, you'll probably find it quite easy to build a trip to the pool into your routine at least three times weekly, if not daily.

The final problem with swimming is the most important: you have to know how to swim. Walking and running are universal, automatic human activities, but swimming is an acquired skill. Most of us learn to swim as children, and with a few tips and some diligent practice we can become competent fitness swimmers. But if you're a nonswimmer or a technically poor swimmer to start with, you'll need to take lessons before you can use swimming for fitness and health.

EQUIPMENT

A nice advantage to swimming is that very little gear is required; unless you are fortunate enough to be able to build your own pool, the most expensive piece of equipment you'll need is your bathing suit. If you go in for flashy designer suits, this can be expensive indeed. But for health and fitness you should be more concerned about function in the water than appearance at poolside. Lightweight, close-fitting suits are best because they don't billow out in the water and hence they produce less drag and resistance. Women should choose one-piece suits with straps that fasten around the neck or cross in the back to prevent them from slipping. Synthetic fabrics are best because they dry quickly, so that one suit is really all you need even if you swim daily. You can prolong the life of your suit by rinsing out the chlorine after you swim in a pool. Men who wish to keep things even simpler can wear close-fitting nylon running shorts to swim, thus cutting equipment cost to an absolute minimum.

Many pools require both men and women to wear a cap. Racing caps may cut down on drag and help speed you through the water, and if the cap is well fitting it can protect your hair from the drying effects of water and chlorine.

The single item that is most important for your comfort is goggles. The chlorine in pools is very irritating to your eyes, but well-fitting goggles will protect you. Prescription goggles are available, but they are much more expensive, and most swimmers find them unnecessary even if they need eyeglasses for land sports. If you wear contact lenses, you can keep them on while you swim if your goggles are very well fitting and secure. Experiment with various goggle styles until you find the one that fits best. Remember to wet your goggles before you put them on to prevent fogging; water, saliva, or special wetting solutions can be used.

Whereas these items are all essential, a few other things are quite optional. Some people find the water irritating to their nose and sinuses and may benefit from nose clips. Inexpensive plastic earplugs can also be purchased, but unfortunately they tend to be less effective at keeping your ears dry. If you have an ear disease that mandates dryness, you should look into having a customized set of earplugs made to minimize water exposure.

Another very optional item is a waterproof watch. Some swimmers dislike lap counting and prefer instead to swim by time. A waterproof watch that has a stopwatch is just as useful in water as on land. There are even models with built-in thermometers, which will allow you to measure water and air temperature.

Some athletes enjoy shopping for new equipment and take delight in trying the newest design in tennis racquets or the latest model of running shoes. If you are a gadgeteer, you may be a bit frustrated by swimming because there is really nothing else to buy. About the only other items you could even consider would be a few simple devices that can be used as teaching or training aids in improving your strokes. Most swim clubs will have these available without extra charge. The most commonly used items are kick boards, which will keep your upper body afloat so that you can work on kick technique and leg strength. Hand paddles can also be used to improve your hand entry and position. Finally, pull-buoys can be used to stabilize your legs, forcing you to depend on your arm stroke, which will improve your technique and strength.

All in all, the equipment you need for swimming is simple, straightforward, and inexpensive. Pack your suit and goggles into your swim bag, add a towel and some soap, and head for the pool to get started.

GETTING STARTED AND TECHNIQUE

Throughout this book, we have stressed the importance of careful, progressive warm-ups and cool-downs before and after exercise and sports. Some swimmers claim that they can dispense with a formal warm-up and cooldown, and they do have a point. Swimmers tend to maintain a good level of joint and muscle flexibility

and they have a low risk of injuries, so supplementary stretching and strengthening exercises are not mandatory. You can use a warm shower before you swim to start warming up your muscles, and you can use swimming itself to warm up your heart if you start out slowly.

Clearly you should not dive into the pool and start sprinting at full speed. However, you can jump in and begin swimming slowly until your breathing is comfortable and your heart rate has slowly risen. You may also wish to vary your strokes in the first few laps to get all of your muscles into gear. And you can reverse the procedure to cool down after hard swimming simply by doing a few easy laps with various strokes or by treading water. Because the water itself is cool, your body will not overheat during swimming, and more elaborate cool-down routines are not needed. If you are used to stretching exercises before any form of sport, you certainly can incorporate these into your pre- and post-swim routine. For swimming we suggest particularly exercises to loosen up your shoulders, upper back, hips, and thighs. Specific examples can be found in Chapter 6 (Figures 6–5, 6–8, 6–9, 6–10, 6–14, 6–17, and 6–18).

To swim for fitness, you must know the fundamentals of stroke technique and breathing. If you are a poor swimmer or a nonswimmer, you'll need lessons. Don't be shy about this; it is an absolute misconception to assume that lessons are intended for children only. True, many Y's and swim clubs offer classes for tots from age three up, but adult classes and private lessons are also available. Swimming is such an excellent form of exercise that you should seriously consider making the effort to learn to swim well. You will acquire a skill that is excellent for fitness and recreation and that will also open the door to safe participation in boating and other water sports.

Even beginners who are just learning to swim can use the pool to get into shape by doing exercises in shallow water. These aquadynamics can also be useful for people who are very out of shape or for those recovering from injuries. Aquadynamics are a relatively gentle form of exercise, consuming perhaps 360 calories per hour, which would be roughly equivalent to a walk/ jog program covering three and a half miles in an hour. In aquadynamics you move your body against the resistance of water in an isokinetic fashion.

At the simplest level of aquadynamics, you can jog or hop across the pool in waist-deep water. Or you can venture into deeper water and tread water using a flotation device or holding onto poolside if necessary. You can also hold on to the side of the pool with your belly down to practice the flutter kick to build up your hips and quadriceps. You can turn over and hold on with your belly up, raising your knees to your chest to build your hip and abdominal muscles. You can bob up and down in chest-deep water to build your thighs and trunk. Remember that they are very gentle forms of exercise and that you'll have to work at them for prolonged periods to get much fitness benefit from them. But they are a good place to start and they will make you comfortable in the water.

Once you know how to swim, you can build fitness simply by swimming, swimming, and more swimming. The basic stroke you'll need to master is the freestyle or crawl. But ideally you should learn at least one additional stroke, such as the breaststroke, backstroke, or sidestroke, so that you can rest your muscles by varying your stroke until your ability to sustain a crawl improves. The sidestroke and, to a lesser degree, the breaststroke are also less strenuous than the crawl because of their glide phase between strokes; hence, they are very useful for beginners. It's quite true that there are "different strokes for different folks," and you may find that you prefer one of these alternate strokes as your major aquatic fitness tool.

Whatever stroke you choose, if you are very out of shape you may have to content yourself at first with swimming back and forth across the width of the pool, resting for a few seconds in between. Soon you should be able to build up so that you can swim a lap down the length of the pool. It's all right to change strokes or even float during your first few laps. But soon enough you'll be able to swim a lap without interruption. Rest if you have to at the end of the pool, turn around, then head down the pool for another lap. At first, pick a lane that is empty or being used by other slow swimmers. As you improve, you'll find yourself swimming more and more laps and also moving into the faster lanes at your pool.

As your strength and endurance improve, you will want to spend more and more time thinking about technique. Even if you haven't had lessons to get you started, you may well want to take a few lessons to improve your stroke efficiency. The basic idea, of course, is to minimize water resistance. Whereas the auto industry is just now emphasizing aerodynamic styling for efficiency, swimmers have spent years figuring out ways to reduce drag, up to and including shaving off all their hair. Mark Spitz collected his Olympic golds with a full head of hair, so you surely don't have to go to extremes.

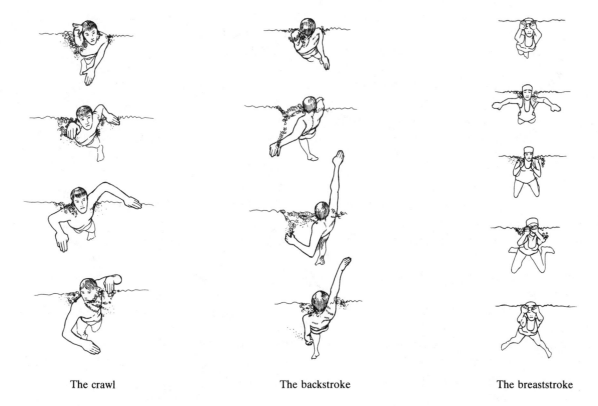

The crawl   The backstroke   The breaststroke

FIGURE 9–2: *Basic Stroke Mechanics*

But you should keep your body as horizontal as possible by keeping your head position low in the water while keeping your legs close to the surface rather than letting them dangle deep into the water. Your arms should enter the water smoothly to prevent turbulence; a lot of white water means wasted energy. Your strokes should be smooth, steady, and strong. Keep your fingers together, but don't cup your palms. Keep your breathing rhythmic and steady, always exhaling through your mouth. Strive for a nice rhythmic stroke as well, coordinating your arms and legs smoothly; most distance swimmers use six flutter kicks to each stroke while doing the crawl. Finally, most good swimmers keep their eyes open so that they will stay on course.

Each stroke has its own technical tricks. It would be very worthwhile for you to have a good coach or teacher evaluate your technique and give you pointers for improvement. We can think of no better authority than James E. Counsilman, the legendary swimming coach at Indiana University. Figure 9–2 shows Doc Counsilman's suggestions for the crawl, backstroke, and breaststroke, as modified from his excellent book *Competitive Swimming Manual for Coaches and Swimmers*.

SWIMMING GOALS AND FITNESS PROGRAM

Once you've mastered the fundamentals of stroke technique, water safety, and comfort, fitness is simply a matter of adding lap upon lap as you slowly improve. However, a few simple guidelines may be helpful. As with any aerobic exercise, the training effect depends on the intensity, duration, and frequency of exercise. It's ideal to swim three to four times per week if this is your basic fitness activity. Although you can use the target heart rate concept to guide the intensity of your swimming, a small modification is in order. The human body retains a very primitive reflex called the diving reflex. Whenever you are submerged in water your heart rate tends to slow down a bit. As a result, it may be a little harder for you to achieve your target heart rate while swimming than it is during land sports. You may want to deduct as many as ten beats per minute from your target to set a realistic goal while swimming. Because of the limitations imposed by rhythmic breathing, you won't be able to use the "talking pace" as your guide, and even breathlessness may be a bit difficult to interpret. Because of the cooling effects of water, you won't even know if you're working up a sweat while you're swimming. Basically, you will simply have to

gauge how your body feels. As in land sports, you ought to feel that you are pushing yourself hard enough to get a workout but not so hard as to produce exhaustion.

One nice thing about swimming is that even if it's a bit difficult to judge intensity accurately, it is extremely easy to judge distance. The standard indoor pool is 25 yards long, so 72 laps equal one mile of swimming.

What should your goals be? If swimming is to be your major fitness activity, it would be ideal to burn up as many as 2,000 calories per week at this sport. Remember that swimming is four to five times more strenuous than running on a per-mile basis. Swimming four to five miles per week will equal running twenty miles per week, which in turn equals your 2,000-calorie fitness goal. So we'd advocate building up to one to one and a half miles of swimming per day, repeated three to five times per week. Whereas these distances are optimal for health, as you really get into the swim of things, you may well find that you want to swim longer and harder. Go right ahead! We've seen many friends and patients make the transition from nonswimmer to truly excellent endurance swimming.

SAFETY AND PRECAUTIONS TO AVOID INJURY

Swimming is great for health, recreation, and competition, but there are hazards to swimming, and the essential first element must always be safety. There are seven thousand accidental drownings in the U.S. each year. In fact, drowning ranks third behind motor vehicle accidents and falls as a cause of unintentional injury deaths.

The cardinal rule for swimming safely is never swim alone. Accidents do happen, and even the most expert swimmer can on occasion get into serious trouble. Although we think of drowning mainly as a complication of ocean swimming, snorkeling, or scuba diving, drownings can and do occur in lakes and pools. The two ways to prevent this are: first, never swim alone. There should always be a lifeguard or other competent individual within easy reach. This rule is so fundamental and elementary that it may be overlooked. We urge you to follow it without exception. The second rule is no less self-evident: use common sense. Don't swim when you are tired, seriously injured, or ill. Always listen to your body, and don't push yourself beyond the limits of strength and endurance.

A particular precaution applies to diving: never dive until you are absolutely certain the water is of sufficient depth. As obvious as this seems, it is often overlooked, with tragic consequences. There are five hundred serious brain and spinal cord injuries in this country each year because of diving into empty pools or shallow water. Be careful even in pools that have a "deep end"; in short pools, the floor may slope upward very abruptly, and a deep, horizontal dive could be trouble. Look before you leap.

How about the safety rule that all of our mothers harped on: never swim after you eat because you could get stomach cramps. Although we hate to pick a fight with all the mothers of America, we know of little scientific documentation for the occurrence of stomach cramps when swimming after meals. However, strenuous swimming requires a tremendous increase in blood flow to your exercising muscles, a fair amount of which is shunted away from your stomach and intestines. So all and all we would suggest only fluids or light snacks within the two-hour period before strenuous swimming.

A final safety consideration is water temperature. If you are swimming in pools, the temperature is generally between 75 and 80 degrees, so you should have no problems. But lakes, ponds, and oceans can be very cold, and anybody with a heart problem should avoid swimming in cold water because of the danger of producing serious disorders of heart rhythm. Even healthy people should approach cold water with great caution. Your performance will be limited at best, and hypothermia is a real risk. Water conducts heat away from your body twenty-five times more rapidly than does air, so even if you are moving your muscles strenuously, your body temperature can fall to dangerous levels if you stay in cold water too long.

If you follow these simple safety rules, swimming should be an extremely safe sport with few serious injuries. The buoyant force of water simply makes it very difficult for you to overdo it and injure muscles, ligaments, and tendons. Even so, a few characteristic problems can occur, as outlined in Figure 9–3. You can find out how to manage these problems in Chapter 12.

Skin and hair dryness are very common in swimmers, because these tissues depend on natural oils for moisture, and repeated or prolonged exposure to water simply washes these oils away. You can prevent these problems by adding back oils after you swim and shower. Various hair conditioners and moisturizers or emollients are available for this purpose.

Eye irritation is another common problem peculiar to swimmers, particularly if you swim in chlorinated pools. You may notice burning, redness, and tearing of your eyes, and your vision may be blurry with halos around bright objects for up to twenty-four hours. These visual halos are caused by irritation and swelling of the corneas of your eyes. Although this is uncomfortable and alarming, it will almost always settle down even without specific treatment. The best treatment, however, is prevention, and we strongly urge the use of well-fitted goggles for serious swimming.

Sinus irritation can also occur if water is forced up your nose into the sinus passages. This will almost always resolve with time, but in some cases decongestant medications may be needed. Here, too, the best treatment is prevention, simply by breathing in and out through your mouth. Nose clips will also provide additional protection to your nasal and sinus passages.

Another minor but irritating problem is swimmer's ear. If moisture persists in the external ear canals, bacteria and fungi that commonly inhabit the skin in this area can overgrow, producing crusting, irritation, and pain. This problem can be minimized by thoroughly drying your ears after each swim. But some people find it hard to get all the water out their ears and may therefore be particularly prone to swimmer's ear. Although this problem can be irritating and even quite painful, it is usually not at all serious and can be readily treated with prescription eardrops such as Vo-Sol or Corticosporin. If you have swimmer's ear, you should stay out of the water for several days until the problem is controlled. Your doctor may also suggest preventive use of eardrops if you are prone to recurrent external otitis, or swimmer's ear.

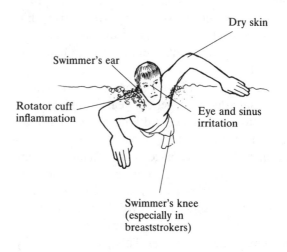

FIGURE 9–3: *Common Swimming Injuries*

Beyond these common complaints, there are several other potential difficulties that are so uncommon we'll merely mention them in passing. A few swimmers have developed erosion of their tooth enamel because of the effects of chlorine. However, this problem seems to occur only in pools that are excessively chlorinated, so don't worry about your teeth — just pick a well-monitored pool. Finally, we have seen several cases of a rare skin infection called "swimming pool granuloma," which can be acquired by contact with pools or even tropical fish aquariums. This condition can be readily treated, but may not be recognized by many doctors because it is rare. So if you develop a skin nodule that slowly spreads over a period of weeks or even months, see your doctor — and remind him or her that you are a swimmer.

ADVANCED TRAINING FOR COMPETITION

Well, you're swimming three or four miles per week and enjoying it. You've never felt better, and you've never looked better. What's next?

From the point of view of health, of course, it's not necessary for you to work out any longer or any harder than you are right now. If you do want to do more, you might be well advised to mix your swimming with another sport such as biking or running, which will give you variety, flexibility, and balanced muscle development by stressing your leg muscles a bit more than swimming does. But if swimming is your thing, you can certainly go beyond swimming for health and fitness and get into competitive swimming. Before you think of turning yourself into a competitive swimmer, you may want to stop and think about how much hard work is involved.

Competitive swimmers are among the most hardworking of all athletes. Over the years, topflight swimmers have gotten younger and younger, so that many of these competitive, highly gifted athletes begin serious training in their early teenage years. Champion swimmers often get up at five A.M. and swim four to six miles even before going to school. And not even four miles before breakfast is sufficient, for young men and women on these training regimens will typically have a second hard workout in late afternoon. This goes on seven days a week for years and years. As with any athletic endeavor, true excellence requires not only a very special body and inborn talent, but also lots and lots of very hard work.

Competitive swimmers use a range of training methods very similar to the techniques used by competitive runners, as discussed in Chapter 8. One of these techniques is over-distance swimming, which is entirely analogous to the long slow distance technique practiced by runners. Most competitive swimming events are basically sprints, but even an athlete who is training for a fifty-meter race is well advised to build up endurance by swimming mile after mile at a slow pace well within the range of his or her aerobic metabolism.

Whereas over-distance swimming builds up endurance, competitive swimmers obviously require speed work as part of their training as well. Sprint training is the way to do this. An example would be to swim for twenty-five or fifty yards at a nearly all-out pace, not once but six to eight times with only a short recovery period in between. Swimmers often refer to this type of sprint training as "repeats," and the basic philosophy is exactly the same as the interval training practiced by runners. The idea is to build those muscles specifically needed for speed, and to improve the body's anaerobic capacities. Repeats should be done after a gradual warm-up period and be followed by a cool-down period as well.

Swimmers should develop a careful plan before they embark upon interval swimming. As with other repetition training, this plan depends on four elements: the *distance* to be swum, the *interval* of rest between repetitions, the number of *repetitions* themselves, and finally the *time* or pace at which they are swimming. Interval training must be done with care to avoid injuries. At best it's hard work. No wonder swimmers commonly refer to their interval schedule by the acronym DIRT (*D*istance, *I*nterval, *R*epetitions, and *T*ime).

Any training schedule must be individualized on the basis of your abilities, the level of your fitness, and your goals. It is important to develop a progressive training schedule so that you will slowly increase the intensity of your workouts to get yourself in shape for a big meet. It's very important to leave time so that you can taper down your swimming in the week before your major race. Progression also is important in each individual workout. You should always start with a warm-up of easy swimming of different strokes and possibly with some stretching exercises on land as well. Warm-up is particularly important for breaststrokers, who may otherwise injure their knees and legs. Many swimmers in addition choose to use a kick board so that they can isolate their kick technique and leg development. Similarly, a pull-buoy can be used to neutralize the legs so that you can work on your stroke and arm development.

Another training technique that is unique to swimming is "hypoxic training." The idea here is to take in less oxygen during your training swim so that your body will become gradually acclimated to the state of relative oxygen depletion. Hypoxic training can be hazardous, and it is very important to carry this out only under carefully controlled situations. Hypoxic training is not a breath-holding contest. Instead, hypoxic training means taking a breath at every second or third stroke instead of at every stroke. If you plan to swim more than one hundred yards during hypoxic training, be sure to take at least two breaths per twenty-five yards. No more than one-quarter to one-half of your total workout should be done under these hypoxic conditions. In addition, during this type of training you should swim at a controlled speed and not at an all-out sprint. Although carefully controlled research has not been done on hypoxic training, Doc Counsilman believes that this is a helpful training technique. We feel, however, that it is best reserved for the highly competitive swimmer who is in a controlled training program under the careful guidance and supervision of an experienced coach.

What is the role of land exercises in training for competitive swimming? Although some swimmers (like runners) believed that their sport is the perfect conditioning activity, most coaches now feel that supplementary land exercises will add additional strength and balanced muscle development. And even if competition isn't your goal, land exercises will help ensure balanced muscle development and total fitness, which will keep you at the ready for most any sport. We must emphasize, however, that if swimming and only swimming is your thing, land exercises are optional.

If you choose to do land exercise, you will want to work on four areas: your shoulders, upper chest, elbows, and wrists. You may also want to do flexibility exercises, including ankle stretches, Achilles stretches, and particularly shoulder stretches. All of these exercises are detailed in Chapter 6.

The Amateur Athletics Union has an excellent competitive swimming program that operates at the local, regional, and national level for all age groups. Because highly competitive swimming has become dominated by athletes in their teens and early twenties, the AAU masters program begins at the tender age of twenty-five. Athletes are grouped into five-year age categories (twenty-five to thirty, thirty to thirty-five, and so forth, right on up). A great variety of events and distances is available, so everyone can find his or her own niche.

Competitive swimming is not for everyone, but it can provide motivation, fellowship, and fun. So if you want to find out what your limits are, investigate meets in your area. You may meet former champion swimmers who still compete to stay in shape or people like Fred Allen, who began competing at age seventy-seven and was still winning national titles at age eighty-five.

It's interesting that marathon swimming is now coming of age. This is really nothing new; just think of the highly publicized assaults on the English Channel and similar bodies of water over the years. Many of these have been solitary, individual efforts in which one man or woman triumphs over distance rather than opponents. Some of these attempts have been truly extraordinary. The most dramatic recent example was Diana Nyad's attempt to swim from Cuba to Key West, Florida, in 1978. Her training program was every bit as spectacular as the effort itself. Diana trained for over a year. At first her schedule included a daily run of ten miles, thirty minutes of rope skipping, three hours of squash, and two hours of swimming. This was just the beginning, however — as her epic swim approached, she was swimming seven hours daily with continuous swimming for as much as twenty-four hours on weekends. Needless to say, this type of dedicated effort left her little time for other activities. She must have put aside a fair amount of time to eat, however, since she estimated her daily caloric intake was 10,000 to 12,000 calories per day to support this training schedule.

Long-distance swimming is also becoming a competitive event. The New York City road marathon began modestly in 1969, but the annual Manhattan Island *swim* marathon began on an even smaller scale; on September 14, 1982, ten men and two women competed in this twenty-seven-mile swim around Manhattan, which is an extraordinary achievement in view of the distances, tides, temperatures, and unclassified biological hazards in these murky waters. The winner was David Horning, who completed the course in seven hours, twenty-five minutes and forty-five seconds. The first woman was Karen Hartley, whose time was 7:37:13. You can see from these two times that women do extremely well in ultralong-distance swimming; in no other sport is there so little intrinsic difference between the sexes. A new record (6:12:29) for the swim around Manhattan, in fact, was set by a woman, Shelley Taylor, in 1985. And if once around Manhattan is not enough for you, in 1983 a swimming untramarathon two times around Manhattan was held. So you thought long-distance *runners* were nuts?

Obviously we are citing these extraordinary examples to point out the limits of human endurance, not to encourage you to train for similar events. All competition, in fact, has negative as well as positive aspects. If you find racing enjoyable and stimulating, go right ahead. However, remember to train carefully and to stay within your own limits at all times. Don't push so hard that you become stale. Remember what Mark Spitz said after his incredible eight-gold-medal performance at the 1972 Munich Olympics: "I'll never swim again."

As you can see, swimming is quite a safe, injury-free sport. It is also an excellent conditioning activity for your heart and circulation and for all of your major muscle groups, building both strength and flexibility as well as coordination. Although a few simple guidelines for safety and injury prevention are important, we can recommend swimming without reservation as an excellent sport for fitness and health.

ROWING

Imagine for a moment that you are visiting Beaver Lake in the Ozark Mountains of Arkansas. If it's early morning, and halfway decent weather, you'll see a solitary oarsman smoothly stroking across the water at a steady pace for eight miles. A closer look will show that this athlete is a sturdy, healthy six foot four. But he is also over eighty years old. He is Dr. Benjamin Spock, America's most famous pediatrician. A member of the Yale crew that won the gold at the 1924 Paris Olympics, Dr. Spock believes that a lifetime of rowing has kept him fit, healthy, and young.

Long considered the preppiest of sports, rowing is now becoming accessible to many more people. Once the domain of highly trained, elite, competitive athletes, rowing is increasingly becoming a fitness activity for people at all levels of performance. Let's look at how this transition has come about and what it can mean for you.

Although Harvard and Yale have been rowing against each other since 1852, the appeal of the sport is beginning to spread. Whereas American and English collegiate crews dominated the sport in its early years, national teams and even some elite boat club entries now predominate. An even more striking development is the boom in women's rowing. When the National Women's Rowing Association held its 1968 regatta, there were fewer than one hundred participants; just ten years later this same event attracted over six hundred fifty competitors in one hundred fifty shells from more than sixty rowing clubs. Rowing became a women's Olympic event in 1976, and current estimates tell us that 25 percent of the oarspeople in America are oarswomen.

When most of us think of competitive rowing, the first image that comes to mind is of the cool and elegant scullers beautifully painted by Thomas Eakins a hundred years ago. The rhythmic beauty and smooth power of rowing have not changed, but rowing itself is making the transition from an aristocratic sport to a modern fitness tool. It's too bad that Eakins can't paint the Head of the Charles Regatta, which is held in Boston each October. Participation in this race has now swelled to seven hundred crews and over three thousand oarsmen and -women — to say nothing of fifty thousand spectators. The U.S. Rowing Association estimates that there are now over ten thousand dedicated rowers in the country. Although the majority of these are still former collegiate rowers who belong to well-organized rowing clubs, more and more individual rowers are joining the ranks.

Rowing is attracting new participants because it is an ideal sport for fitness, offering excellent cardiovascular conditioning. When performed at a modest to moderate pace for prolonged periods of time, rowing is a fine aerobic sport. As competitive crew racing is basically a sprint event involving shorter periods of all-out effort, rowing is also an excellent way to build anaerobic capabilities. Because of this combination of aerobic and anaerobic effort, rowing will decrease your body fat and build muscle strength and endurance. Rowing also enhances both flexibility and coordination. Best of all, rowing involves almost all of your major muscle groups, including your legs, back, shoulders, arms, and even wrists and hands. In all of these respects, rowing is an excellent conditioner for your whole body. Moreover, although rowing can be very hard work, it is basically nontraumatic, so major injuries are relatively infrequent.

Not surprisingly, elite rowers are among the best conditioned of all athletes. They are lean, have a low percentage of body fat, have very high scores for both aerobic capacity and anaerobic threshold, and rank very high in power and strength. One look at a top competitive crew will convince you: the 1979 Yale crew *averaged 6'4"* in height and 200 pounds in weight.

Although elite rowers are obviously highly gifted athletes, much of this superior performance can be attributed to extremely intensive training regimens, which are probably more demanding than any other collegiate program. Happily all of this hard work pays off in health as well as in strength and fitness; a medical study followed the Harvard class of 1914 over a sixty-year period, and found that crew members lived significantly longer than did their nonrowing classmates.

While the physical benefits of regular rowing are truly impressive, rowing is still the least popular of the lifesports listed here. Actually, the disadvantages of rowing do not relate to the exercise itself, but to logistics. To run, you need a road and shoes; to swim, you need twenty-five feet of water; to row, you need open water, calm conditions, reasonable temperatures, and a boat. In many parts of the country, rowing is strictly a seasonal sport confined to the months between late spring and early fall. Additional disadvantages are the considerable expense of your boat (the average price of a racing shell, for example, is three thousand dollars), to say nothing of the need for launch facilities and regular maintenance. However, modern innovations are starting to overcome some of these disadvantages. For one thing, rowing machines allow you to stay in shape for rowing by rowing year round. In addition, newer fiberglass shells are less expensive and more durable, require less maintenance, and are also easier to use. Finally, an increasing number of boat clubs are opening their ranks to oarsmen at all levels so that you can get instruction and fine fellowship, and rent equipment at a relatively modest cost.

EQUIPMENT

Racing shells have come a long way since the early days of this sport, and technical innovations are still being introduced each year. The earliest shells had fixed seats like today's ordinary rowboats. With fixed seats, only your back and your arms generate the power to propel your boat through the water. The rolling seat was invented in 1871, and rolling or sliding seats have been used ever since. From the point of view of fitness, the sliding seat allows you to integrate your legs and abdomen with your back and arms, so that all of your major muscle groups are at work with each stroke. From the point of view of the sport, the sliding seat allows greater fluidity, smoothness, and speed.

Rowers can be characterized as scullers or sweepers. Scullers use two oars; often they row alone in single sculls or open rowboats fitted with sliding seats, but there are also two-, four- and even eight-man sculls. Sweepers use both hands to pull on a single oar, with alternate oars rigged on opposite sides of the boat. Eight-

oared crews are steered and directed by a ninth, nonrowing teammate, the coxwain; smaller crews can row with or without a cox.

Until recently, racing shells were handcrafted of cedar. Because lightness is at a premium, this wood was only one-sixteenth of an inch thick, and was so fragile that if an oarsman stepped on the hull instead of the small stepping platform at each seat, he'd go right through the shell. Most modern shells are now made of fiberglass or newer carbon fiber synthetics, which are lighter and more durable. But the basic structure is otherwise the same. You'll strap your feet into foot stretchers, shoes that are screwed to a platform to allow you to push and generate tremendous power with your legs. The seat slides on two steel tracks, and you'll be facing backward, rowing with one twelve-and-one-half-foot-long sweep, or two nine-and-one-half-foot skulls; the oars are surprisingly light despite their formidable length.

Many of the recent innovations in rowing have taken place in the single shell, forty pounds in weight, thirty feet in length, but only twelve inches wide. The novice will find these shells tippy even in calm water, and even the most experienced oarsman runs the risk of capsizing in rough conditions. Since the mid-1960s, however, designers have been experimenting with new hull designs. The Alden Ocean Shell is a good example; this fiberglass boat is a cross between a kayak and a racing shell and has a twenty-four-inch beam, giving it much greater stability. Because the hull can be decked over, this craft is much less likely to take on water and is much more secure for beginners. Aldens are now the largest class of recreational shells in the United States, and other wide-bodied models are usually represented at regattas as well. Whether you live near a bay, harbor, river, lake, pond, reservoir, or even a flooded strip-mine pit as do rowers in central Illinois, rest assured that you can find a shell to match both your abilities and the water conditions in your area. Although racers and other purists still extol the traditional cedar shell, more and more modified fiberglass designs are now available, including ultrastable twin-hulled catamarans.

A final noteworthy development is the rowing machine. Because of the seasonal nature of rowing, competitive oarsmen have always trained indoors in winter, traditionally in large rowing tanks sequestered in the nether regions of the athletic building. Although rowing tanks are still used by teams who need to coordinate their timing and endlessly practice stroke technique, you can get all of the fitness benefits of rowing without so much as touching an oar to water by using a rowing machine. Chapter 6 discusses the use of these machines in your home or fitness club.

In addition to this relatively sophisticated equipment, you can get fitness benefit from traditional watercraft as well. The old-fashioned flat-bottom, fixed-seat rowboat can be used for cardiovascular conditioning and will build strength in your arms, shoulders, and upper back, but will not do much for your abdomen and legs. Canoeing and kayaking are also good sports, but safety precautions are particularly important when you take your kayak or canoe from the relative safety and calm of a lake into the turbulent and exciting but hazardous white water of a fast-flowing river.

GETTING STARTED AND TECHNIQUE

Surprisingly little skill is required as a prerequisite for rowing. The basic technique (see Figure 9–4) is a smooth, continuous movement, described by Stan Pocock, the dean of American shell builders, as a "symphony of motion." You'll begin to generate power with your legs and back, and then smoothly transfer the bulk of your effort to your shoulders and arms toward the end of your stroke.

The movement can be divided into four components:

1. *The catch.* At the beginning of your stroke, your legs and trunk are flexed, with your arms extended. Your low back should be stabilized as the blade enters and catches the water.
2. *The drive.* This is the power component of the stroke. Your legs extend and your back straightens simultaneously. Your arms are brought inward to your body. All this power propels your oar through the water, generating the force to move the boat.
3. *The finish.* Your hands drop to elevate the oar from the water. Your wrists pivot and drop to feather the oar, so that it is parallel to the water, lessening air resistance as it moves forward into the next stroke.
4. *The recovery.* Your arms extend and your legs and back flex to get ready for the next stroke. At the end of the recovery, your hands and arms pivot to position the blade for the next catch.

Though this sounds incredibly smooth and easy, when you first try rowing in a shell you'll probably find that the technique does take a while to master. But once you achieve a smooth stroke, you are ready to begin a balanced program to make progress with your rowing.

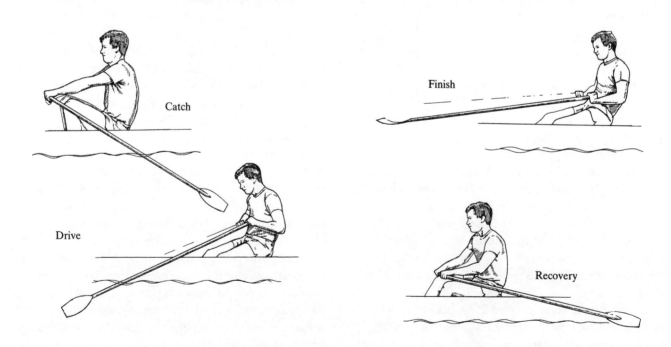

FIGURE 9–4: *Basic Rowing Technique*

GOALS AND FITNESS PROGRAM

Elite oarsmen are in wonderful shape. Alas, relatively few of us are 6 feet 4 inches in height and twenty years of age, although a distressing number of us may weigh 200 pounds. Fortunately, the fitness benefits of rowing apply to the beginner as well as the acomplished performer. One of the nice things about rowing is that it can be done at all levels of intensity. You can begin at low levels, rowing by yourself and using rowing as the foundation of your fitness program. As you get into shape, you can increase the intensity and duration of your effort so that you will improve more. You can row alone for fitness, you can join others to form a two-, four-, or eight-member crew, or you can enter competition either by yourself or as a crew member. And as demonstrated by the octogenarian Dr. Spock, you can continue rowing as long as you remain healthy and fit.

The caloric costs and metabolic benefits of rowing are a bit hard to quantitate because the intensity of effort is so variable: external conditions such as tide, waves, and wind play a major role in determining the amount of work you'll do while you row. Rowers can consume as few as 300 calories per hour if they are moving at a leisurely pace. At the other extreme, at high stroke counts and full power oarsmen may burn more than 900 calories per hour, making it one of the most intensive sports. At full output, elite lead oarsmen may be working twice as hard as comparably gifted runners. As a rule of thumb, thirty minutes of hard rowing will have approximately equivalent fitness benefits of five miles of hard running.

At first you'll be rowing as far as your technique permits, usually one to three miles at most. You'll begin with easy rowing for short intervals. Your stroke count should be low, generally less than twenty strokes per minute. In addition, each stroke will be modest in intensity, pulling at perhaps one-half of your full pressure.

As you improve, you'll increase both the power and the tempo of your strokes. After you've warmed up with slow, easy rowing, build your tempo by increasing your rate to thirty strokes per minute for periods of perhaps thirty seconds. When you can sustain this comfortably, gradually increase the duration of higher-cadence rowing. When you feel you can row all day at a respectable cadence, it's time to increase the pressure or power of each stroke from one-half to three-quarters to full. Again, this is best done not in one fell swoop, but by intermittent training — add first ten, then twenty,

and finally thirty strokes at full pressure. When you can row for twenty to thirty minutes continuously at three-quarters pressure, you will have achieved an excellent fitness base. From the health point of view, we'd recommend twenty to sixty minutes of such rowing three to four times a week as optimal for fitness.

Because rowing trains most of your major muscle groups at the same time as it gives you a good aerobic workout, rowing can stand alone in your exercise prescription. However, bad weather will force you to use your rowing machine to stay fit during winter. For variety, you can substitute swimming for upper-extremity strength and running and biking for your legs. And if you've got the bug, you should do supplementary strength and flexibility work to train for competitive rowing (see Advanced Training for Competition, below).

SAFETY AND PRECAUTIONS TO AVOID INJURY

In all sports, safety must come first, but this truisim is nowhere more true than in water sports.

The first safety rule for rowing is, in fact, swimming — don't take up rowing unless you swim well. So if you skipped our section on swimming at the beginning of this chapter, but are enthralled with rowing, turn back to page 203 and start all over again.

Even excellent swimmers must, however, observe fundamental safety rules when they row. First, you should never row alone. Ideally, there should be a launch nearby with appropriate safety equipment. At the very least, there should be other boaters or land observers nearby who can summon help. Except when you are racing, be sure to have an efficient flotation device in your boat; unfortunately, many rowers find that life jackets or belts interfere with smooth technique. If you capsize, always stay with your boat. Even if you can't clamber back in, you can hang on and float. Should the boat sink or be swept away, grab on to an oar; all oars float and standard oars can support a weight of up to 195 pounds.

The greatest hazard of capsizing is hypothermia. In cold weather, consider wearing Gove-tex or kayaking garments that are loose fitting but waterproof. You should always choose a life jacket or flotation device that has some insulating properties. If you capsize in cold water, try to overcome the shock of immersion and avoid panic. Stay with your boat and try to climb on it to get out of the cold. Unless land is within *easy* reach, it is better to float quietly instead of swimming around. It is true that muscular activity generates heat, but the average person wearing a life jacket and light clothing can cover only .85 miles in 50-degree water before developing severe hypothermia, so it's best to avoid tiring yourself with wasted motions. Keep your head out of the water, because a great deal of heat is lost from your head. If several people fall out of the same boat, huddle together as you float to preserve body heat. If you are alone, assume the *heat escape lessening position* — the so-called HELP position — which is basically a float in the fetal position with your head out of water.

Above all, of course, try to prevent capsizing in the first place by using prudence and common sense. Never row under adverse conditions such as choppy water, high wind, or when a storm is threatening. And until you become very proficient and confident, always stay near the shore.

Rowing is an excellent conditioning activity, but even at the competitive level injuries are uncommon. This is because rowing is a nontraumatic, self-paced, progressive activity that distributes work and force among all of your major muscle groups. Oarsmen can develop injuries including blisters and calluses of the hands, and tendinitis, strains, and sprains of the wrists, forearms, and back. When these injuries occur, they are entirely comparable to similar injuries from other sports; we'll discuss them along with other athletic injuries in Chapter 11.

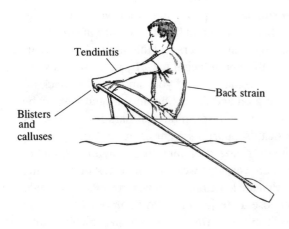

FIGURE 9–5: *Common Rowing Injuries*

ADVANCED TRAINING FOR COMPETITION

Because of the brutal amount of work involved in truly hard rowing, it is very rare for oarsmen to sustain this level of effort for prolonged periods; most rowing events are basically anaerobic sprint races of one thousand to two thousand meters, lasting from three to eight minutes. During these sprints, rowers must exert as much strength as possible, with pauses between strokes of perhaps 1.5 seconds. In fact, crew races *begin* by sprinting: in just ten strokes, eight men must bring a one-ton shell and crew from a dead start to a top speed of about thirteen miles per hour. No other sport that calls for more than two minutes of effort begins with an all-out sprint. No wonder you have to be fit to row competitively! Imagine the amount of effort that goes into the annual four-mile Harvard-Yale race, which has been held yearly since 1852 in New London, Connecticut. This long course requires approximately twenty minutes of all-out effort and is a profoundly exhausting event. Remember, however, that for fitness *per se* we'd like to see you rowing four to eight miles at a much more leisurely pace.

Before you set your sights on competitive rowing, you may want to reflect for a moment on the effort and sacrifice involved. Collegiate oarsmen begin training in September for a short racing season, which does not begin until the spring. Stephen Kiesling, a member of the 1980 U.S. Olympic crew, who wrote an excellent book about his experiences called *The Shell Game,* estimates that during his career he spent approximately twenty-four *hours* of training for each *minute* of racing! And this is hard training indeed. Although even an expert like Stan Pocock felt that training could be accomplished strictly with the three R's (rowing, rowing, and rowing). virtually all modern programs incorporate intensive land exercises as well. In spring, summer, and fall, rowing is the predominate training activity. Crews use over-distance training at moderate intensity to build endurance, and also intervals, sprints, and tempo drills to build speed and strength. They must also use this water time to master the coordination, technique, and teamwork that make racing such a beautiful sport.

But grace and rhythm aren't everything, and rowers also work very hard at strength and power. Although land training goes on year round, it is most intense in the winter, when water time is not available in most climates. Winter training involves rowing in tanks and using rowing machines, and is also the season for supplementary work. Most programs incorporate running for endurance and speed. Typically this involves both road running and also sprinting up stadium or gymnasium stairs, not once but over and over again. Strength training is also very important. In general, rowers design their routine so that they will train with the ratio of three leg exercises to two back exercises to one arm and one stomach exercise. The basic lifts, which are illustrated in Chapter 6, include the clean, the bench pull, the squat or leg press, the French press, and the dead lift. Calisthenics are also very helpful, with sit-ups being particularly important.

Finally, although rowing itself builds flexibility as well as strength, all of this weight work should be counterbalanced by regular stretching exercises to develop flexibility for balanced fitness and to minimize injuries. It is particularly important to stretch your ankles, calves, hamstrings, lower back, and also your shoulders. Appropriate exercises are illustrated in Chapter 6.

How is the formidable training program put together? Stretching is useful daily, both during the racing season and in the winter. When you are training on the water, your weight work will probably drop to one or two days per week. In the off-season, you may choose to do weight work on three days, endurance work on two days, and speed work on one day each week. Believe it or not, this schedule will allow you a day off — even the most avid competitive rower is, after all, human.

AEROBIC DANCE

Let's join Louise Boland in her aerobics class. Louise has a master's degree in language but switched from teaching reading to teaching aerobics in the early 1980s. Aerobic dance keeps the teacher fit: Louise ran a very respectable 3:47 in the wet, windy 1984 Boston Marathon, known to all of us who ran it as the Monsoon Marathon. And now Louise is using aerobics to improve the flexibility and endurance of her students. The music is upbeat and the atmosphere in the gym is warm and friendly. Louise herself is a trim 5 feet 2 inches, but her students in this particular class hardly fit the stereotype of the small but shapely aerobic dancer. In fact, the shortest student is 6 feet 4 inches and the tallest is 7 feet — Louise is teaching aerobics to the Boston Celtics.

For centuries dance has been classified as an art form or as a social activity. These functions of the dance are as valid today as they ever were, but during the past fifteen years dance has also become a fitness activity. Although dance itself is certainly not a sport, rhythmic gymnastics is a specialized dancelike sport, which was added to Olympic competition in 1984. And aerobic dance rivals and exceeds many sports in its ability to promote balanced fitness. Let's look at how dance spans the spectrum from art to exercise, and how you can use dance to attain and maintain optimal fitness.

Classical ballet is certainly the most time-honored and traditional dance form. Ballet dancers look like terrific athletes: they are slender, supple, and strong, and their performances seem to require substantial endurance as well. But in terms of cardiopulmonary fitness, ballet dancers are generally not quite as fit as they look. The reason for this is that ballet training places a heavy stress on isometric, or static, exercise mixed with short bursts of dynamic exercises similar to sprinting. While this is an excellent formula for developing strength and speed, it tends to be a bit lacking in dynamic, aerobic exercise, which builds cardiopulmonary fitness and endurance.

Ballet dancers are very strong, flexible, and well coordinated, but have only moderate levels of aerobic fitness. The VO_2 max of ballet dancers averages between 40 and 50 ml/kg/min. This is very similar to non-endurance athletes such fencers, gymnasts, and volleyball and basketball players, but is substantially lower than the aerobic capacity of trained endurance athletes such as swimmers, cross-country skiers, and runners. Confirmation of this difference has been obtained through medical studies of the "coeur de ballet," or "dancer's heart." Ballet dancers have increased muscle thickness in their heart walls, similar to athletes who do isometric exercises but different from the increased chamber volume found in the hearts of endurance athletes such as runners, swimmers, and bikers.

How do other forms of dance stack up? Dance marathons of the 1920s and '30s notwithstanding, ballroom dancing is no more taxing than walking at a modest pace of three miles per hour or bicycling at a leisurely six miles per hour. Whereas ballroom dancing rates higher for nostalgia than exercise, today's modern disco dance is a bit better for fitness, producing demands similar to walking at four miles per hour or biking at ten miles per hour. This level of exercise certainly can be a great help for fitness, particularly if you were to disco dance three to five times each week, for an hour each session. Even if this schedule is good for your heart and your muscles, it may have some deleterious effects on your ears, so you might want to consider square or folk dancing. These lower-decibel forms of dance are roughly equivalent to disco, and can be helpful for fitness. In addition to being moderately helpful to cardiovascular or aerobic fitness, these forms of dance can also produce modest gains in muscle strength, flexibility, and coordination.

Figure 9–6 summarizes the relative strenuousness of these dance forms by looking at the number of calories you will burn during one hour of dance. But as you can see, an entirely different form of dance heads the list. Aerobic dance is an excellent fitness activity. In terms of calorie consumption and cardiovascular conditioning, aerobic dance rivals jogging; one hour of brisk, continuous aerobic dance can burn up to 650 calories and is equivalent to jogging six ten-minute miles. Because of this, aerobic dance is a good way to decrease your percentage of body fat and to attain the other metabolic benefits of fitness. Aerobic dance is also a very good way to develop musculoskeletal fitness, while building strength, flexibility, and coordination. Moreover, because your whole body is used in aerobic dance routines, you will attain these benefits for all your major muscle groups, including your legs, your trunk, and, to a somewhat lesser extent, your arms.

You won't find aerobic dance on the program at Jacob's Pillow or Lincoln Center. Aerobic dance, in fact, is much less an art form than a type of exercise; although the technique is dance, the emphasis is very much on the aerobics. The aerobic dance movement began to gather momentum in the late 1960s and early '70s and is still growing in popularity. Aerobic dance is a blanket term for a variety of exercises, calisthenics, and dance

steps performed to music. The individual motions include running, jumping, hopping, bending, stretching, and skipping, but instead of a goal-oriented sequence of movements focused around a ball or track, these body motions are choreographed into dances set to musical accompaniment. Aerobic dance is the form of dance most suited to fitness.

Even admitting that aerobic dance is an excellent fitness activity, why go to the bother and expense of signing up for a pre-scheduled class indoors when you can simply step out the door and run or bike on your own? As compared to other lifesports, the thing that makes aerobic dance unique is its social context. In a sense, aerobic dance is the diametric opposite of long-distance running, because dance is essentially a group activity rather than an individual effort. For people who enjoy the support and encouragement of a group, this is clearly an advantage. Scheduled classes three or four times a week provide structure and discipline, which may be very helpful, especially when you are getting started. A well-trained instructor can provide motivation and also supervision to be sure that your program is both safe and effective. Finally, most aerobic dance classes have an invigorating, upbeat atmosphere, which can take the drudgery out of exercise. Some cardiac rehabilitation programs have even added dance to break up the "monotony" of walking, running, and biking. The music itself may be helpful in this regard; although the music played at aerobic dance classes varies from jazz to rock to pop, it is uniformly fast paced and bright and tends to take your mind off your aches and pains to help you keep moving faster and longer.

The Boston Celtics notwithstanding, most aerobic

FIGURE 9–6: HOW MANY CALORIES YOU USE BY DANCING FOR ONE HOUR

Type of Dance	Your Weight 100	120	150
Aerobic dance			
Low intensity	200	230	275
Moderate intensity	325	370	450
High intensity	480	550	650
Ballet, modern (advanced)	350	420	520
Ballroom	200	250	350
Disco	300	350	450
Folk, square (strenuous)	275	325	425

dancers are women, which can be an advantage or disadvantage depending on your sex and your point of view. But an increasing number of men are finding aerobic dance a stimulating and enjoyable form of exercise. If you desire privacy, you can try aerobic dance at home by following directions on a videotape, but this is generally much less successful than organized class activities.

EQUIPMENT AND CLOTHING

You'll need very little in the way of gear for aerobic dance. The only really important item is your shoes. Don't bother to bring your ballet slippers to class — remember that aerobic dance is actually a form of exercise rather than a dance form. The ideal aerobic shoe will be well fitting and supportive, while still allowing lots of room in the toe box. The sole should have good traction on the outside and provide plenty of cushioning on the inside to absorb shock. It is also very important to choose a shoe that gives you good lateral support; whereas runners land on their heels and roll forward, dancers start and stop abruptly and execute quick lateral movements, which can cause ankle sprains unless good support is available. Because of this, you should never wear running shoes during aerobic dance. High-quality tennis shoes can work well, but best of all are special shoes designed for aerobic dance. These are now manufactured by a number of high-quality athletic shoe makers, including Adidas, New Balance, Nike, and Reebok. They tend to be less expensive than running shoes, generally costing between twenty-four and thirty-eight dollars a pair. If you pick your shoes carefully, they will last for many classes and are well worth the investment.

In terms of clothing, comfort is the watchword. Most dancers wear leotards, but gym shorts and T-shirts are certainly perfectly acceptable. In cool weather, tights or leg warmers can be helpful.

The rest of the equipment will be provided by the class. Although music is the only essential, you should try to pick a class with a well-lighted, well-ventilated, room. Ideally, the dance floor should be wood, which is much more resilient and forgiving than concrete. The room should be large enough to give each dancer plenty of floor space. Air-conditioning is a plus during summer months.

GETTING STARTED AND TECHNIQUE

Even before you enroll in aerobic dance, you should consider the question of medical screening. Once more we remind you that this is exercise rather than art, and you should therefore follow the same precautions as you would for any sport. If you are young and healthy and feel fine, you can jump right in; if you are over forty, if you have any adverse symptoms, or if you are overweight and very out of shape, you should check with your physician and discuss possible screening studies (see Chapter 5).

The next issue is selecting an appropriate class. Over the past fifteen years, the fitness boom has helped make aerobic dance a big business. Everyone is trying to get into the act. Aerobics classes are now offered in the names of TV personalities, movie stars, figure skaters, and athletes, as well as dancers. Aerobic dance is offered at most Y's and community centers, at many colleges and other educational institutions, and at traditional dance schools.

Don't let all this variety confuse you. Although there are subtle differences among these programs, they are all physiologically sound. You should pick a program based on its convenience and accessibility, its cost, the quality of its facilities, the size of its classes, and above all on the skill of the instructor. Most instructors are very well trained. They are generally good dancers who "come up through the ranks" in an aerobics program and then attend workshops and clinics to learn fundamental exercise physiology as well as advanced dance techniques. Most programs require physical fitness tests for their instructors, and many demand cardiopulmonary resuscitation training. Find out the background of your instructor before you sign up for the class. Some instructors have been certified by the American College of Sports Medicine as fitness instructors, which is an excellent credential. Various university programs also provide certification. Finally, there are independent organizations, such as the American Aerobics Association (AAA) or the National Dance Exercise Instructors Training Association (NDEITA), which provide certification, though their standards are somewhat less rigorous than the American College of Sports Medicine fitness instructor program.

The most important thing of all is to pick a class that is appropriate for your level of fitness and dance ability. You wouldn't take on Joan Benoit in a marathon one month after buying your first pair of running shoes, and you shouldn't attempt to join an advanced class for your first exposure to aerobics. Find a program that offers beginner, intermediate, and advanced classes. Visit each so you can find the level that is appropriate to you.

GOALS AND FITNESS PROGRAM

Aerobic dance classes follow physiologically sound principles. You will begin by learning your target heart rate and how to take your pulse. Each session will start will gradual stretching exercises and warm-ups to slow music. Your instructor will demonstrate the steps before each dance and will lead and demonstrate during each dance. After five to ten minutes, the intensity of your dancing will gradually increase. At first you may have only three or four fairly rapid dances, separated only by a very brief pause to check your pulse. As you get into shape, your routines will become more demanding and the number of consecutive dances will increase; eventually you will keep moving for as long as forty or fifty minutes. Finally, each session will conclude with a cool-down period of slower dancing and stretching.

Although programs vary, a typical aerobic dance class will last for eight to twelve weeks, meeting two to three times weekly. We suggest that you try to dance at least three times a week; if this is not possible, add some other form of endurance workout to fill out your schedule. Remember that endurance training is best achieved with at least three or four workouts each week.

This type of steady progression will usually get you into shape over three or four months. But a problem may occur if there is a disparity between your physical fitness and your coordination or dance ability. Admittedly this is not a common problem, but it is of particular interest to me since I (HBS) have it. I can say honestly that I am physically fit; however, I can't dance. I am assured that with patience and persistence I could conquer this sport too. But I secretly think that there may be an undiscovered type of coordination that I lack, an occult ear-to-foot reflex that has somehow gotten tangled up in my nervous system. I have no cause to envy the fitness of dancers, but I certainly envy their skill. For now, I'll have to stick with running, but for many others aerobic dance is an ideal mix of invigorating exercise, supportive companionship, and enjoyable self-expression to music.

If you have even a modicum of rhythm, regular aerobic dance will help you attain a high level of fitness. But once you've reached an advanced class, you'll find that you have to move faster and harder to attain your target heart rate; with continued training you'll be able to maintain your pulse in the target range for thirty to sixty minutes nonstop. This is an excellent fitness goal

in and of itself. If you can dance for three to four hours a week, you'll be able to burn about 2,000 calories and attain medically optimal fitness while having lots of fun.

Many people stick with advanced aerobic dance to maintain fitness. New music and new dance steps are introduced in each session so that boredom shouldn't be a problem. But aerobic dance can also be useful as one element of a more diverse fitness program. Jacki Sorensen has been called the founding mother of the aerobics movement. She started Aerobics Dancing in the late 1960s and now heads an organization that includes four thousand instructors and one hundred fifty thousand students throughout the country. She still dances and choreographs new routines for her instructors, but she also swims, bikes, walks, and runs, and she includes successful completion of a marathon among her achievements. In terms of her fitness, her leadership, and her success, Jacki Sorensen is the Bill Rodgers of aerobic dance. If this petite blonde represents one end of the physiological spectrum, at the other end is Carl Elkern, a 6 foot 3 inch, 225-pound player for the Los Angeles Rams. Elkern and some of his teammates found that ninety minutes of aerobic dance twice weekly during the off-season was a useful part of a balanced fitness program, improving flexibility and coordination as well as maintaining endurance. So whether you grunt on the gridiron or preside over a business empire, you can include dance in a balanced program of exercise, sports, and recreation.

Another outlet for aerobic dancers are exercise classes that use similar group techniques to build other skills. Many programs are available; an increasing number of them can also be purchased as books or video cassettes. Often named after media stars ranging from actress Jane Fonda to bodybuilder Arnold Schwarzenegger, these lessons are excellent ways for you to improve your muscle strength, body tone, posture, and flexibility. But remember that these workout classes can be very strenuous; to avoid frustration and injury, begin at a level that is suited to your abilities. Move yourself along gradually, always remembering to warm up and cool down before and after each workout. And don't forget that these workout classes are *supplements* to aerobics but should not *substitute* for endurance training; calisthenics and stretching are great for strength and flexibility, but you should still continue aerobic dance (or other endurance training) for cardiovascular fitness.

SAFETY AND PRECAUTIONS TO AVOID INJURY

Aerobic dance is exercise, and if you dance you are prone to injuries similar to those sustained by other athletes. The causes of injuries are usually poor technique, muscle imbalance, and inflexibility. Faulty shoes or hard floors can certainly cause their share of problems. But the major factor is simply doing too much, too fast, too soon. To prevent this problem, begin each session with a gradual warm-up; you may even want to do some stretching on your own before the class starts. Always join a program at your appropriate level of skill, and give yourself a chance to progress in a slow, steady, gradual fashion. Be particularly careful if you are exercising alone with a tape or video cassette. A good instructor will force you to warm up and to stay within your limits, but if you're on your own you may overdo it — resulting in a case of "VCR" back or a similar injury.

Because of the injury problem, a new type of aerobic dance is gaining popularity. Low-impact aerobics shares all the basics with ordinary aerobics — except that one foot is on the floor at all times. Hence, low-impact aerobics relates to standard aerobic dance just as walking does to running. Traumatic injuries to feet and legs are less common, but low-impact aerobics is less intense, so you will have to spend more time at it to get fit. To compensate for the lack of jumping motions, low-impact aerobics increases upper-body movements.

This will increase your flexibility — but carries an increased risk of arm and shoulder tendinitis and back strain. All in all, the relative merits of this new form of aerobic dance are not yet clear, but low-impact aerobics is certainly worth considering, especially if you are starting out overweight or very out of shape.

The injuries experienced by dancers are fundamentally similar to those experienced by runners except that they tend to be less frequent and milder in dancers. Figure 9–7 shows some common dance injuries, and Chapter 12 reviews the management of these problems. But the best management of dance injuries is prevention. The prevention, recognition, and management of dance injuries are exactly the same as for other sports medicine problems (see Chapter 11).

ADVANCED DANCE

One of the nice things about aerobic dance is that it's totally noncompetitive. You can progress at your own pace until you are maximally fit, and then you can stay with advanced dance classes to maintain fitness. But if you wish to progress further, you can become an instructor yourself, or you may want to branch out, using your dance skills to learn modern or jazz dance or your stamina to take up competitive sports.

BICYCLING

Just as aerobic dance is the fitness sport of the 1980s, and running was the major fitness activity of the '70s, bicycling was the rage in the 1960s. For a time, there was actually a shortage of good ten-speed bicycles. By 1979, a Nielsen survey indicated that more people still biked regularly (about seventy million Americans) than ran (about thirty-six million). The enthusiasm leveled off for a while, but with the stellar performance of the U.S. Olympic gold medalists in 1984, interest in the sport has picked up again. If you live in most major cities, the bicycling commuter is commonplace, and vacation touring in groups can be arranged in many rural areas of the U.S. and Europe.

The popularity of bicycling attests to one of its major features. It can be done by people of almost all ages, body types, and levels of conditioning. It can be enjoyed by beginners as well as by experts. Biking can be done by fat and thin, muscular or weak. It is enjoyable when

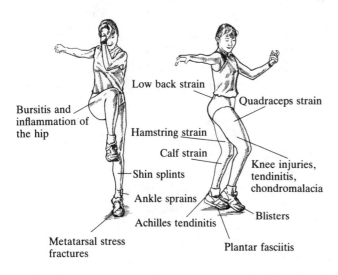

Low back strain
Quadraceps strain
Bursitis and inflammation of the hip
Hamstring strain
Calf strain
Shin splints
Knee injuries, tendinitis, chondromalacia
Ankle sprains
Achilles tendinitis
Blisters
Metatarsal stress fractures
Plantar fasciitis

FIGURE 9–7: *Major Aerobic Dance Injuries*

done leisurely and when done fast; in this respect, it combines the appeal of walking and running. Bicycling is also truly recreational. It can be done solo or in groups; at a very easy pace while touring or at a very intense pace when training or racing. It is not surprising that biking is one of Americans' favorite recreations.

From the point of view of cardiovascular fitness, bicycling is an excellent aerobic sport. If done with intensity, it is ranked just behind jogging and cross-country skiing in its energy expenditure, and is about equivalent to swimming (see Figure 9–1). If you bicycle at thirteen miles per hour (about four and a half minutes per mile), you will burn about 50 calories per mile and about 650 calories an hour. That means bicycling also contributes nicely to weight control. And because biking is less sensitive to the weight of the rider, it is an excellent sport to try if you are overweight or out of shape and want to begin an exercise program.

Bicycling is also an excellent way to train for other sports. It calls on the leg muscles (primarily quadriceps, hip extensors of the buttocks, and, especially if you use toe clips, the calf and anterior shin muscles). The quad provides the major force, and this muscle is highly developed by bicycling. Furthermore, depending on your use of the gears and grade, you can bicycle at very low resistance or relatively high resistance. Bicycling is thus an excellent sport for building knee strength and endurance, complementing running in terms of a balanced fitness program. It helps prepare for downhill skiing and skating, both of which depend on the strength and endurance of the quadriceps muscles.

Bicycling also makes significant demands on the back, shoulders, and arms because of the need to maintain a static upper-body posture while controlling the bicycle. The sport contributes to balance and quickness (the average pedal speed is about sixty to seventy rotations per minute), but very little to flexibility, coordination, or kinesthetics.

EQUIPMENT AND CLOTHING

This is either the beauty of bicycling or its bane, depending on your point of view. Cycling is enormously sensitive to equipment, and even a novice will notice the difference between a low-priced frame and a good touring bike. Add the various gear mechanisms (derailleurs), brakes, seats, and hubs that are available, and it is a gadgeteer's delight. If you are interested in equipment, are willing to spend the time talking about it and learning about it, love tinkering and adjusting,

oiling and assembling, your local bike shop will become your second home. If not, you will have to compromise and find a bike shop that you can trust to sell you an appropriate bike for your level of skill and involvement, and then maintain it in respectable shape. Nonetheless, you will still have to learn to do minor adjustments on the road.

But don't be dismayed. The relationship between human and machine is one of the aesthetic delights of bicycling. You should allow yourself to be wooed within the constraints of your time and money. Unlike running, bicycling *can* cost big money. But for fitness and recreational bicycling, there are less expensive bikes that provide a good ride and enjoyment, allow you to get into shape, and to tour modest distances. So there's no need to spend a lot of money in order to enjoy biking.

When shopping for a bike, it is the frame that is the main determinant of quality and price — better frames are lighter and more rigid. Rigidity opposes the torque you generate when you pedal, some of which turns the wheel and some of which tends to twist the frame. The more rigid the frame, the more your torque goes into turning the wheel and the less into unproductive effort twisting the frame. As you become a better cyclist, such considerations make all the difference in the world.

There are more than one hundred million bikes on the roads (or in the garages) of America. Most are sold by department stores, discount chains, or catalogs. We suggest that you buy your bike from a bike shop instead. You may pay a few dollars more, but you will be able to choose a machine suited to your needs, it will be well assembled, service will be available, and you can get all the accessories you need.

A few other things should go into your choice of a bike. Weight is important: try to find a model that weighs less than thirty pounds. Size is crucial, and here's where a bike shop can really help. You are probably used to picking a bike for your kids based on wheel size (twenty, twenty-four, or twenty-six inches), but almost all ten- or twelve-speed bikes have twenty-seven-inch wheels. These bikes do come in sizes, but the frame dimensions determine the size. Choose carefully — only one size is right for you, and as little as one inch can make a difference. To tell if a bike is the right size for you, straddle the tubing in front of the seat while standing flat on the floor; there should be one or two inches of clearance between the tubing and your crotch. Finally, select a bike with the proper gearing — the larger gear on the rear wheel should have at least twenty-eight teeth and the smallest gear on the pedal crank should have at least forty-two teeth. You'll be glad to have chosen good gearing when you ride hills.

In most cases, a good ten- or twelve-speed touring bike will be all you need. But if you get into biking, you can explore alternatives. All-terrain bikes, called ATB's, are very sturdy "fat tire" bikes that can be ridden over rough terrain in the city or country; these bikes are a cross between a sleek Italian racer and your old Schwinn, giving you ten speeds and relatively light weight, as well as strength and durability. Or you can move in the direction of a racing bike, sleek greyhounds that are amazingly light. You can even have a bike custom-built to your measurements and specifications; Cinelli of Italy will assemble the eleven hundred pieces needed — if you have about two thousand dollars to spend and three months to wait.

Although the bike is your major investment, some other equipment is important. A high-quality helmet is absolutely essential, and you should wear it anywhere you ride, no matter how short a distance. The U.S. Cycling Federation has underscored the importance of helmets by requiring bikers to wear hardshell helmets in all USCF-sanctioned races beginning in 1986. A good bike lock is worth the money it will cost to protect your investment.

Clothing presents many options. If you are going to do some serious bicycling, a pair of chamois-lined pants is a good bet. It's amazing how much they can reduce the wear and tear on your groin, especially if you are just beginning to develop calluses in the important areas. Gloves are also very helpful in reducing the pressure on the palms of your hands from leaning on the handlebars. Toe clips with or without biking shoes position your toes over the pedals and give you more pumping leverage. Special biking shoes add stability, but can be reserved for the accomplished cyclists. Finally, a good jersey gives you color, warmth, and a comfortable pocket in the back. A water bottle is inexpensive and its own reward.

New advances in materials, construction, gearing, and so forth occur all the time. An example is the recent "Funny Bike" developed by Huffy Bicyles for the very successful U.S. Olympic team. It has a small front wheel, a large, solid, plastic back wheel, and odd-shaped handlebars. Not surprisingly, it is now available to the public. If cycling is to be your main sport, new equipment can be part of the challenge and enjoyment of the sport. If cycling is a part-time pursuit, get a decent bike, helmet, small set of tools, a good book on bike maintenance, and don't worry about the rest.

Biking has one obvious drawback — wet and cold weather. Because of the wind, ideal cycling weather may be as much as fifteen to twenty degrees warmer than running weather, despite the comparable energy expenditure. Cyclists may need long-sleeved shirts below 60 degrees Fahrenheit and gloves and leg covering at 45 degrees. Layers of clothing will protect you when the temperature drops below this level; remember, though, that your face is vulnerable, so you'll need a mask sooner than when jogging to avoid frostbite. Note that wind chill rapidly becomes a factor when traveling at fifteen miles per hour, and frostbite can be a serious concern.

However, gear and equipment do very little for wet weather. Ponchos help, but only marginally, since the forward movement drives rain into every slit. Worse, brakes don't hold very well, and extreme caution is necessary when your hubs become wet. In snow and ice conditions, most of us prefer to hang our bikes up for the season and turn to a winter sport or indoor exercise to stay fit. Or you can bike indoors, by putting your ten-speed on rollers or using a stationary bike (see Chapter 6).

GETTING STARTED AND TECHNIQUE

Once you have learned how to ride a bike, you will never forget. The combination of balance and movement that characterizes riding becomes truly a reflex maneuver, even if the last time you mounted a bike was twenty years ago. Of course, if you've never biked before, you may have to overcome some psychological hurdles to learn.

If you are too old for training wheels, try this trick. Find a bike that allows you to reach the ground with both feet while sitting (you may have to lower the seat temporarily). Point down a very gentle hill and allow yourself to coast down slowly, with both feet acting as outriders to catch you if you tilt to one side or the other. Do this repeatedly until you have learned how to balance yourself comfortably. Next, do the same thing with your feet resting on the pedals without turning them. You have now solved one-half of the problem. The other half is to maintain your balance while pushing the pedals around. If you are fairly strong, reverse the process and pedal uphill. That way, you won't go too fast while learning to pedal and balance. If your legs are weak, pedal downhill, but first learn how to control your speed with your hand brakes.

One of the common concerns about technique has to

do with the use of the curved handlebars. If you have never used them, they are awkward and the so-called drop-down position may bother your back. In fact, you'll notice a lot of bicyclists with curved handlebars will ride upright holding the bar rather than the handles. The main virtue of the drop-down position is lower wind resistance. Dropping down also shifts your weight forward and allows you to get a more forceful thrust from your hips. For many situations, such as commuting or touring, especially if there are few hills, the reduced wind resistance and added thrust are not significant factors, and any comfortable handlebar is fine. Once you have gotten used to the curved ones, however, you will be surprised at how comfortable they are.

Biking, running, and skating complement each other very well, because they emphasize the use of different leg muscles. For many of us, bicycling will be recreational, rather than our main fitness sport. If you run regularly, you should be able to bike long distances fairly easily, although you won't keep up with someone who trains regularly on a bike. We've found, for instance, that you can bike about ten to twelve miles in the time you would ordinarily run seven and a half miles, while someone of equivalent athletic ability who has been training on a bike would cover fifteen to eighteen miles — without becoming nearly as sore as a part-time biker.

Supplementary strength exercise is very important in cycling, focusing on hands (grip strengtheners), arms,

upper back and shoulders (Figures 6–37 through 6–61), and lower back (Figures 6–63, 6–65, 6–89 through 6–101), and groin (Figures 6–71 through 6–76). Since your knees are such prime candidates for overuse injuries, strength work using the squat (Figure 6–68) or with resistance machines (Figures 6–77, 6–79) is very worthwhile. Because much of your body is relatively rigid during biking, our special program for your lower back (pages 158–159) as well as stretching exercises for your upper back and shoulders (Figures 6–14, 6–17, 6–18), your groin and quads (Figures 6–4 through 6–8), and extra lower-back stretches (Figures 6–10, 6–21, 6–24) comprise a good cool-down routine and are very helpful in preventing soreness.

GOALS AND FITNESS PROGRAMS

Weather aside, bicycling is an ideal sport for fitness. If you are overweight or are not very athletically inclined (as yet), biking is a great place to start. The first month or so should be devoted both to getting your legs used to continuous biking and to developing your "wind" (aerobic power). Find a nice area with a minimum of hills to start with, over which you can ride five to six miles without worrying too much about traffic, potholes, or dogs. Plan to ride about thirty to forty leisurely minutes per day, four or more days a week, getting used to the bike, allowing your seat to toughen up, and familiarizing your body with its new task. Ride at a seven- to eight-minute-mile pace or slower for the first week (i.e., thirty to thirty-five minutes for a four-mile course). Avoid any sensations of breathlessness or strain. Unlike walking or jogging, you are training your balance, reflexes, instincts, and ability to handle gears, brakes, and traffic, at the same time. So take it easy.

When this seems comfortable and your initial stiffness has disappeared, you can begin pushing up your pace somewhat. Your speed will depend a great deal on the terrain, on your facility with gears, and on your leg strength and aerobic capacity. As a rule, avoid breathlessness and pick a speed that leaves you slightly sweaty, somewhat tired, and faintly exhilarated. A six-minute pace (ten miles per hour) is a good one to start serious training. Maintain the same distance, but twice a week increase the pace to ten miles per hour, and the rest of the time go about one minute per mile slower. Each week, maintain a pattern of two fast and two to five slow days and gradually increase the pace five to ten seconds per mile per week until you can handle five miles at a four-and-a-half- to five-minute pace. You are

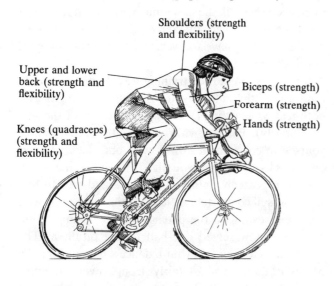

Shoulders (strength and flexibility)

Upper and lower back (strength and flexibility)

Biceps (strength)

Forearm (strength)

Hands (strength)

Knees (quadraceps) (strength and flexibility)

FIGURE 9–8: *Key Areas for Conditioning for Bicycling*

now functioning at a good intermediate range for cycling.

At this point, your goal should be to develop endurance, muscle strength, and maximal cardiovascular function by gradually extending the distance you go on slower days. If you can handle a five-minute fast pace and a six-minute slow pace, try to increase your distance by about 10 percent per week on your slower days, i.e., from thirty minutes to thirty-three minutes to thirty-six minutes, etc., while continuing your short fast rides. Your short rides will develop increased leg strength and aerobic capacity; the longer rides will increase your endurance. As with all aerobic sports, resist the temptation to increase speed and endurance at the same time. That combination leads to overuse injuries.

Many people who stay in shape with other aerobic sports (running, cross-country skiing) will be able to begin at about this level and ride for about one hour at a five- to six-minute pace, feeling somewhat sore in the rump and stiff for the first week or so, but thereafter finding cycling a good supplementary sport, offseason training aide, or just good enjoyment.

SAFETY AND PRECAUTIONS TO AVOID INJURY

Unfortunately, biking can be a hazardous sport. The National Electronic Surveillance System tells us that there were 556,682 biking injuries in 1984 — far more than in baseball (423,126), football (390,267), or basketball (440,293). Most cycling injuries occur because the operator of the bike was careless about automobiles, traffic laws, or road conditions, and 75 percent of biking accidents occur among children. These figures tell an important story. Most injuries are preventable, especially in noncompetitive situations, by a combination of proper equipment (gloves and a good helmet), common sense, obeying traffic laws (riding with traffic and stopping at lights), and defensive bicycling (anticipating and giving way to automobiles). Avoid hazardous conditions (bad roads and wet roads) and exceeding speeds at which you can control the bike. Use adequate reflectors and lights at night. Many bikes can use a long vertical pole with a flag to increase visibility on cross-country trips. This should be considered if you are doing a lot of touring or commuting.

There are many special situations that are dangerous. Avoid narrow, two-lane country roads. When passing parked cars, be alert for doors opening into your path. Watch for road hazards, such as sewer grating bars that can trap your tires, objects in the road, slippery pavement, hot tar. And, of course, drinking and driving is as bad for the cyclist as it is for the motorist.

Dogs represent a special hazard, more dangerous to the cyclist than to the runner. Short of using a chemical spray or outracing the dog, the most effective way of halting an attack is to stop and dismount, keeping the bike between you and the dog. You can usually walk away and resume riding a few hundred feet later.

We have already mentioned cold and frostbite (pages 176–177) but a word on heat injuries is appropriate here. Cycling can, like other intense, aerobic sports, produce so much body heat and sweating that dehydration and dangerously high body temperatures can occur with little warning. (See Chapter 7 for ways to prevent this.)

Besides trauma, there are a few characteristic, minor injuries associated with bicycling that everyone will meet sooner or later. Among those likely to strike sooner is *saddle soreness*. This can be reduced by altering the position of the saddle during long rides, or by shifting your position on the saddle. A chamois-lined pair of biking pants helps dissipate some of the pressure. Ultimately, the area toughens up and you will no longer have the problem. Women, however, have special problems because their pelvic bones are wider and the usual seat may not give them adequate support. Special saddles are now made for women and can be ordered through ads in cycling magazines if your bike shop does not carry them.

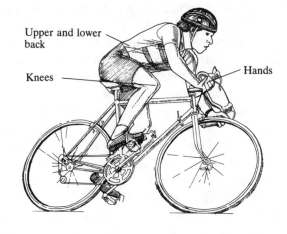

FIGURE 9–9: *Common Areas of Injury in Bicycling*

An analogous problem in men can cause the *numb crotch syndrome*. A long ride without shifting position has left many a rider with an absence of sensation in his crotch and the end of his penis, caused by nerve compression. The nerve damage is reversible, however, and sensation returns in minutes to weeks depending on the degree of damage.

Similar nerve damage can affect the hand, leading to the *numb finger syndrome*, in which riding with your weight on your hands can compress the ulnar nerve as it leaves the wrist and enters the palm. It usually affects sensation and strength of the fifth and fourth fingers and is likewise reversible. Padded gloves help dissipate the pressure and avoid the problem.

The most common biking injuries (Figure 9–9) are caused by overuse, and can be managed like other athletic injuries (see Chapter 12).

ADVANCED TRAINING

If you choose to go beyond fitness, to cycle for sports and even competition, you should build up to an average distance of one hundred to one hundred fifty miles per week, with short rides of five to ten miles alternating with longer ones, including at least one of thirty or more miles each week. Some of your cycling should be at a twelve-miles-per-hour pace or faster. Continue your supplementary conditioning and flexibility exercises. And plan to continue your sport year-round on an indoor biking device.

More advanced cycling depends on a mixture of technique, equipment, and conditioning. Gearing and pedaling frequencies become important, the weight and durability of your components and bike frame become crucial, and serious conditioning programs are necessary. This is true in part because of a unique factor in cycling: you have to overcome not only the resistance of friction and gravity (a lesser factor), but also wind resistance, which rapidly becomes the limiting factor as your speed moves beyond twelve to thirteen miles per hour. Dropping down on the handlebars reduces wind resistance and the energy cost of cycling.

If you decide to race, you are going to have to make a serious commitment. Racers, even sprinters, train very intensively, often averaging over three hundred miles a week. Because of the growing popularity of racing, many clubs now offer clinics in racing techniques and sponsor regular trials, which will help you develop the necessary skills. Finally, if your taste runs toward triathlons, remember that most are won by cyclists.

Biking in America is undergoing an interesting transition. In many parts of the world, biking is a primary mode of transportation, but in our affluent society four-wheel vehicles hold sway. Biking for health and fitness really began in the U.S. with the sage advice of Dr. Paul Dudley White, who captured popular attention after he treated President Eisenhower's heart attack. Even today, thirty years later, the bike path along the Charles River in Boston is named after Dr. White. But in the late 1960s and '70s we began to forget biking; the Arab oil embargo produced a flurry of renewed interest, but biking began slowly to drift back to its traditional role as a childhood pastime. Even in the fitness boom, biking has received less attention than it deserves. But this is changing, as biking is getting a boost from a new direction: racing. Americans fared brilliantly on bikes in the 1984 Olympics, and — wonder of wonders — the 1986 Tour de France winner was not a Belgian, Italian, or Frenchman, but an American — twenty-five-year-old Greg Lemond. You certainly don't have to race to bike for fitness, but we hope these marvelous achievements will inspire you to find your own level, and bike for fitness, fun, and even sport.

CROSS-COUNTRY SKIING

When people think of skiing, what often springs to mind are snow-covered peaks and chair lifts reaching up to the clouds. Unfortunately, however, downhill skiing rarely offers much in the way of aerobic fitness. The Alpine skier relies more on the forces of gravity than on his own muscle power for the thrill of the sport. And since this book emphasizes the aerobic benefits of lifesports, we find cross-country, or Nordic, skiing the more physically beneficial sport. And the quiet independence of cross-country skiing can't be beat, offering the skier a more controlled and less injury-prone sport.

Cross-country skiing can be enjoyed by people at all fitness levels. Beginners will find it an excellent recreational sport, requiring little more than basic fitness. Alternatively, cross-country skiing can be one of the most demanding competitive sports. Champion cross-country skiers must be among the most physically fit of all athletes, expending as much as 1,000 calories per hour during race conditions.

From casual touring to racing, cross-country skiing represents a unique pleasure, combining the exhilaration of sports with beautiful and always changing terrain and climate. It is one of the fastest growing sports in America today, benefiting from the general boom in fitness and the rising price of downhill skiing. Even with the trail "donation" of two to five dollars, it is an inexpensive sport. As a means of conditioning, cross-country skiing promotes excellent, all-around fitness — and at a time of the year when, at least in northern climates, there are few outdoor alternatives.

I (SRL) had skied downhill in the mountains of Colorado since I was a toddler, but after moving east in my teens, I had little opportunity to ski and began to run regularly. When the opportunity came to spend a long weekend cross-country skiing at Jackson, New Hampshire, the premier cross-country ski area in the Northeast, it seemed like a good idea. After all, I knew how to ski and I was in pretty good shape. After a few days of learning technique, I decided to try the Ellis River trail, about five miles of intermediate skiing. I was moving along pretty steadily, actually passing many people, and working up a good sweat. Just as I began to feel pretty proud of myself, I heard a soft "track" from the rear, and before I knew it, I was passed by a gray-haired woman of sixty, who looked forty and skied as if she were twenty. Her form was flawless, and she looked as if she were dancing. In contrast to my clatter, her skies barely whispered. Where I was sweating and breathless, she was hardly working. And in a second, she was by me and gone around the next bend. *That* is cross-country skiing.

Fitness *and* technique dominate this sport. Regardless of the fact that beginners can start touring with only a modicum of fitness, they will quickly reach limits that prevent them from taking on more difficult trails or even spending more time on easy trails. These limits are determined by their physical condition and, as I found out, by technique. Conversely, cross-country skiing is an excellent means of developing fitness, if you can spend enough time at it.

Cross-country skiing, as an aerobic sport, demands and produces a very high degree of cardiovascular fitness. In part because you use both upper and lower extremities, the energy demands range from 600 to 900 calories per hour, which is greater than any other sport except for competitive road racing. Cross-country skiing also demands and produces excellent endurance. Citizen races (see page 232) may be as short as five to ten kilometers or as long as sixty-five to seventy-five kilometers. Obviously, such energy demands have major effects on metabolism, burning calories at a rapid rate, helping you stay lean, and reducing blood lipid levels.

Muscular fitness requirements for this sport are equally arduous. As the beginner soon finds out, cross-country skiing uses all the muscles in the body. Proficiency requires high degrees of both muscular endurance and strength in these muscles. These are developed only with long months of practice. Cross-country skiing also requires good flexibility, especially in your lower back (because of the nature of the kickback), Achilles, and shoulders. Finally, balance, rhythm, and coordination are important corollary skills that cross-country skiing promotes. For most of us, the requirements for good fitness mean that we will have to be in shape to ski rather than expect to be able to ski ourselves into shape.

On the other hand, once mastered, skiing combines the grace and pleasure of dance with the vigor of running and the exhilaration that comes with the beautiful winter mountains. Of all the lifesports, it demands the most work. But there's no question it rewards the effort.

EQUIPMENT AND CLOTHING

What cross-country skiing demands in the way of conditioning, it forgives in equipment. Cross-country skiing can be almost as inexpensive as running. A good pair of cross-country skis can be had for the price of a pair of top-quality running shoes, and the skis should last for years. Poles, boots, wax, and gloves cost a modest amount more, and the rest is a matter of comfort. Since, during cross-country skiing, your body generates a great deal of heat, it's best to dress in layers so that you can shed or add clothing depending on your body's need for warmth. Some skiers begin their cross-country skiing experience in a pair of jeans, long underwear, turtleneck shirt, old sweater, and a knit hat, adding T-shirts for layers if the weather is very cold. That's fine for short tours (under five kilometers), but if you're going to ski greater distances — and most cross-country skiers do — it's sensible to dress in certain basic garments designed especially for the sport. Polypropylene long johns have been proven to have better wicking ability than ordinary cotton, silk, or woolen ones, and will keep your skin drier, and thus warmer, even on the coldest days. A turtleneck shirt (preferably polypropylene), nylon or corduroy knickers with woolen kneesocks, a lightweight hooded nylon or Gore-tex shell, a hat, and lightweight insulated cross-country gloves are all you will need to remain comfortable during most tours. For rest stops it's wise to carry a sweater or fresh turtleneck, and if you plan to ski a great deal on ungroomed trails, a pair of nylon gaiters will keep snow from accumulating around your boots, and thus are a sensible purchase. In all, you can dress and equip yourself for cross-country skiing for under two hundred dollars — considerably less than what you would spend for downhill gear.

What else? Unless you buy *waxless skis* (more in a moment), you'll need waxes and a means of applying them (corks, torches, etc.), of removing them (scrapers, rags, and solvents), and of carrying them along with your extra supplies, including trail snack (fanny or backpack).

Additionally, if you'll be traveling any distance to cross-country ski, a lightweight car rack makes sense: this, again, costs considerably less than an Alpine model.

The type of ski you buy depends largely on the kind of skiing you'll be doing. For most people, a good pair of *touring skis* allows them to negotiate most terrain at a typical cross-country touring center, and yet are also wide enough for easy touring through field and forest. As you improve, you may want to try citizen racing, using a pair of *racing skis,* which are lighter and narrower than touring ones and therefore faster and less fatiguing to use.

Once you've picked your skis, you'll need to select appropriate bindings and boots. Whichever boot you choose, make sure it fits you comfortably from heel to toe. Nothing is worse on the trail than an ill-fitting pair of cross-country boots and the blisters they can cause.

In the case of touring skis, new developments in *waxless bases* allow the beginner simply to snap on his skis and go. But for maximum performance both up and down hills and in all snow conditions, *waxable skis* remain the better choice. In principle, ski waxes work by creating a surface smooth enough for gliding forward while providing purchase against the snow's crystal structure, retarding slippage of the ski during the "kick" phase of cross-country's stride (more on technique in a moment). Different temperatures and snow conditions require different waxes. Your local cross-country touring center can give you helpful pointers on how to apply wax, and in most cases will cheerfully do the job for a fee. In general you should not be cowed by the seeming mysteries of waxing — it's really a fairly straightforward skill if you approach it in a logical way. As you ski during the course of a day, you'll find that snow conditions change, even in a matter of hours. What was correct wax for a bright midday sun no longer works at 4 P.M. with the sun slanting through the pines. Thus, to be able to ski independently all day, you should master the art of waxing. Fortunately, many good guides are available.

Even more than hiking, cross-country skiing is one of those sports during which eating and drinking are essential. For tours longer than two to three hours, bring a bottle of water and a variety of trail snacks, combining seeds, nuts, raisins, chocolate bits, and other goodies.

Enough advice for now: it's time to get skiing.

GETTING STARTED AND TECHNIQUE

By now you know that cross-country skiing is a skill sport. Touring with waxless skies on groomed trails at your local golf course can provide a wonderful winter's afternoon of pleasure for the beginner, but to progress to twenty-kilometer trips on mountain trails, you'll need both fitness and finesse.

We advise beginners to take lessons. Choose a ski area that offers lessons for all skill levels. The so-called diagonal stride — the kick and glide — and various poling and skating techniques are not natural movements and require guidance and patience. Even if you have downhill skiing experience, you will also need to learn how to turn and how to stop in deep snow.

Until you've had lessons, you can get started on relatively flat trails on your own. First, get used to walking on snow wearing your cross-country skis. Notice how your heel comes off the ski on your trailing foot. Place

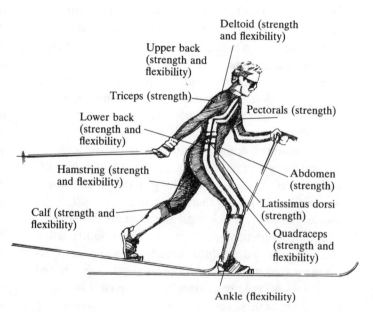

FIGURE 9–10: *Key Areas for Conditioning for Cross-Country Skiing*

your pole ahead of you on the side opposite the trailing foot (you alternate poling in rhythm with your stride). Next, push off lightly with the trailing foot. As your heel comes off the ski, put your weight on the ball of your foot and push your ski forward, at the same time pushing with the pole on that side. Slide the trailing foot to catch up once you've given yourself a little forward momentum. Alternate sides, pushing the rear ski and pole rhythmically to get your momentum. Then you are ready for the characteristic cross-country skiers' motion, the kick (see Figure 9–10). Instead of just pushing off, push and then lift your leg and foot slightly from the hip, to unweight the ski before gliding it forward. The kicking action uses your lower-back, buttock, and hamstring muscles. The backward kicking phase takes practice, but is the essence of the diagonal stride.

Terrain deserves a word, especially when you are ready to get off the flat trails. Many towns in the Snowbelt have golf courses that double as cross-country ski courses in the winter, and have some gentle hills. As your skill improves, you will want to travel to specialized cross-country ski areas. The best ones provide groomed trails, warming huts, lessons, and waxing services. They also mark trails, from beginner (flat) to expert (steep hills that demand good waxing and good technique). There is a natural tendency to overestimate your skill and level of conditioning, so try a short run first.

Even if your access to snow is limited, you can use one of the special cross-country exercise devices to learn the rhythm and timing of the cross-country stride while also improving your fitness. Among the best is the cross-country ski trainer (see Chapter 6 for details). A more portable (and less-expensive) machine, but which works only the upper muscles used in skiing, is the Exer-Genie, which you attach to a doorframe so you can practice the poling motion while pulling against resistance. Roller-skis allow you to "ski" outdoors all year round. They are long, roller skate–like devices that combine wheels with an aluminum track and binding. They have a ratchet on the wheels, which prevents them from rolling backward, allowing you to feel a real kick. However, while they are the next best thing to New Hampshire in February, they are expensive (one to two hundred dollars a pair) and a bit difficult to use correctly at first. In addition, falling on a paved road while using roller-skis can be a far more injurious experience than falling in fresh snow while skiing. We recommend you use roller-skis in the off-season only after you've learned to ski on real snow.

GOALS AND CONDITIONING

Developing your technique requires practice and instruction. Developing the stamina necessary to be able to ski for two to three hours requires hard work. Since cross-country skiing uses so many of the body's muscles, conditioning has to be multifaceted. Figure 9–10 shows all of the various areas of the body used in cross-country skiing.

As cross-country skiing uses practically every muscle group, you have to train each of them specifically to prepare yourself. The major muscles include: (a) the quads, calves, and hamstring muscles of the leg used in uphill skiing and in the diagonal stride; (b) the trunk muscles, including the abdominals, used in trunk bending and pulling, and the lower-back muscles, used in the kick; and (c) the muscles of the upper body, including the trapezius, the deltoid, the latissimus dorsi, the pectorals, and the triceps, all used in poling.

Cross-country conditioning begins with cardiovascular fitness and endurance. While all aerobic sports contribute to cardiovascular fitness, running is probably the best because it more closely mimics every part of skiing action. As alternatives, biking (because it relies on the quadriceps muscle) or swimming (because it emphasizes the upper body) are good supplementary aerobic conditioning sports.

Add to these workouts a variety of lower-extremity exercises with weights (Figures 6–51 through 6–59) or use resistance equipment and concentrate especially on doing leg extensions (Figure 6–61), hamstring curls (Figure 6–60), and calf raises (Figure 6–64).

Your trunk muscles — abdominal and lower back — will likewise benefit by a combination of sports, calisthenics, and stretch routines. Kayaking, rowing, and canoeing are excellent conditioners for the back and upper body. Sit-ups, both conventional bent-knee and twisting ones (Figures 6–80, 6–81), remain the primary strength builders for your abdomen. It can make sense to use an incline board or a small weight held behind your head to increase the resistance, thereby building increased strength (Figure 6–82). Leg raises will help build the lower abdominals (Figure 6–83). To achieve greater levels of back strength, do "good morning" exercises (Figure 6–57) and clean and press (Figure 6–58). As with all trunk exercises, don't do them if you have back pain.

Your upper body — shoulders, upper back, lats, chest, and arms — also requires strength training if you are to ski at your best. Swimming is the best complementary sport, using all of these muscles. For the rest, you should rely on a full array of upper-body exercises. Be sure to include various press exercises for your chest and triceps (Figure 6–54 through 6–56), pull-down exercises for your lats (Figure 6–52, 6–53), dips for arms and shoulders (Figure 6–75), and exercises for your upper back (Figure 6–34). Use free weights to concentrate on key exercises such as bent-over rowing, one of the most important arm and back exercises in cross-country skiing (Figure 6–37), and side lateral and front dumbbell raises (Figures 6–45, 6–46).

Just as cross-country skiing requires general muscular conditioning, it requires a thorough stretching program as well. Using Chapter 6 as a guide, spend ten to fifteen minutes going through the following stretches: calf, hamstring, and quad stretch of the leg (Figures 6–1 through 6–4), careful toe touches (Figure 6–11), back extensions (Figure 6–90), William's and cat's back exercises for the back (Figures 6–12, 6–13), lateral side bends (Figure 6–18), windmills (Figure 6–77), shoulder stretch (Figure 6–14), and the leaning chest stretch (Figure 6–17). All the advanced, yoga-style stretches are useful (Figures 6–20 through 6–27).

Finally, to achieve improved balance, practice Bob Woodward's "stationary diagonal": stand on one leg and start the other leg and opposing arm swinging. Do this on each leg for about two minutes, swinging your arm and leg backward and forward easily (Figure 9–11).

We have stressed conditioning so much because cross-country skiing is as sensitive to your level of fitness as it is to technique. For that reason, conditioning should be a year-round effort. Of course, cross-country skiing is an ideal component of a balanced fitness program.

In the winter months cross-country skiing substitutes wonderfully for running or other aerobic exercises. But if skiing is your focus, develop a year-round training program. During the spring, focus on aerobics by running, biking, jumping rope, or swimming. During the summer, maintain your aerobics and add (or increase) upper-body sports such as swimming, canoeing, and calisthenics, as well as some muscular conditioning one day per week. During the fall, supplement the aerobics and muscular conditioning with hill and interval training and a cross-country ski trainer. Then, when the snow hits, you should be ready to go.

SAFETY AND PRECAUTIONS TO AVOID INJURY

Cross-country skiing may be a cold-weather sport (although some of the most remarkable runs will come in 40 degrees during spring thaws), but it is far from a chilling experience. In fact, it is quite the opposite, and that represents yet another challenge. Cross-country skiing generates as much or more heat as competitive running, once you are able to maintain a sustained stride. It may be 10 degrees below zero on the thermometer, but inside your shirt it is pushing 100 degrees plus as your muscles burn up enormous quantities of energy, much of it going into heat production.

Generally speaking, you have to deal with this heat just as you would for other sports, but with even more attention and care since you may be out for four or more hours, and cold air and rest stops add to the problem by cooling you down. Resourceful dressing, flexibility, and planning are the keys:

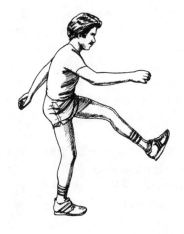
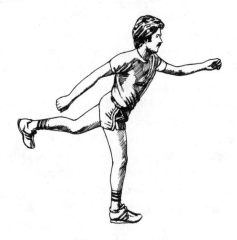

FIGURE 9–11: *The Stationary Diagonal Exercise*

1. Dress in layers for insulation and so you can peel down or dress up as your activity and the climate dictate.

2. Your clothes should have zippers or be made of stretch fabric, so that you can change quickly when necessary.

3. Carry lightweight duplicates of essentials, such as your hat, mittens, and socks, whenever you plan excursions lasting more than two or three hours. Lives are saved by a few extras.

4. Dress for wetness. You'll be wet from perspiration and, if you fall, from the snow. Moisture will produce rapid cooling if you are suddenly confronted by adverse conditions, such as falling temperature, a headwind, disappearing sunshine, or anything that forces you to slow down or stop. Heat is lost most quickly through cotton or older synthetic garments. Make sure you wear *wool* socks, hats, gloves, and sweaters. Or consider the new synthetics such as polypropylene (see pages 191–192) — like wool, they have the ability to insulate even when wet. Insulating, heat-retaining garments save lives.

5. Plan. Planning doesn't only mean choosing a route, but also providing for rest and food stops and checking the weather, paying special attention to the "wind chill factor," in order to calculate your clothing needs.

6. Advertise your route and leave your estimated time of arrival with a responsible party. People do survive unexpected nights on the trails, but never wish to repeat the experience.

7. Prepare for accidents. In particular, this means broken ski tips. An easy glide on three feet of powder can turn into an exhausting nightmare if you break a ski tip, since the snow won't support your weight off skis. Along with extra clothes and food, a temporary snap-on ski tip belongs in your backpack for any trip away from well-traveled trails.

Among the more unusual problems with climate, frostbite is often forgotten. Just because you are soaking your shirt with sweat does not mean that your ear tips, out there in a twenty- to thirty-mile-per-hour breeze, can't begin to freeze. Keep vulnerable areas covered. Likewise, don't forget your fluid needs. You will lose water as fast skiing in the winter as you will running

in the summer. So carry fluids, and stop and drink often (see Chapter 7).

Cross-country skiing is reputed to be a sport low in injuries; compared with downhill skiing, the injuries tend to be less serious but they do occur, usually from falls. One of your first lessons should be how to fall safely — a relaxed fall can prevent many injuries. Prevention also means attention to muscular conditioning of the knee and lower leg, as well as the recognition that the downhill component of cross-country skiing poses hazards.

Another type of traumatic injury occurs during tours in the woods, where wayward branches can prove dangerous to hands, head, and eyes. Again, caution is the only way to prevent injuries.

And don't neglect overuse injuries. In cross-country skiing, overuse can affect arms, shoulders, back, knees, or calves, and is similar to the tendinitis, bursitis, and muscular pulls seen in other sports (see Chapter 11). One unique type of overuse injury occurs in cross-country skiing because of the "kick." That motion uses the muscles of the lower back and buttocks, which are difficult muscles to condition and are very susceptible to overuse and inflammation. Pain usually occurs in the area midway between the thigh and the hip. Ice, anti-inflammatory medications, and stretching will help. To prevent further injuries, the back-kick routine taken from aerobic dance and described in Figure 6–95 can be helpful.

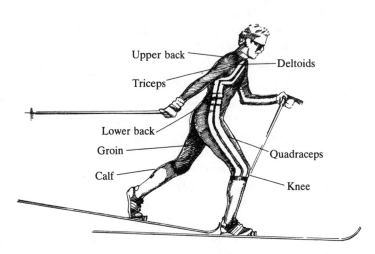

FIGURE 9–12: *Common Areas of Injury in Cross-Country Skiing*

ADVANCED TRAINING

Advanced training for cross-country skiing involves skill drills for technique, and even more conditioning. We have already addressed the proper method of basic, year-round conditioning, but if you want to race, your conditioning work will have to be longer and more frequent than we described earlier. You probably should add upper-body exercises and light weight workouts even in the spring. Use every opportunity to ski, whether on the slopes or on machines.

Like other aerobic sports, cross-country skiing requires speed training for anyone who wants to compete (see Chapter 6). More advanced skiing also requires an aggressive approach to hills and the ability to tolerate anaerobic conditions briefly.

Hill running and hard biking will help in this regard. Hill running means literally charging hills in a manner and at a pace similar to what you will need to ski. As your strength improves, pretend you have poles and are using them up the hill or, better yet, use a pair of old poles with broken tips and bound up the hill.

Obviously, skill training requires that you ski as often as possible. Off-season, the cross-country ski trainer will help develop the coordination, timing, and balance vital to this sport. Advanced techniques such as skating, double poling, charging hills, and downhill skiing require on-snow instruction and practice, practice, practice.

Because of its intensity, conditioning for cross-country skiing can be all-consuming. Since it involves so many different types of training, burnout can occur. Moderation is the key. Think in terms of seasons and years, not in terms of days and weeks. Avoid burning out by paying attention to your body; when you are fatigued, lessen the intensity of your training. If you have had a very hard day, follow it with an easy day. Use a training log to help yourself progress. Move forward in small increments, not giant leaps. And try to achieve balance between your training and the rest of your life.

When the time comes to race, the best plan is to begin by joining one of the many citizen races organized by local clubs. Citizen races exist in most areas in the United States and are held all winter long. These shorter races (usually ten to thirty kilometers) offer local competition combined with good skiing, scenery, and good fellowship. These are the races to begin with, building later on to the longer-distance races.

The most notorious citizen races make up the "Great American Ski Chase," which is a series of races conducted in different areas of the country. They are roughly fifty kilometers in length, and the United States Ski Association can provide information on these. A longer race, sometimes as long as ninety kilometers, is the U.S. Birkebenier, part of a worldwide series. Famous ski races, like running marathons, attract upward of ten thousand participants and are as much of a spectacle as a sport. Like marathon runs, entering with a goal to finish is the ambition of most of the skiers; with proper conditioning, this is an attainable goal.

Whether you join in a mass race with thousands of fun-loving outdoor enthusiasts from eight to eighty years old, or whether you ski simply to escape into a peaceful, silent forest miles from anyone else, you will find Nordic skiing a beautiful, very satisfying sport.

ICE SKATING

Who could watch Scott Hamilton performing one of his spectacular routines during the 1984 Olympics and not dream of learning how to skate like that; or cheer for Eric Heiden's unique triumphs in the 1980 Olympics, and not look around for a pair of speed skates? For a sport so especially photogenic, skating engenders an unusual impulse to participate, not just watch.

But ice skating is really four sports, not one. True, the skates and the ice are common, but beyond that, recreational skating, figure skating, speed skating, and hockey (see Chapter 10) are very different sports, as far from each other as downhill skiing is from ski jumping. Recreational skating is a sport for all ages and all levels of athletic ability. Speed skating is a high-speed sport for highly conditioned athletes. And if sports had personalities, hockey would be the milltown roughneck, while figure skating would be the elitist aesthete. Each type of skating has special conditioning requirements as well.

But all varieties of skating demand good aerobic conditioning. In fact, speed skating is one of the most demanding aerobic sports; Eric Heiden, who won every speed skating competition at the 1980 Olympics, was probably one of the best-conditioned athletes in the world. His feat, equivalent to a runner winning every distance between the 100-yard dash and the 10,000-meter, demanded anaerobic conditioning and speed for the sprint and aerobic conditioning for distance, a very rare combination. Hockey, on the other hand, with periods of one to ten minutes of intense activity followed by inactivity, is akin to basketball in its requirements. Figure skating is similar to dance and requires stamina, strength, speed, flexibility, and superb body control. That leaves recreational skating, which can be anything you want. But as with so many sports, the better shape you are in, the more you can enjoy it.

As a lifesport, skating, when done regularly, contributes to cardiovascular conditioning and endurance. It falls between running and bicycling in its energy demands, though of course the intensity at which you skate will be a major determinant. Its musculosketetal demands are very similar to bicycling, depending extensively on quad strength. It's no surprise that Heiden went on to win the first U.S. Professional Cycling Championship five years after skating to the gold. Unlike cycling, however, skating involves the upper extremities as well, and is thus a more balanced form of exercise.

The aesthetic features of skating — its demand for balance, rhythm, coordination, and timing — are what make it such a unique sport and so enjoyable for participants of all ages. As with bicycling, once you have learned, you can always skate. You have only to go to your local rink to see people well into their seventies enjoying it. And recently noncontact hockey has become a major recreational game for adults over forty.

EQUIPMENT AND CLOTHING

All you need are skates. What kind you get depends on what kind of skating you do and/or your level of expertise. Hockey and speed skates have a smooth blade, primarily designed for a smooth, stroking stride. Figure skates have a variety of different tooth patterns at the front of the blade, allowing spins, turns, and jumps. If you are serious about the sport, buy the boot separately from the blade. Look for proper function and ignore fashion and endorsements. A good boot should be high enough to support the ankle without enclosing the calf. It should have a well-padded tongue and provide good padded support at the toes, arch, and ankle. Make sure it fits well at the ankle bones, arch, the small toe, and the Achilles — the major pressure points when skating.

The blades for figure skating should be bought separately and attached by an experienced fitter. The alignment of the skate on the boot will differ from person to person. Figure skating blades have many particular features depending on the type of figure skating you do; free skating, for example, uses a different blade than does dancing. Most people begin figure skating with a good all-around blade.

Comfortable, loose-fitting or stretch clothing is all the additional equipment necessary, unless you skate outdoors and need gloves, hat, and scarf. Of course, as with all aerobic sports, you generate a lot of heat and will have to be able to adjust your clothing as you warm up.

The most difficult (and potentially expensive) requirement for the sport is rink time. While rinks are available year-round even in the deep south, for most people skating means competing for relatively scarce ice time, which is a particularly severe problem when you need an entire rink for hockey or figure skating practices. This leads to two A.M. practice sessions and other types of behavior reasonable only to devotees.

Recreational skaters tend to wait for the cold weather. Skating weather usually arrives at about the time when it is difficult to ride bicycles and so it fits neatly into a year-round fitness program.

GETTING STARTED AND TECHNIQUE

Skating requires coordination, speed, strength, flexibility, grace, body control, and agility. To skate well, you need to be in the same good shape as to participate in any rigorous aerobic sport. Since skating is a seasonal sport, this means you will need to get into shape and stay fit using other forms of exercise. For skating, the best complementary sport is bicycling. Besides the aerobic benefit, cycling develops the quad and hip extensor strength and endurance that skating requires. While running will condition your heart, it differs mechanically, so that some skating coaches recommend it for supplementary training only as a last resort.

The next step is to define your goals. Do you want to be a casual recreational skater, content to go out and skate circles around the rink? Or are you the dedicated amateur skater, developing some of the skills of hockey, speed, or figure skating? Or the competitive skater, training diligently for top-level efforts?

If you want to play hockey, much of your effort will have to be directed toward puck handling. If speed skating attracts you, you will have to find a suitable rink and work on style and conditioning. The most structured training exists for figure skaters. Once you have developed a reasonably smooth skating style, the next step involves lessons. Under the guidance of a coach, you will learn "compulsory figures," groups of two to three symmetrical circles with precise turns, and free skating techniques, including jumps, spins, positions, and combinations.

For the dedicated figure skater, progress means passing a series of well-defined, progressively harder tests. These are administered by the Ice Skating Institute of America (ISIA), a network of twenty thousand members and three hundred clubs around the country, or the U.S. Figure Skating Association (USFSA), comprised of forty thousand members and four hundred fifty affiliated clubs. Over one hundred thousand skaters a year take these tests, but many others enjoy skating for fitness and for fun.

For all skaters, careful warm-ups are necessary, because on-ice maneuvers make unique demands on your muscles. Go through a good stretching routine, emphasizing your groin, legs, and lower back. Then skate easily for five to ten minutes to get the blood flowing and your muscles warm.

GOALS AND CONDITIONING

Basic aerobic fitness is necessary for skating, but on-ice conditioning is essential if you want to become reasonably proficient. The recreational skater must train for three to four hours per week to achieve good aerobic capacity, and at the highest levels of competition, skaters train for four to six hours per *day*. The figure skater will have to divide his or her time between the practice of skills (compulsory and free skating) and speed and endurance training. Special drills are used to develop both speed and endurance.

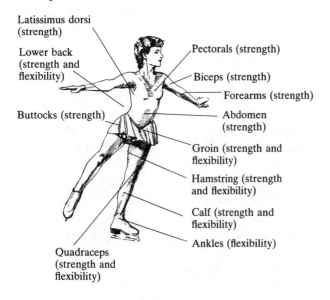

Latissimus dorsi (strength)

Lower back (strength and flexibility)

Buttocks (strength)

Quadraceps (strength and flexibility)

Pectorals (strength)

Biceps (strength)

Forearms (strength)

Abdomen (strength)

Groin (strength and flexibility)

Hamstring (strength and flexibility)

Calf (strength and flexibility)

Ankles (flexibility)

FIGURE 9–13: *Key Areas for Conditioning for Skating*

Off-ice training focuses on strength and flexibility. Skating requires good strength at the extremes of motion, and Nautilus equipment helps toward this end. Skating demands strong quads, buttocks, hamstrings, groin, and ankles. Less obvious, but no less important, is the contribution of upper-body strength. See Chapter 6 for regimens to strengthen all these areas.

Pay particular attention to your groin muscles, which are stressed by skating's unique stride; jumping jacks (Figure 6–93) are an excellent way to condition them. For increased strength, try straddle hops (Figure 6–66) or use Nautilus equipment designed to exercise the abductors and adductors of the hip (Figure 6–70). This is especially useful for hockey's many quick stops and starts.

Ankle strength is built by skating, of course, as well as by systematic exercises with foot and ankle weights. In addition, do regular heel-and-toe walking. Perhaps one of the most useful devices to build ankle strength is a tilt board made up of a 3-foot by 4-foot section of plywood balanced over a 3- to 4-inch round log or dowel. Standing evenly and tilting back and forth develops good balance and ankle strength. It is, incidentally, a good way to rehabilitate from an ankle sprain. Build up until you can tilt from side to side for ten to twenty minutes at high rates of speed.

Upper-body strength, especially back, shoulder, and upper arm, is very helpful in "power skating," which refers to the quick start and quick changes in direction that hockey demands. Conventional programs of muscular exercises for the upper body are sufficient, and are discussed in Chapter 6.

Except for figure skating, skating develops very little flexibility. The lower extremity and back muscles of skaters are often tight, leading to a high prevalence of groin, hamstring, and lower-back strains. Prevent these by very aggressive stretching programs for your groin, calves, hamstrings, and lower back. If you are going to play hockey, spend twenty minutes a day on a full series of these stretches. Finally, we recommend dance and rope jumping in addition to bicycling as good exercises to complement skating. They develop good aerobic fitness, good ankle, foot, groin, and upper-extremity conditioning, and help with balance, timing, and coordination.

SAFETY AND PRECAUTIONS TO AVOID INJURY

There are, of course, the usual overuse and overstress injuries. For skaters these commonly involve the groin, ankles, and back. A study of elite figure skaters for example, revealed that nearly half suffered a significant injury during a one-year period. The reason may be found in another result of the survey: on average, these skaters spent only one *minute* doing flexibility and warm-up exercises for each 2.2 *hours* of skating. Avoid similar problems of your own by careful warm-ups, supplementary strength training, and careful flexibility exercises.

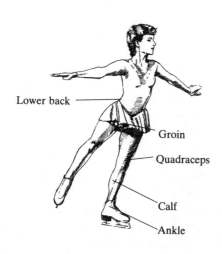

FIGURE 9–14: *Common Areas of Injury in Skating*

Carefully fitted boots will prevent pressure sores over the heel, arch, or front of the foot, the other areas of common disability. Good boots will also support your ankle and help avoid sprains and fatigue.

The major cause for injury is, of course, falling. The better you skate, the less likely you are to fall. Turning, starting, and stopping correctly will keep you out of trouble and will decrease your risk of falling. However, learning the proper way to fall is essential for skating; rolling, relaxed falls will prevent many injuries.

More important are hockey-related injuries. While this discussion properly falls into the section on competitive sports (see Chapter 10), we want to emphasize the importance proper safety equipment plays in any sport using a ball or puck. Don't play hockey without a helmet and face protection. This equipment has already made a dramatic difference in the injury rate in junior hockey players. In addition, we'd prefer to see the contact aspect of the sport eliminated, focusing instead on the skill of the game: skating, puck handling, and shot making. There are senior hockey leagues that have adopted these rules, and it has made hockey for adults a safe, enjoyable, and highly beneficial sport.

ADVANCED TRAINING

The competitive figure skater is in the small minority. Advanced skating puts a premium on athletic skill. The enterprising beginner starts as a youth, and develops slowly with years of training. The skater may need an hour of lessons per day, spending an additional two hours on compulsory figures, one to two hours on free skating, and another hour conditioning for speed and endurance. The speed skater likewise will put in long hours. Eric Heiden's training included biking, practice on the ice, and supplementary exercise for hours each day. Except for hockey, there is not very much formal skating competition available for the adult. For most skaters, then, personal improvement becomes the goal. For them, skating well is its own reward.

In the last two chapters, we've discussed a large sampling of "lifesports," sports you can participate in all your life, which in turn contribute significantly to your good health and fitness. They range from the most basic (walking) to the most elegant (figure skating). They share a common foundation in good aerobic fitness, and if you can do one, you can try any of them — and we hope you do.

10

Competitive and Team Sports: Racquet Sports, Basketball, Soccer, and Hockey

Our focus is on fitness and health. Until now, we have emphasized lifesports, which all contribute significantly to cardiovascular and musculoskeletal fitness. While lifesports require skill to perform at an advanced level, they can all be enjoyed by beginners and by people of all ages.

However, lifesports are only part of the picture. Most Americans watch competitive team sports, and many have played them — or would like to. Even a dedicated runner will want to help out when her company plays a rival in softball, or help his kid make the basketball team by playing some one-on-one with him (and then try out for the senior league himself). The number, variety, and popularity of competitive sports attest to their importance. The question is, what is the role of team sports in fitness?

First of all, team sports are *fun*. They provide companionship; they reward talent as much as perseverance; the payoff comes in hours and not in years; and the preparation and post-game activities are almost as much fun as the games themselves. *Games*. That's what competitive sports are. And games are not just for kids. Games provide recreation, and recreation helps us live our adult lives more fully. A hard, long run may provide satisfaction and a sense of accomplishment; a hard match of tennis also provides exhilaration. Winning a tough game adds to the fun of competitive sports, if you avoid developing an obsessive thirst for victory. You are not playing for a silver trophy or a multiyear contract — a competitive spirit can add to the fun of sports but if

"winning is the only thing," it can be a decided drawback (see Chapter 3).

Besides their recreational and social characteristics, competitive sports have one other unique characteristic — they call on such neurologic and physiologic skills as eye-hand coordination, spatial orientation, and the ability to react quickly to changing circumstances. Team sports require that the participant function in traffic and know where his teammates are and what they are likely to be doing. Games require thought, strategy, planning, and intuition — often in the face of physical fatigue. Team sports also frequently ask the participant to subordinate his personal goals to those of the team.

To be played effectively, team sports require considerable amounts of learning and coaching. You don't need a mentor to learn how to run, but few people can play good tennis without lessons. And once you've joined a basketball or hockey team, coaching and practice sessions will concentrate on finesse rather than fitness. Thus, unlike the lifesports, you won't be able to play yourself into shape — but if you get into shape, you will play better, with fewer injuries.

Despite important differences, team sports make certain common demands on the athlete. Many competitive sports require both aerobic and anaerobic conditioning; they demand rapid bursts of intense activity interspersed with periods of lower intensity in a start-and-stop, push-and-pull pattern. Thus, they require interval training techniques (see Chapter 6, Speed Training) to allow you to accelerate to very intense levels and then to drop back for a while and recover. Of course, some of the intensity is mental, produced by the enthusiasm of competition.

The same change of pace that challenges your cardiovascular system also asks a lot of your muscles. Besides good basic conditioning, you'll need explosive strength and quickness, relying on anaerobic, high-energy, fast-twitch muscle fibers. Similarly, you'll need good dynamic flexibility to handle sudden movements and changes of direction.

But most of all, these sports demand highly developed neuromuscular control — that is, coordination, timing, balance, quickness, and kinesthetic sense. Your basic FAS(S) program can help in each of these areas, but the principle of specificity demands that the specific skills of each sport be practiced on the playing field. Hitting against a backboard in tennis, dribbling in soccer, and shooting baskets in basketball are essential training methods, developing technique and coordination while conditioning specific muscles.

Figure 10–1 highlights selected competitive sports and the demands they make on your body and Figure 10–2 lists some other properties of these sports. In general, you will choose a team sport for recreation rather than for fitness. Use these tables to tailor a fitness program around your sports and your goals. In most cases, you'll need a supplementary aerobic program for cardiovascular conditioning and systematic speed drills to build up your peak capacities. You will also need specific flexibility, strength, and endurance training to maintain balanced fitness and to do your best at each sport. Use these tables and the FAS(S) program to design a personal program for total fitness and sports.

GETTING STARTED

Starting out in any sport depends on your fitness and skill level, the demands of the sport, and the need for partners, teams, and coaching. For example, archery requires little fitness besides upper-body strength, but does require good eye-hand coordination and enough coaching to bring you up to a skill level that allows

---

FIGURE 10–1: FITNESS REQUIREMENTS OF SOME COMPETITIVE SPORTS

Scale: 0 (none) to 4 (high)

Sport	Aerobics	Speed	Strength Upper Body	Strength Lower Body	Endurance	Flexibility	Neurophysiological Skills and Coordination	Skill Level Required*
Archery	0	0	3	0	0	2	4	2
Baseball/softball	2	2	3	3	1	3	4	1
Basketball	3	4	3	3	3	4	4	2
Bowling	0	0	2	1	2	2	3	1
Fencing	3	3	3	3	3	4	4	3
Football, touch	3	3	3	3	2	3	2	1
Golf (walking)	2	0	2	1	1	2	4	2
Gymnastics	3	3	4	4	4	4	4	3
Hockey	3	4	3	3	3	3	3	2
Martial arts	3	3	3	3	4	4	4	3
Skating, figure	3	3	3	3	3	4	4	3
Skiing, downhill	3	4	3	4	4	3	4	2
Soccer	4	3	3	4	4	3	4	2
Tennis and other racquet sports	2	4	3	3	3	3	4	2
Volleyball	2	3	2	3	3	3	3	1

Italicized are discussed in the following pages.
*Skill level: 1 implies that even beginners can play with enjoyment. The higher numbers imply that full participation needs coaching, practice, and talent.

competition. Touch football requires moderate general fitness, but you can have fun at it even while you are a beginner — if you get a group together. Tennis requires modest cardiovascular fitness, but good coordination and a moderately high level of skill.

Because competitive sports all require a mix of coaching, camaraderie, competition, and equipment, most are organized around clubs and leagues. Clubs allow you to meet others with similar interests, find partners or teammates at your skill level, and get coaching or instructional help. So if you decide to become actively involved in sports, look around for a club or team nearby.

Coaching can be tricky. It can be hard to find a good coach or instructor, particularly since the player-coach chemistry is so important. A world-class player may be a poor teacher: knowing how and showing how are very different skills. Avoid the drill-sergeant type unless you know that's what you need to get off your duff. Don't be afraid to experiment. Ask around. Find someone who has already helped others; this is the best indication of successful coaching.

Finally, don't neglect warm-ups and cool-downs in all team sports. The sudden demands of the game mean that your muscles have to be warm and loose *before* you play. As a general rule, do a thorough regimen of stretching, then five minutes of aerobics and five minutes of technique-specific drill. Whether it is tennis, hockey, or basketball, starting cold leads to poor play and frequently to injuries.

After the game, cool down to help avoid the muscle soreness and aches that intense play produces. Jog or walk for two to five minutes to keep your circulation moving, flushing waste products from your muscles, and go through another round of stretching exercise to keep your muscles and joints loose.

CONDITIONING

Basic conditioning for all team sports calls for your own version of the FAS(S) program described in Chapter 7. A good aerobic base is the cornerstone. Muscular endurance should be developed as well, by the use of calisthenics, exercise equipment, and complementary aerobic sports. Strength conditioning for all muscle groups is important, but team sports demand especially high levels of arm, shoulder, back, neck, abdominal, knee, and ankle strength. Flexibility in these areas and in the groin should be correspondingly high. Professional teams

are finally incorporating flexibility training, realizing that the sudden changes in a player's direction and speed can lead to injuries unless a player's flexibility is ideal.

In general, we suggest aerobic workouts of forty-five to sixty minutes at least three times a week in the off-season; during the season, supplement practice and game sessions with aerobics as needed. Muscular strength work should be done twice a week after your other workouts. A year-round program of this sort will provide a superb level of conditioning, sufficient for the basic demands of all amateur competitive sports.

In addition to a program of flexibility, aerobics, strength, and speed, high-level conditioning will also work on areas specific to competitive sports. Speed or sprint training is one of these. Many of these sports require explosive and intense effort interspersed with periods of rest. You will have to train yourself for this. Many hockey, basketball, and soccer practices include "wind sprints." But they are also important for tennis or even softball. If you want to compete at a high level, speed conditioning is necessary (see pages 159–160).

As you recall from Chapter 2, many important neurophysiological skills (balance, coordination, kinesthetic sense, reaction time) are not sport-specific. In this regard, playing tennis may well help your basketball, and rope jumping may help your softball game. Just because your sport is seasonal doesn't mean you should retire for the rest of the year. On the contrary, if you don't play a competitive sport each season, take up a lifesport to keep you fit year-round.

Competitive and team sports provide remarkable rewards for those who stay in shape. As I (SRL) have found out, being able to ski better at age forty than at age fourteen, solely because you are in shape, is a powerful motivator. And the rewards of top-flight tennis, especially if you are already a super senior, make the hours of conditioning worthwhile. The rewards of these sports not only supplement your fitness regime but, more importantly, enrich your entire life.

SAFETY AND PRECAUTIONS TO AVOID INJURY

Competitive sports pay many dividends. But intensity and enthusiasm also set the stage for injuries. About 5 percent of all basketball and soccer players are injured each year; in hockey, the figure approaches 10 percent.

Unfortunately, some are injured seriously enough to require hospital treatment.

Injuries in team sports differ from those in lifesports. While endurance athletes often develop tendinitis from intensive training (the "too much" part of the overuse syndrome), competitive athletes tend to get strains and sprains from intensive play without enough conditioning (the "too soon" part of the equation). And even non-contact play, as in racquet sports, can produce unexpected collisions with the ball, racquet, wall, floor, or even an opponent. Thus, *trauma* is a large part of the injury pattern in competitive sports.

Fortunately, these injuries are caused by factors that can often be controlled:

- the "enthusiasm factor," when that extra effort you put out for your teammates in reaching an unreachable ball results in a torn hamstring;
- the "absent coach factor," when poor form, poor play, and excessive physical contact result from insufficient instructions;
- the "bad habit factor," when behavior such as mixing beer and basketball produces problems on court or field;
- the "poor conditioning factor," when you try to make your body perform in early April the way you can in July;
- the "poor equipment factor," when faulty fields, racquets, balls, or shoes cause disasters, both minor and major;

- finally, the "absent equipment factor," when the missing headgear in hockey or the eye guard in squash can lead to tragedy.

Proper coaching, conditioning, habits, and equipment, combined with some common sense — that's the prescription to prevent many of these problems.

And while trauma is impossible to eradicate, restricting the contact in competitive sports will reduce injury greatly. The elimination of spearing in football and the spread of noncontact hockey and touch football are good examples of ways in which organized sports have dramatically reduced injury rates.

SPECIFIC SPORTS

In this section, we discuss a typical competitive sport (tennis) and three representative team sports (basketball, hockey, and soccer). These sports are prototypical, popular, and can play a role in your conditioning program. Tennis is a good example of *"ball-and-stick"* sports. It combines start-and-stop play with requirements for eye-hand coordination, strategy, and good overall conditioning. Other sports in this category include squash, racquetball, handball, Ping-Pong, and badminton.

Basketball, though it puts a premium on height, is the ultimate *"team sport"* in which anticipation, passing skills, and the importance of teamwork are as important as individual skills. Very high level cardiovascular

FIGURE 10–2: OTHER ASPECTS OF COMPETITIVE SPORTS

| | | | Injury rate | |
| | | | contact injuries | noncontact injuries |
Sport	*Seasonal*	*Requires coaching*		
Archery	−	+	Low	Moderate
Baseball/softball	+	±	Low	Moderate
Basketball	−	+	High	Moderate
Bowling	−	±	High	Moderate
Fencing	−	+	Moderate	Low
Football, touch	+	±	Moderate	Low
Golf	+	±		Low
Gymnastics	−	+	Moderate	Moderate
Hockey	+	+	High	Moderate
Martial arts	−	+	High	Moderate
Skating, figure	±	+	Moderate	Moderate
Skiing, downhill	+	+	Moderate	Moderate
Soccer	+	+	Moderate	Moderate
Tennis and other racquet sports	−	+	Low	Moderate
Volleyball	−	+	Low	Low

Italicized sports are discussed in the following pages.

fitness is necessary for basketball, as well as as for hockey, soccer, and other team sports.

The features of some other sports are outlined in Figures 10–1 and 10–2. These sports can also be classified functionally. Downhill skiing is the best example of what might be called *"challenge sports,"* in which the competition is between nature and yourself. Companionship, yes; teamwork, no. Talent, technique, and conditioning are equally important; natural beauty, exhilaration, and the enjoyment of conquest are the rewards. Sports as diverse as mountain climbing, waterskiing, skydiving, and, at the tamer end of the scale, orienteering and golf share some of these attributes.

Other sports, such as baseball and softball, are *"role sports,"* in which each player has a defined task and offensive and defensive modes alternate, so activity is interrupted frequently. Conditioning and skill requirements for these sports depend very much on the player's position, and coaching is very important. For these sports, we emphasize only the need for conditioning and the potential for injury.

The *"devotional sports,"* including martial arts, gymnastics, and figure skating, share the need for long-term, intense devotion to develop the requisite top-level skills and total conditioning. These sports are relatively easy for beginners, but improvement requires coaching, practice, and commitment as well as fitness. These activities can be very worthwhile and rewarding, returning dividends in proportion to the time invested, but they are not for the weekend athlete.

Last and, from the health point of view, least are the *"contact sports."* Football, rugby, boxing, and lacross are representative of this group. They are enormously popular sports, particularly for spectators. They have some merits, but health and fitness certainly cannot be numbered among them. Injury is a risk run by all athletes, but sports that require contact are clearly out of place in a health and fitness guide.

TENNIS (AND OTHER RACQUET SPORTS)

Racquet games are among the most popular sports in America, with more than forty million participants. Whereas squash retains a faintly elitist flavor, tennis underwent a popular boom in the 1960s, and racquetball became immensely fashionable in the 1970s. Although the racquet boom has leveled off (8.6 million tennis racquets were sold in 1976, versus 2.7 million in 1984),

the broad-based popularity of these sports is assured.

What accounts for such popularity? Stick-and-ball games have been part of human society since the beginning of civilization, with variations in every culture. Games involving competition, skill, strategy, and exercise appear necessary for man, and racquet sports are one of the easiest and most acceptable ways for adults to play games in our society.

Tennis is a prime example of a competitive sport as compared to an aerobic or lifesport. Tennis does contribute to fitness, but its recreational and social aspects account for its popularity. In fact, skill can compensate for poor fitness — a wily, skilled fifty-year-old player with a potbelly can triumph over a twenty-three-year-old triathlete who tries to substitute endurance for technique. However, fitness *is* important — in games between players of comparable skill and motivation, the player who is in better shape will win every time.

Tennis can even be your major aerobic exercise — if you play *vigorous* singles at least three times each week. Doubles, in contrast, is no more intense than moderately paced walking. Squash and racquetball can be very intense and beneficial — if you are fit enough to play for an hour and skilled enough to sustain rapid action. The same is true for an old standby that resembles racquetball without the racquet or the sex appeal: handball. And if racquets are your thing, you can get a surprisingly good workout from badminton or even Ping-Pong. Here, too, you must be fit, skilled, and determined if these sports are to be helpful aerobically.

EQUIPMENT AND CLOTHING

Tennis does not require a major investment in equipment. A good racquet can cost $60–$80, a good pair of tennis shoes, $30–$40, and the rest of the outfit can be assembled from your bottom drawer if need be. Granted, you will have to buy balls, but many communities have public courts that enable you to bypass steep club dues and court fees. Not so for indoor tennis, squash, and racquetball, unfortunately. Many Y's provide good courts at reasonable prices but you will most likely have to pay some sort of court fee in any event.

Your *racquet* should be well balanced, and should have the largest grip that you can comfortably handle. Many frames are available, but no one material is superior to the others. Midsized or oversized racquets are an advantage, especially to the novice, because of the larger "sweet spot." We recommend that you avoid extremely tight strings; in a standard-sized racquet, 16-

gauge gut string between 52 and 55 pound is usually best. Avoid playing with heavy, dead, or wet tennis balls — a case of tennis elbow is more expensive than a dozen cans of new balls.

The most neglected equipment for racquet sports are the shoes. Except for running, skiing, and skating, athletic footgear is generally built for style rather than for proper play and injury prevention. The situation is improving, but there is no substitute for careful shoe selection. For racquet sports, the primary characteristics to look for are a sole that provides proper traction, forefoot construction that is flexible enough for you to get up on your toes, and good lateral stability to prevent your foot from turning over as your weight shifts side to side. Don't wear your running shoes for racquet sports — they simply don't have enough lateral support.

GETTING STARTED AND TECHNIQUE

Tennis is a wonderful sport, but it is very technique-intensive. If you've never played, you will have to invest time and money in lessons. There is no other effective way to learn how to hit properly, keep the ball in play, or master basic strategy. Your enjoyment from tennis is proportional to your skill. If it is going to be an important game for you, make the effort to learn good technique. Squash and racquetball are a bit easier for beginners, but still require coaching and practice.

Racquet sports rely on superior eye-hand coordination, balance, and the smooth transmission of power to the ball, all of which must occur while you are in motion. To develop adequate skill, you will have to practice your strokes intensively, find a coach, a partner, a ball machine, or a backboard, and hit, hit, hit. But always remember to warm up thoroughly — racquet players are the most negligent of all athletes, and they pay the price in injury.

CONDITIONING

Exercise training is very important for racquet sports. At first glance you might assume that tennis involves only a little running and a small amount of arm motion, but in truth, tennis places great demands on your cardiovascular system, shoulders, arms, wrists, hands, upper back, lower back, abdominal muscles, groin, quadriceps, hamstrings, calves, and feet.

Tennis requires total conditioning, and playing it well demands high levels of conditioning. Aerobic training and calisthenics are necessary for endurance, and speed training is necessary to get you from baseline to net quickly. Use running, biking, or other aerobic exercises to build stamina, and interval training to build speed (see Chapter 6).

Here's an example of one tennis player who understood the necessity for conditioning in his game. Immediately after unseeded Boris Becker stunned the tennis world by winning the 1985 Wimbledon at age seventeen, his coach announced that he would start a mountain running program to build endurance and balance before the U.S. Open Tennis Championship. Boris Becker obviously knows that in sport, winners don't rest on their laurels — or on their duffs.

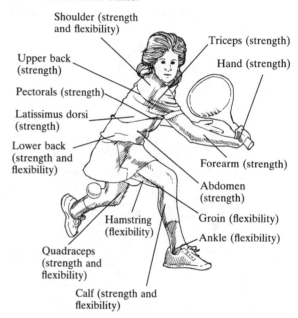

FIGURE 10–3: *Key Areas for Conditioning for Tennis*

For top-notch tennis, muscular strength should be built by a combination of calisthenics and weights. Resistance equipment can be helpful, but for most players dumbbells or barbells will be more than enough. Similarly, stretching exercises will increase your range, and protect you from injury. Supplement the FAS(S) program in Chapter 6 by grip exercises using a spring-loaded hand exerciser.

SAFETY AND PRECAUTIONS TO AVOID INJURY

Tennis is better known for its "elbow" than for its "leg," but any part of a player's body can suffer from overuse injuries. Tennis elbow is provoked by bad form on the backhand or serve, as well as by overuse and forearm weakness.

Another area of major concern in tennis is the lower back. The number of weekend tennis buffs who have back trouble is legion. Nor does this injury spare the professional; even someone as young as Tracy Austin can have serious back trouble. Tennis leg is also common, occurring when a sudden forward surge tears the muscle under the calf. Even the foot can be injured, as the name "tennis toe" suggests.

Eye injuries are important but often neglected. They are more prevalent in squash and racquetball, but occur in tennis as well. Just as a helmet is essential for biking, proper eyewear is essential for racquet sports, meaning safety glasses or goggles. The prevention and management of all these problems are detailed in Chapter 12.

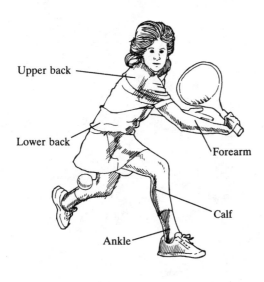

FIGURE 10–4: *Common Areas of Injury in Tennis*

STRENUOUS TEAM SPORTS: BASKETBALL, SOCCER, AND HOCKEY

Despite their obvious differences, basketball, soccer, and hockey are all examples of team sports that require both fitness and skill. And, like the other sports in this category, the whole is more than the sum of its parts. Teamwork means subordinating individual play to the requirements of strategy, role-playing, and cooperation. A pickup game of basketball will have relatively little of these elements, while a well-coached team will emphasize them. Coaching, then, is the crucial unifying element in team sports. But don't despair, even if your team consists of a self-coached, Sunday morning collection from the over-the-hill gang. Playing together for a while will develop teamwork and allow you to enjoy camaraderie and competition, even if you don't win often.

These sports also share another requirement — the need to function in traffic. They are fast-moving games in which the puck or ball is being passed back and forth between rapidly moving players in shifting patterns of offense and defense. Highly specialized neurophysiologic adaptations (balance, coordination, kinesthetic sense) distinguish the superstar from the substitute in team sports.

Each sport, of course, has unique requirements. Soccer is one of the world's most popular sports and can be one of the most demanding. In the last several years, it has begun to catch on in the United States as well. It is played by children and adults, men and women, with varying levels of skill. Your ability to control a ball with your foot (or head) improves with practice, and makes enormous demands on your neck, upper and lower back, groin, and leg muscles. Combine a large, uneven field, intense bursts of sprinting with only short rest periods, and the need to integrate your play with that of your teammates, and you have one of the ultimate team sports.

Although professional basketball is dominated by the tall, the game is played by men and women of all sizes in gyms and playgrounds all around the world. Dribbling, ball movement, passing, and good defense are as important as good shooting. Full-court basketball, too, is a running sport, with brief periods of rest punctuated by spurts of high speed. A half-court game demands less speed and stamina, but still calls for great coordination and teamwork.

The most dominant characteristic of hockey is speed, greater than that in any of the other amateur team sports. Add sudden stops, a loose puck, passing, and nonstop action, and you'll see why hockey is such a challenging and exciting sport.

EQUIPMENT AND CLOTHING

As with most competitive sports, footwear is the most important item for individual players. Though important, there is nothing daunting about shoes or skates — but a hardwood court, a grassy field, or a frozen rink are indeed impressive bits of equipment. In fact, the need for specialized facilities is the greatest drawback of team and competitive sports.

Other equipment is specific to each sport, but we should emphasize the importance of helmets and face protectors for hockey. Since their introduction into junior league play, the injury rate has fallen dramatically. Without this protection, a puck traveling at one hundred miles per hour is a lethal missile indeed.

GETTING STARTED AND TECHNIQUE

To get started in any team sport, you need a team. Pickup games are enjoyable but unpredictable. To develop individual and group skills — and, indeed, to play with enough regularity and intensity to improve fitness — a core of regulars is best. With the growth of leisure time, teams for basketball, soccer, and hockey exist in most major urban centers and are often divided by age groups. In fact, there is even a senior (over fifty) national men's hockey tournament. Most important, join a team at your own skill and fitness level. If you are a novice, look for an instructional league, or check to see if your local YMCA/YWCA or JCC sponsors beginners' teams or provides instruction. If not, it will be difficult to get started; you may even have to learn from your own kids.

CONDITIONING

All three sports require the three basics of fitness: flexibility, endurance, and strength, and in all three there is nothing optional about the fourth type of fitness train-

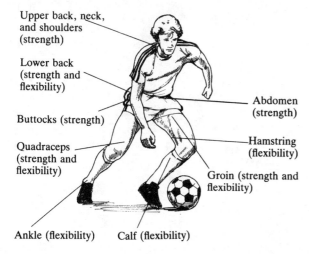

FIGURE 10–5: *Key Areas for Conditioning for Soccer*

ing — speed. But each sport goes beyond balanced fitness to require special skills. In soccer, these include heading the ball and dribbling. Proficiency requires lots of practice and special exercises. Running at an aerobic pace does not prepare you for the quick start-and-stops, cuts from side to side, and the back-and-forth leg movements that you use in dribbling a soccer ball. The same obviously holds true for your neck and upper-back muscles. Coaching drills will help you, but you have to do extra work to strengthen these crucial areas. Do a full set of groin exercises, including jumping jacks (Figure 6–93). Practice running backward as well as forward,

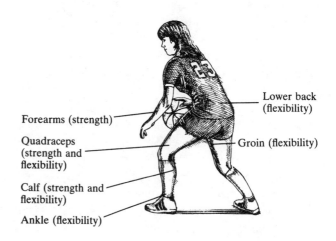

FIGURE 10–6: *Key Areas for Conditioning for Basketball*

and run patterns to prepare for lateral moves. Do careful leg, groin, and lower-back stretches (Figures 6–1 through 6–13, 6–15, 6–16, 6–18), and add our special program for your back (pages 158–159). Work hard at your abdominal muscles as well. And find a good Nautilus training center where you can do abductor and adductor exercises for your groin muscles (Figure 6–70).

Basketball also demands special skills, especially jumping, dribbling, and quick side-to-side and twisting motions. Since much of your running is backward or to the side, do the same running drills suggested for soccer. Lower-extremity strengthening programs will help your jumping, and should include special work for your quads and exercises to build your calf muscles. The smaller muscles of the feet and ankles can be helped by rope jumping. Once you are in shape, vigorous full-court play will itself provide excellent exercise and training for fitness — if you play two or three times a week and play a running game. Shooting alone won't suffice. But even if you play an NBA schedule, supplementary exercises can enhance some of your skills and help prevent injuries. Warm-ups and cool-downs, which involve full stretching programs as well as shooting baskets, are essential.

Conditioning for hockey means developing the capacity for bursts of high-intensity play on the ice. Assuming that you have developed your aerobic base, add interval training and skate your speed drills if you can get enough ice time. If not, the best alternative for interval training is a stationary bicycle. Another method is to run hills, charging up and jogging down. Hills and the bike will concentrate your training where you need it — on your quads.

The major muscular demands of hockey are on the groin, quads, and hamstring muscles. Nontraumatic injuries affect these areas, and betray a lack of attention to good strength and flexibility training. In addition, upper-body strength contributes a good deal to acceleration or "power skating." So a program to stengthen the shoulder, trunk, and back is very important. Knees, of course, are a major problem in hockey, largely from the trauma of checking, and quads require extra work.

The final point about hockey is that it seems the least advanced in terms of pre-game warm-ups. Skating for a few minutes may get the blood circulating, but does little to loosen up all the injury-prone areas we have discussed. It's hard to sit and do groin stretches on the ice, so you'll have to do these exercises in the dressing room.

SAFETY AND PRECAUTIONS TO AVOID INJURY

In team sports, injuries come from the problems we discussed in the introductory section — too much enthusiasm, too little conditioning — but also from trauma. Soccer and basketball have managed to keep physical contact from becoming a goal in itself, and although contact occurs, it is not generally applauded (and is even penalized). Unfortunately, contact, or checking, is part of the mystique of hockey and a variety of injuries are specifically caused by this. Hockey has a very high incidence of knee injuries caused by checking, and unfortunately torn meniscal cartilages do not heal. We strongly favor noncontact hockey, where finesse and skating skill are emphasized. Many of the adult amateur leagues have adopted these rules and we strongly support this trend.

Safe hockey also requires that you learn to skate well, both forward and backward. Since your risk of injury is strongly related to falls, you will play a much safer game if you learn how to fall in a relaxed manner. And again, we strongly urge the use of helmets and face protectors.

Groin pulls are one of the most common injuries for both soccer and hockey. Their prevention and treatment are detailed in Chapter 12. Basketball, while it has its share of groin pulls, is more likely to cause knee trouble of the tendinitis, bursitis variety, and ankle strains. They too are discussed in Chapter 12.

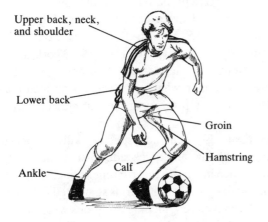

FIGURE 10–7: *Common Areas of Injury in Soccer*

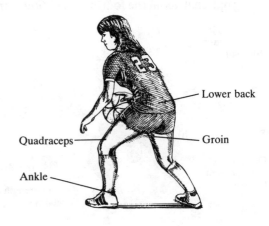

FIGURE 10–8: *Common Areas of Injury in Basketball*

This survey of typical high-intensity team sports is not meant to be all-inclusive, but rather it should provide some models for this type of recreation. Team sports offer the fun of playing games, the need for teamwork, the reward of camaraderie. They require good conditioning for adequate play and to prevent injuries. And they supplement either pure conditioning exercises or the lifesports as a means of staying fit and healthy.

IV

SPORTS MEDICINE

The Prevention, Recognition, and Treatment of Common Athletic Injuries

11

The Basic Approach to Athletic Injuries

Sports medicine is perhaps the fastest-growing new medical specialty. Not surprisingly, the growth of sports medicine directly parallels the popularity of physical fitness and exercise in this country. Even the most fanatical fitness advocate would have to acknowledge that there is a causal link between exercise and injury; we, too, must admit that even with the most diligent preparations and precautions, injuries will still occur in the course of exercise and sports. In Part IV we discuss the diagnosis and treatment of common sports injuries, and we stress rehabilitation, which is both a tool to speed your return to sports and an important technique to prevent recurrent injuries. So prevention is one of our major themes.

In discussing these injuries, we will emphasize the most common problems and highlight the relatively mild difficulties that you can manage yourself. We will not attempt to be encyclopedic, and we will certainly not try to turn you into doctors. We hope that our guidelines will help you deal effectively with any minor injuries; however, if you do not improve according to schedule, get additional help. We ourselves follow this rule when dealing with our own aches and pains — if they seem more severe than usual, or if they simply don't come along quickly, we seek the advice of a colleague rather than treating ourselves. The doctor who treats himself has a fool for a patient, and the athlete who persists in self-treatment beyond the point of common sense is no less foolish.

WHAT IS SPORTS MEDICINE?

If you do need expert medical help, what kind of doctor should you see? A good general physician should be able to handle 50 to 60 percent of sports-related medical problems (see Chapter 5 for guidelines on selecting a physician). Unfortunately, many doctors haven't kept current in exercise physiology and tend to refer sports problems to orthopedists. Orthopedists, or "bone doctors," have long been the backbone of sports medicine, as indeed they should be. However, even among orthopedic specialists important differences exist. Perhaps an anecdote from my own (HBS) experience will help illustrate this. When I first began marathon running, my left knee developed a rather sizable joint effusion ("water on the knee"). My knee was only slightly painful, and the swelling did not interfere with my running. However, I wanted to be sure that continued running would not damage my knee. I sought a consultation from a very experienced and widely respected orthopedist, who examined me carefully and did blood tests and X rays. The results were encouraging: he could find no clearcut evidence of joint damage. His advice, however, was the epitome of common sense: since your knee is swollen, there must be some subtle injury, and since it's injured, you should not run on it. Fortunately, the fluid went down quickly, so I did not have to stop running. However, when the problem recurred a few weeks later, I consulted with a younger but no less respected orthopedist who is himself an athlete. The examinations were similarly negative and the basic diagnosis was the same. But the advice I got was slightly different: unless it gets worse, cut down on your mileage as much as possible and try to avoid hills and hard running. Again my knee improved, only to swell again as I resumed intensive marathon running. My third consultation was with an orthopedist who specializes in sports medicine. For the third time the examinations were negative, but now the advice was geared to the athlete: keep your knee lightly wrapped, ice it down after you run, and use common sense — but unless the problem gets worse you can stick as close as possible to your training schedule.

Today I run more miles than ever without any knee problems at all, probably as a result of extra exercises for flexibility and strength. But this story may help illustrate why sports medicine is becoming a new specialty. The bone, joint, and muscle problems that complicate sports are subtly different from the aches and pains that occur in people who don't exercise. Even more important, dedicated athletes require special handling. Sports medicine specialists recognize this and gear their treatment plan toward continued participation in sports if at all possible. If rest is required, alternate forms of exercise are prescribed so that the athlete can keep fit even while he is recovering from his injury. Likewise, a major emphasis is put on rehabilitation and prevention of future problems. Finally, psychology plays an important role in sports medicine. Athletes will often disregard advice to rest an injured limb unless they are given a prescription for other activities that can fill their need to exercise. And if true rest or immobilization is absolutely needed, a sports medicine specialist who understands the athlete's psyche may even put him in a cast or brace just to be sure the advice is followed, even if that cast is not essential for healing.

Although orthopedic surgeons remain the key figures in sports medicine, one of the nice things about this field is that it is becoming a truly multidisciplinary endeavor. Sports medicine clinics often include internists or cardiologists to help with exercise prescriptions, general aspects of fitness, and cardiopulmonary complications of exercise. Podiatrists are integral members of the team, dealing with problems of the foot and prescribing orthotics, which may even help alleviate problems of the leg, hip, or back. Physical therapists play a crucial role in directing rehabilitation programs and in prescribing exercises for flexibility and strength. Athletic trainers may assist in this process, and are often the most knowledgeable individuals when it comes to practical matters such as taping. Finally, coaches are often involved in the sports medicine process, because they are best able to identify areas of technique that can lead to injury, and they can help plan training regimens designed to improve performance with fewer injuries.

Needless to say, we hope you never have injuries. In the real world, however, minor problems are almost inevitable from time to time if you exercise strenuously. Hopefully, you can manage these yourself with the aid of the advice in this chapter, but for problems that are persistent or more serious, see a doctor. If you need help, you can start with your personal physician or internist. If your problems persist, or if your situation is complicated to begin with, you should see an orthopedist who is interested in sports medicine or go directly to a multidisciplinary sports medicine clinic.

THE APPROACH TO SPORTS INJURIES

As much as we enjoy seeing athlete-patients, we'd rather have you spend your time running on a track or court instead of running to your doctor every time you get an ache or pain. So let's look at a five-point program that can enable you to take the first steps toward managing your own problems.

1. *Recognize your injury or impending injury as early as possible.* This may seem like very obvious advice, but athletes are notorious deniers and often overlook and ignore important early warning signs of trouble. Don't do it. Early recognition will allow you to get early treatment, and may help you avoid more serious problems later on. The most obvious symptom of most sports injuries is pain, but the pain of an early injury can be easily mistaken for the "normal" aches and discomfort of intense training or competition. Other telltale symptoms of injury may be stiffness or decreased mobility, abnormal swelling, or even audible crackles and creaks when you move an injured joint. Or the first signs of an injury may be extremely subtle, including fatigue, loss of desire, or simply diminished performance. Most confusingly of all, an injury to one part of your body may show up first as pain in an altogether different area. A good example is knee pain; knee injuries are among the most common problems of athletes, but knee pain may sometimes occur in healthy knees as a result of

underlying difficulties in the foot or hip. We don't want you to be obsessed with your aches and pains, or to fret about every subtle nuance of athletic performance, but we do want you to listen to your body so that you can promptly identify illness or injury.

2. *Identify the cause of the injury.* It's well and good to know *what* hurts, but it's just as important to know *why* it hurts. If you can identify the cause of the injury, you'll be able to treat it most effectively — and also to prevent similar problems in the future.

The most common cause of athletic injuries is *overuse*, the cumulative effect of repetitive motions, which eventually produce excessive demands on your body. Clearly, overuse injuries mandate a change in your training schedule, with a prompt decrease in the intensity and frequency of exercise and then a slow, gradual buildup to the levels you desire.

Another common cause of injury is *overstress*. Here the problem is not the gradual, repeated trauma of overuse, but a single, sudden, excessive force. For example, runners may develop ankle problems through overuse because of running mile after mile, day after day. In contrast, an overstress injury can occur in the briefest instant: a false step into a pothole may twist your ankle, resulting in a sprain or even a fracture. Overuse injuries are typically gradual and subtle, whereas overstress injuries are often both abrupt and dramatic.

Trauma is a special form of overstress that accounts for many athletic injuries. Although we have not emphasized contact sports in this book, because they are basically not good for your health, falls and other forms of direct trauma can occur inadvertently in any sport. You won't be likely to overlook traumatic injuries, but you should know how to treat them promptly to contain the damage.

Less dramatic, but no less important causes of sports injuries are *muscle imbalance, lack of flexibility,* and *biomechanical problems* such as flat feet, a short leg, or an abnormal stride. These problems usually don't begin to bother athletes until they move from the beginner to the intermediate or even advanced stages. The reason is that continued training may exaggerate a muscular imbalance because certain muscles may develop more than others during training, particularly if you are emphasizing only one sport. Similarly, as muscles become stronger they tend to become stiff and tight, so if you don't stretch diligently, you may develop injuries caused by lack of flexibility. Exercises for strength and flexibility are the key to correcting these problems. Sometimes shoe inserts called orthotics can be ex-

tremely helpful for biomechanical defects such as a slightly short leg or flat foot.

The other major causes of sports injuries are *faulty equipment* and *improper technique.* You can often make this diagnosis yourself by simply inspecting your running shoes and finding that they are excessively worn, or by checking your tennis racquet and discovering that the grip has been too small for all these years. Or you may think back and discover that your problems first began when you switched to a new shoe or racquet. Even if you can't identify an obvious problem with your equipment, it's always a good idea to bring your gear with you when you go to a sports medicine clinic. Similarly, even if you can't spot your own error in technique, a knowledgeable friend may be able to watch you closely and pick up the flaw. Sometimes your opponents are the best source of this information. Best of all, return to basics by checking in with a coach or a teaching pro — your injuries may disappear even as your game improves.

3. *Estimate the severity of your injury.* If your problem is mild, you may well be able to keep on playing with the aid of a modified schedule, special exercises, and simple treatments or medications. If, on the other hand, the problem seems more serious, use common sense and back way off or turn to another sport that will allow you to rest the injured area until you are better. Finally, if the problem has even the potential to be more serious, get professional advice instead of fiddling around with self-treatment. This applies particularly to any of the sort of difficulties that may affect your heart, circulation, or lungs, as discussed in Chapters 1 and 12.

4. *Initiate early treatment.* This is the key element to self-management of athletic injuries, but it's not as complicated as you may think. The secret to success is PRICE. No, we're not being mercenary doctors, and you won't need to show anyone your Blue Cross card to follow this advice. Instead, PRICE is an acronym for the five steps that will allow you to realize a savings in the cost of medical treatment — and even more important, a reduction in pain and disability.

Protection is the first principle. An injured area must be protected against further damage. Protection can take many forms, ranging from a sterile dressing to cover a cut or scrape, to an elastic wrap for a mild sprain, to a splint or even a cast for a severe sprain or fracture. Although your doctor will have to apply these fancy protective devices for serious injuries, you should always think of simple ways to protect minor injuries from further damage.

*R*est is of central importance in the early management of sports injuries. An injured tissue simply cannot be expected to go on doing the same things as healthy parts of the body. Rest, of course, is the enemy of the athlete in training and is often the treatment principle that is overlooked or ignored. But remember that rest need not be absolute, and is certainly not a one-way ticket to your easy chair. Sometimes rest can be very brief — if, for example, you turn your ankle during a tennis match, you may have to retire for the afternoon and rest for as little as a day or two before you resume playing. In addition, rest can be *selective*, so you can maintain overall fitness even while you are resting an injured part of your body. For example, Joe Namath swam one and a half miles per day using arm strokes only while resting his injured knees — and went on to win a Super Bowl. Alberto Salazar rested a running injury but was still able to use his legs strenuously on a stationary bike — and went on to set a world record in the New York Marathon. In a curious way, an injury can sometimes be a blessing in disguise, in that it can force you to develop balanced fitness. You may even develop new skills and discover new sports that you can enjoy long after your original injury has healed and the "rest period" is over.

*I*ce is the cheapest, simplest, and yet the most effective treatment for many sports injuries. This is particularly true for mild to moderate injuries that involve tissue trauma or inflammation (see below). Ice can be helpful in many ways. You'll appreciate it at once, because the application of cold will deaden pain. You'll appreciate it even more later on, because ice will decrease swelling and inflammation to help limit tissue damage and allow earlier rehabilitation and recovery. We'll describe various methods for applying cold when we discuss basic treatment modalities for athletic injuries (see pages 257–258). For now we'd just like to emphasize the importance of acting immediately. In the case of an acute overstress injury, apply an ice pack or cold compress as soon as possible after the injury occurs, keep it on for fifteen to twenty minutes, and apply cold repeatedly four or five times a day for the first twenty-four to forty-eight hours after your injury. In the case of chronic overuse problems, you may want to apply cold after each and every time you exercise. For example, a runner with chronic Achilles tendinitis may ice down his ankle after each run.

*C*ompression is also important for the early management of many athletic injuries. Pressure will help reduce swelling and inflammation, and can therefore be very helpful to limit tissue damage and speed recovery. For most minor problems, compression is simply a matter of wrapping the injured area in an ace bandage as soon as possible.

Compression will also provide helpful protection and support for your injured region. However, you must be very careful in applying any form of compressive dressing. The goal is to provide gentle pressure on the injured area *without* pressing so hard that you interfere with your circulation. The tricky thing is that swelling can progress for many hours after the injury has occurred; the bandage which is only slightly snug at first may become downright hazardous if it is not loosened as the tissues underneath become more and more swollen. So remember to apply your compressive bandage with care, and to loosen and rewrap it if it seems tight later on. Another trick is to place a small piece of foam rubber directly on the site of the injury and then wrap the bandage over this bit of foam rubber. This approach may allow you to produce just a little pressure on the precise area that needs it, without clamping down on your healthy tissues or circulation.

*E*levation is the fifth and final component of the PRICE approach to the early management of athletic injuries. Elevation is a simple strategy that will enlist the force of gravity to drain fluid away from the injured region so that swelling, inflammation, and pain will be reduced. You don't have to stand on your head any more than you have to go overboard with our other principles of treatment. To elevate an injured foot, for example, you may want simply to prop your leg up on a hassock or foot stool, or to rest in bed with a pillow or two arranged comfortably under your leg. You won't cure a sprained ankle merely by elevating your foot, but every little bit helps.

PRICE is the key to the self-management of athletic injuries, particularly in their earliest phases. But even this five-point program may not do the trick. Simple medications such as aspirin or other anti-inflammatory drugs can provide additional benefit, and we'll discuss these on pages 262–263. For more serious injuries, your doctor may prescribe stronger medications or a wide variety of additional treatments. But even if you suffer a severe accident or injury, you'll make your doctor's job a lot easier if you follow the PRICE program on your way to the office or emergency room.

5. *Rehabilitation* is the final element in your program for the self-management of athletic injuries. Rehabilitation should begin where PRICE leaves off; as soon as the early acute damage subsides, you should begin

to work toward restoring motion and strength so that you can return to sports. Ultimately, the goal of rehabilitation should be to build yourself up so that you are stronger than ever before and, hence, less likely to have recurrent injuries. We just cannot accept such traditional teachings as "Once sprained, always sprained" — you *can* prevent recurrent or chronic problems of this sort by gradually building yourself up.

Active rehabilitation involves many components. Exercises are the key. Begin with isometrics, so that your muscles can contract and build strength without moving injured tendons, ligaments, or joints before they are ready to be mobilized. As you improve, you can gradually add range-of-motion exercises and finally isotonics to build muscle strength over their entire range of motion. Specific exercises, of course, depend on the part of your body that is injured; we'll talk about some of these when we review individual injuries in Chapter 12.

Another helpful element in rehabilitation is heat. We are not contradicting our enthusiasm for ice when we prescribe heat, because we are prescribing these thermal extremes at different times in the injury-recovery process. Ice is crucial early on, but when it's time to mobilize injured tissues in the recovery phase, heat can be very helpful. Heat can also be extremely useful during the warm-up period when you return to play. There are many ways to apply heat, ranging from simple warm packs to elaborate diathermy treatments, and we'll outline these on pages 258–259 when we discuss basic treatment modalities.

We've stressed the importance of early rehabilitation, but it's equally essential to be patient and persistent — rehabilitation is something that just can't be rushed. As a rule of thumb, it is reasonable to allow yourself three days of rehabilitation for each day that you miss because of an injury. Athletes tend to become very frustrated by a long-drawn-out process of rehabilitation; remember, however, that your goal is to be better than ever before, so patience and hard work will eventually be amply rewarded.

COMMON SPORTS INJURIES AND WHAT TO DO ABOUT THEM

". . . ITIS"

Even a casual reader of the sports pages will recognize "itis" as one of the important common denominators of sports injuries. Indeed, throughout these pages we have referred repeatedly to "itises" of various sorts, including tendinitis, bursitis, and arthritis. If you are already an athlete and have experienced some of these injuries, you may well regard "itis" as a four-letter word. In fact, this simple suffix can be applied to so many different types of problems simply because it connotes inflammation.

Although more than twenty years have passed, we clearly remember intoning the five cardinal signs of inflammation with our fellow first-year medical students: *calor, dolor, rubor, tumor*, and *functio laeso*. Happily, you don't have to study medicine or even Latin to understand the major manifestations of inflammation; we've all had "itis" of the tonsils or sinuses, and anyone who has trained for the Boston Marathon has most likely had at least a little "itis" of tendons or joints. So we can all recognize that inflammation causes warmth, pain, redness, swelling, and diminished function of the body area involved. In fact, these simple terms are the exact translations of the fancy Latin names we learned in medical school, and they are the exact symptoms experienced in many common sports injuries.

Inflammation is common to so many different types of injuries and illnesses because it's the body's final common response to various insults. When an injury occurs, blood flow to the damaged tissue increases. This increased blood flow may make the tissues warm to the touch, and may produce a reddish hue if the injured tissue is close enough to the skin surface. The blood vessels in the injured area are engorged, and they also leak fluid into the surrounding tissues. This accounts for the swelling that you'll notice with even a moderately severe injury. The fourth symptom, pain, is no surprise when you consider that all of the swelling will put pressure on delicate nerve endings in the area. And it's also easy to see how this combination of factors will impair function of the injured tissue, which is the final major symptom of inflammation.

In a sense, all of these symptoms can *help* the body: increased blood flow and heat can promote healing, and pain and swelling should prevent a premature return to activity, which could cause further injury. It is true that for mild-to-moderate sports injuries, time alone will promote healing, and the inflammation will subside of its own accord. But athletes are not notably conspicuous for their patience, and none of us should put up with unnecessary pain. Furthermore, prolonged activity can certainly lead to problems, including stiffness and muscle weakness. So one of the major strategies of sports medicine is to shorten the inflammatory process so that healing will occur faster and rehabilitation can restore normal function sooner. We'll tell you how this can be done when we review methods of treatment in the next section of this chapter; but first, let's look at the common varieties of "itis."

Tendinitis

Tendons are bands of fibrous tissue that anchor muscles to bones. Fibrous tissue is strong, simple material, not unlike the scar tissue that forms to heal a deep cut in your skin. Every time a muscle contracts, it transmits its force through its tendon to the bone. No wonder tendinitis is one of the commonest sports injuries, since a great deal of force can be concentrated on a relatively small structure.

The familiar symptoms of tendinitis are pain, swelling, warmth, and redness. The pain is typically most severe when you first start exercising; if you keep going, however, the pain typically eases up, and may even go away entirely — only to return with a vengeance after you've cooled down.

Bursitis

Bursae are small fluid-filled sacs that cushion joints, muscles, or bones like miniature hydraulic shock-absorbers. Although the most infamous form of bursitis involves the shoulder, there are many bursae all over the body, and any one of them can become inflamed. Nor is the problem restricted to athletes; "housemaid's knee" is a good example of simple bursitis caused by excessive pressure on the knee joint.

Arthritis and synovitis

You may be used to thinking of arthritis as a chronic disease of the elderly, but in fact young athletes often develop arthritis from sports injuries. The bone surfaces meeting in a joint are covered with a smooth, shiny tissue called cartilage, which allows smooth movement of bone upon bone. Joints are surrounded by a thin membrane called the synovium, and the entire sac is filled with fluid, which acts as a lubricant and shock absorber.

Sports injuries can cause inflammation of the joint lining, which may be called either arthritis or synovitis. When joints become inflamed, the amount of fluid they contain increases, and this can produce very obvious swelling known as a joint effusion. The most commonly recognized example of a joint effusion is "water on the knee."

Fasciitis

Fascia is a type of fibrous or connective tissue that overlies many muscles and tendons to provide protection for these more delicate tissues. "Itis" can strike even this tough, fibrous tissue. A good example is the painful inflammation of the sole of the foot, which can develop in runners as a result of overuse; this particular type of fasciitis is called "plantar fasciitis."

Myositis

Myositis is nothing more than an inflammation of muscles themselves. Pain is the major symptom; it becomes more severe when the inflamed muscles are put to work.

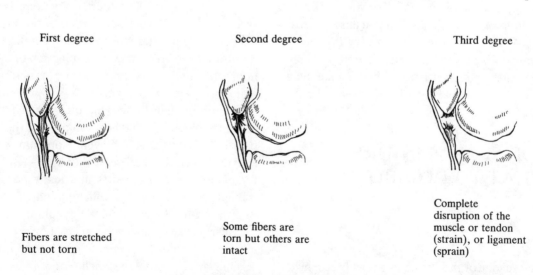

First degree

Second degree

Third degree

Fibers are stretched but not torn

Some fibers are torn but others are intact

Complete disruption of the muscle or tendon (strain), or ligament (sprain)

FIGURE 11–1: *Strains and Sprains*

Periostitis

Bones are surrounded by a thin membrane called the periostium. Inflammation of this membrane, periostitis, causes a deep, nagging pain, which can be quite severe.

The common element in "itis" is inflammation, and the common goal in treating all of these sports injuries is to fight inflammation. For first aid, the PRICE program (see pages 251–252) is best. Afterwards, the various treatment modalities and medications discussed later in this chapter can be used to fight inflammation, restore function, and get you back to sports.

STRAIN

Strains or "muscle pulls" are injuries to muscles or tendons (Figure 11–1) resulting from excessive pulling. Mild strains that involve nothing more than a pulling of fibers are called first-degree strains. Second-degree strains are more severe, because they involve an actual tearing of some of the fibers. Third-degree strains are the most serious of all, because they involve a rupture or disruption of the majority of fibers in the injured muscle or tendon. In general, first-degree strains produce only pain and swelling, whereas second-degree injuries produce at least some degree of weakness, and third-degree injuries produce a dramatic loss of power and motion. Strains are most common when muscles are stiff, cold, or overtired — this is yet another reminder of the importance of prevention in sports medicine.

SPRAIN

Very similar to strains, sprains involve damage to ligaments (fibrous tissue connecting bone to bone). Sprains also come in first-, second-, or third-degree varieties. Sprains are most common at the ankle joint, but the knee, shoulder, or any other joint can be sprained if excessive force is applied to the ligaments that hold the joint together.

Typically, strains and sprains do not result from direct trauma, but from a misstep or fall that places excessive force on a tendon or ligament so that fibers are stretched or torn. The result is pain and, if the injury is severe enough to tear a significant number of fibers, a loss of power and mobility as well. Within minutes, swelling will start; there may also be some discoloration of the skin if the tissue damage is severe enough to cause bleeding.

Mild or first-degree injuries will respond to rest alone, but anything more serious than a minor ankle turn should at least mean an end to competitive play for that day. First-aid management will be very important to limit the swelling and inflammation; PRICE is the key. Aspirin or other anti-inflammatory drugs will also help ease the pain, and may reduce swelling and speed recovery. If there is loss of motion or strength, or if the swelling or pain is severe, be sure to get prompt attention — strains and sprains can be severe enough to require expert care, even including casting or surgery in some cases.

DISLOCATION

Dislocations are among the most painful and disabling of all sports injuries. A dislocation means that the bones slip out of their proper alignment in a particular joint. Pain is the most common symptom; in addition, a deformity is usually visible, and there is an abrupt and marked impairment of joint function. X rays will confirm the diagnosis of a dislocation. Although some athletes who have had recurrent dislocations can reduce ("relocate") the dislocation themselves, we strongly advise *against* any attempts by untrained personnel to do this on the playing field. Ice and a trip to the emergency ward are the best way to handle a dislocation. Further treatment is necessary, however, to prevent recurrent injuries. Sometimes this involves only rest, protection, and support, followed by exercises to strengthen the joint. But in more serious cases, surgical repair may be necessary.

FRACTURES

A fracture is an actual disruption in the continuity and integrity of a bone. Although all fractures are painful, some of them can be relatively minor problems. For example, some runners and other athletes develop hairline or "stress" fractures, usually involving the small bones of the foot or the lower leg. Stress fractures are so small that they may not show up on ordinary X rays, but bone scans can detect them. Stress fractures can be very painful, but they will heal with nothing more than a period of rest, and never require splints or casts (unless that's the only way to stop a fanatical runner from running despite the painful injury).

Unfortunately, many other fractures are much more serious. Simple fractures don't break the skin, whereas compound fractures involve penetration of at least part of the bone through the skin. Obviously, compound fractures are much more serious, because the exposed tissues can become infected. Complex fractures involve multiple breaks in the bone, sometimes resulting in many small fragments. All major fractures require prolonged immobility so that healing can occur. Usually a cast or splint will suffice, but sometimes surgery is necessary so that screws or plates can be used to hold the broken bone together.

Fractures are, of course, most common in contact sports, but they can also occur with any bad spill, whether it be on a ski slope, basketball court, or track. It may be hard at first to distinguish an incomplete fracture from a severe strain or sprain; more serious fractures are often fairly obvious because of severe pain and swelling, or because the alignment of the limb is clearly distorted. No one can expect you to diagnose a fracture on the playing field, but if there is any suspicion of a broken bone, you should treat the injury as a fracture. The key element is getting the patient to expert medical attention as quickly as possible, so that X rays can be obtained and the treatment plan formulated. On the way to the emergency ward, however, a few simple first-aid measures can be very helpful. The injured bone should be rested and protected; even the most macho athlete must not be allowed to walk on a potentially fractured leg or foot. Ice can help limit swelling, as can elevation of the injured area. Immobilization of the injured part will also help limit damage. This can be accomplished with an ace bandage or tape in some cases, but in other situations you may want to improvise a splint by taping the injured limb to a firm object. If you are at a club with a good first-aid kit, you may have some splint material available; if not, you can try gently to tape the injured area to a tennis racquet or other similar object until more definitive treatment is available.

In handling a fracture — as in handling any other first-aid situation — remember that your major job is to get expert help, rather than to attempt fancy treatment on your own. Don't attempt any involved manipulations or immobilizations. Instead, simply try to provide some protection and support for the injured area until trained help is available.

CONTUSION

This is yet another example of how doctors can use fancy names for everyday events: a contusion is merely a bruise or "black-and-blue" mark caused by direct trauma to muscles or bones. The injury damages blood vessels, so that blood leaks into the surrounding tissues, producing the black-and-blue color, which gradually lightens, fades to yellow, and finally disappears. Deep contusions can involve a lot of bleeding and can be painful and disabling; fortunately, most contusions are more superficial and less serious. To treat a contusion, apply ice as soon as possible, but avoid pressure or massage, which can increase the bleeding. After one to two days of ice treatments, switch to heat, which will help your body heal.

CRAMPS

Cramps are strong but temporary contractions of muscles. Although a cramp (sometimes known on the playing field as a charley horse) can be very painful and can pull you up short, it will not last long, and it will resolve without leaving permanent injury to the muscle. However, in some cases cramps can be recurrent and disabling. The trick is to find out why you get cramps, so that you can prevent them. Most cramps are caused by excessive muscle fatigue, dehydration, or, less commonly, by a derangement in one of the body's chemicals such as potassium, calcium, or magnesium. Try to prevent cramps by warming up before you start hard exercise and by doing stretching exercises for flexibility. Stay well hydrated and avoid getting chilled during or after play. If you get a cramp, stop playing and gently stretch the muscle; when the cramp is gone, stretch for another minute or so and then resume play gradually. If you get lots of cramps, ask your doctor to check your blood chemistries. In some cases, a prescription for quinine may be worth a try.

MUSCLE SPASMS

These painful, prolonged muscle contractions can be thought of as sustained cramps. Whereas muscle cramps last for seconds or minutes, spasms can last for hours, days, or even weeks. Almost any type of muscle injury can provoke spasms; strains, inflammation, and trauma are the most common causes. Any muscle can be involved, but the strong muscles of the back and neck are most prone to spasms. Muscle spasms produce pain and stiffness; the muscle may also look enlarged and feel very hard. Spasms should be treated with rest and heat; medications such as anti-inflammatory drugs, painkillers, and muscle relaxants (see page 264) can be very helpful. When the spasms have eased up, use gentle stretching exercises to begin rehabilitation and prevent recurrences.

ATROPHY

When muscles are not used, they weaken; eventually the cells decrease in size — they atrophy. Hence, any significant injury that causes prolonged immobility will produce at least some muscle atrophy. Fortunately, the process is reversible. Obviously, it's best to prevent or at least minimize atrophy by early rehabilitation exercises whenever possible.

LACERATIONS AND ABRASIONS

Lacerations are cuts, and abrasions are scrapes; both require appropriate treatment to prevent infection and to allow healing. You may not need anything more than soap and water and a Band-Aid to deal with small lacerations or abrasions, but don't overlook even this elementary first aid — otherwise, a small problem could become a large one. Gentle pressure should help control bleeding. Careful cleansing of any wound is extremely important; soap and water are excellent for this purpose, but a variety of commercially available antiseptic solutions will also do an excellent job. A clean bandage will complete the management of most cuts and scrapes. However, if the cut appears deep, it's very important to be sure that there is no injury to a nerve, muscle, or tendon. If there is numbness or loss of strength in the tissue beyond the cut, or if a joint is involved, a trip to the emergency ward is important to see if stitches are needed. You should also be checked to see if you need stitches if any cut is more than an inch or two long, or if the edges don't come together very nicely and easily with a simple Band-Aid.

If you have a dirty cut or abrasion that can't be thoroughly cleansed with simple measures at home or in the clubhouse, you should have it checked by a professional to be sure there are no residual foreign materials that could predispose toward infection. In the case of deep or contaminated wounds or abrasions, your doctor may even suggest antibiotics to help prevent infection.

Finally, any injury in which the skin is broken deserves a tetanus booster. Even better, you should keep your tetanus immunizations up to date with a booster every ten years, so that you won't need another shot each time you are injured during sports.

TREATMENT METHODS

Almost all athletic injuries require a multifaceted approach to treatment and rehabilitation. Treatment may be administered by a physician, nurse, physical therapist, or trainer — but the most important person in treating an athlete's injury is the athlete himself. Whereas most patients have only to follow their doctor's instructions in order to recover, the injured athlete must also work hard at rehabilitation in order to recover full function as rapidly as possible.

CRYOTHERAPY

Cryotherapy is the local application of cold to treat injuries. We've already pointed out that ice is one of the most important "drugs" for the treatment of injuries. It is best to apply cold as soon as possible after an acute injury to help reduce swelling, and also to decrease pain. Repeated applications of cold four times a day for twenty to thirty minutes each can be very helpful for the first forty-eight hours after an acute injury. Thereafter, heat is often useful for rehabilitation, but cold packs applied to the injured area immediately after exercise may still be very helpful once you have resumed your activities.

There are many ways to apply cold. The simplest and least-expensive method is as good as any of the fancier techniques: ice cubes or crushed ice in a plastic bag should do the trick very nicely. But if you want to apply cold directly to a small area, and particularly if you want to perform an ice massage of the injured area, a bag full of ice cubes can be awkward. You can make

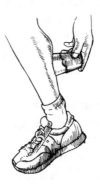

Styrofoam cup. Fill with water, freeze, then peel back to expose ice.

FIGURE 11–2: *How to Use a Homemade Ice Massager*

your own ice massager very simply by filling a Styrofoam cup nearly to the top with water and freezing it overnight. Next, peel back the upper half of the cup so that a generous portion of ice will be exposed, but leave the base of the cup to use as a handle. You can then hold the insulated cup while massaging your injury directly with the exposed ice (see Figure 11–2).

Cold is most helpful when applied immediately after an injury, yet refrigerators are not standard on most playing fields. You have undoubtedly seen a trainer run onto a baseball or football field to spray the skin of an injured athlete. All he's doing is applying cold by spraying on ethyl chloride or another volatile substance that evaporates rapidly, thus cooling the skin. These chemical sprays are a very good way to provide superficial cooling, but most of the cooling effect is confined to the skin and does not penetrate to deeper tissues. As a result, chemical sprays can be helpful for early pain control, but should not be relied on for deeper cooling of injured tissues. You can get more lasting cooling on the playing field by using a chemical cold pack. These devices are simply plastic bags containing chemicals that are inert when they are separate but that interact when they are combined, to produce cold. You can store the cold pack at air temperature until you need it; then press the bag so the chemicals flow together and produce cold.

All cold treatments must be applied with caution, so that you don't suffer frostbite. This can be a bit tricky, because cold produces numbness; on the one hand you'll get welcome pain relief, but if you keep the cold on for too long, you may damage your skin or even your deeper tissues without being aware of it. As a rule of thumb, we'd suggest applying cold packs for no more than twenty to thirty minutes; however, after your skin has warmed up you can reapply these treatments four or five times a day for the first two days after your injury.

As a final precaution, we'd advise you against immersing an injured limb in an ice water bath. Such intensive cooling is simply too much of a good thing, and you run the risk of injuring your tissues. Also, ice baths make it very difficult to elevate the injured area, which is another important part of early treatment.

Use cold with care, but don't let all these precautions deter you from relying on cold for the early treatment of athletic injuries. Although often overlooked by physicians who are not trained in sports medicine, ice is really the hottest thing in the early treatment of athletic injuries.

HEAT TREATMENTS

For the physicist, heat is the opposite of cold; for the athlete, however, these thermal extremes are not opposites, but are complementary ways to treat injuries. Cold treatments are most useful early on, whereas heat is very important later in the rehabilitation from injuries.

Heat treatments are helpful because they relax muscles, which will reduce spasm and increase mobility. Heat will also increase the circulation of blood and can stimulate the flow of lymph fluid in the injured region; both effects can be helpful in the later phases of the healing process.

The relative merits of moist heat and dry heat are often hotly debated in the athletic trainer's room. We won't add fuel to this controversy by taking sides; there is little scientific data to support one side or the other, and in our experience both types of heat can be very helpful.

The simplest way to apply heat at home is with an electric heating pad. This will give you dry heat, but if you cover the injured area with a towel before applying the heating pad, you can retain some perspiration which will give you the effect of moist heat. You can also buy heating pads which allow you to add water to a specially insulated compartment to produce moist heat. But *don't* try to "do-it-yourself" by wetting down an ordinary heating pad — the results can be shocking. Instead, for moist heat simply soak bath towels in hot water; remember, though, that they tend to cool down rather quickly and are messy and cumbersome to use. Hydroculator packs can be used to obtain moist heat conveniently at home. Hydroculators are cloth bags containing a silicone gel filler that absorbs water and retains heat. The hydroculator is warmed in a pot of hot water, wrapped in a hot towel, and then applied to the injured area. The ultimate in moist heat, of course, is simply to immerse the injured area in a hot bath, remembering to refill the tub with warm water if prolonged heat is necessary.

One of the most popular ways to provide heat is by rubbing liniments into the skin. The popularity of liniments is readily apparent from the many brands that are widely advertised and sold. Indeed, liniments are convenient, and they can make you feel good when you rub them over an injured muscle. Unfortunately, they are rather inefficient ways to produce heat, since their effect is only skin deep; skin blood flow and warmth increase, but the temperature of deeper tissues does not change very much. We are not trying to discourage the use of liniments, but we certainly don't feel that you can rely on them for deep heat. Similarly, infrared lamps will make your body feel warm, but they tend to dissipate heat over a large area and are inefficient in providing heat where it's needed, deep in injured tissues.

All of these techniques are available for home use. A well-equipped clubhouse, trainer's room, or hospital physical therapy department will be able to offer you alternate types of heat treatment as well. Diathermy machines are perhaps the most precise way to deliver deep heat to injured tissues. These machines generate either shortwave, microwave, or ultrasound energy, which penetrates into your injured tissues to provide deep warmth. All of them are safe and, although few scientific studies are available, all seem about equally effective forms of deep heat treatment. Ultrasound is the newest form of diathermy, and it's becoming the most popular. If your home heating pad or hydroculator treatments don't seem to be doing the trick, ask your physician or physical therapist about diathermy. It should not be necessary to invest a great deal of time or money in these treatments; if you're not getting the effect you want in six or eight treatments, look for alternate approaches instead of simply persisting.

Another form of heat treatment is the whirlpool bath. Whirlpools can be set at a wide range of temperatures, ranging from 55 to 110 degrees Fahrenheit, so they can be used for either cold or heat treatments. Most whirlpools, however, are set between 100 and 106 degrees to provide heat treatments. Whirlpools also provide moisture and a gentle massaging effect, which can be both pleasant and helpful. Finally, whirlpools are ideal during rehabilitation because you can move an injured joint through its range of motion with the aid of the relaxing effects of heat and the buoyancy and cushioning effects of water. Jacuzzi baths will provide similar benefits; because Jacuzzi may be unsupervised, it is very important not to overdo it in terms of the temperature or the duration of your treatment. If twenty minutes at 105 degrees doesn't do the trick, there is little reason to think that more heat or longer periods will help.

You can also heat yourself up in a sauna or steambath. We won't debate the pros and cons of either, but we must point out that both methods heat up your entire body rather than just the injured area, so they should not be used as a rehabilitation treatment for athletic injuries. If you choose to use a sauna or steambath simply to feel good, remember not to overdo it, or you'll feel bad. Be sure to avoid dehydration, and be particularly careful if you have any potential problems with your heart or lungs, which could be exacerbated if you stress your circulation by getting overheated. Although many people do feel that a sauna after exercise is relaxing and enjoyable, we prefer a systematic cool-down routine, including some stretching for your muscles and some walking or jogging to allow your heart to slow down and your body to cool down gradually (see Chapter 7).

In general, heat is best in the later or rehabilitation phases of recovery. Heat is also useful to help an injured muscle or ligament warm up before exercise, and is particularly helpful to relax tired or cramped-up muscles. All heat treatments, however, must be used with care. Although we speak of using heat, we are really recommending warmth — the idea is to increase local temperatures without broiling your tissues. Temperatures of 100 to 110 degrees should be plenty, but even in the 105- to 110-degree range you have to be careful not to sustain superficial burns of your skin. It is always a good idea to place a towel between you and a hot pack, and above all never fall asleep with a heating pad in place. In general, twenty to thirty minutes should be plenty for each heat treatment, but you may need to repeat these treatments four or five times per day.

MASSAGE

Don't get your hopes up: it may seem suspicious that we are taking you from the steambath to the massage parlor, but although this book has plenty to say about racing, there is nothing racy about it. In fact, the type of massage we are talking about originated not in Times Square, but in China five thousand years ago. In contemporary terms, massage is a perfectly legitimate technique for the treatment of various muscular injuries.

Massage has many potential benefits, including relaxing muscles, increasing blood flow, and promoting the drainage of lymph fluid away from injured tissues. As with so many physical therapies, there have been few scientific studies of the pros and cons of massage, but many athletes find massage extremely helpful for stiff, sore muscles. There may well be a psychological element to the relaxing effects of massage, but as long as your muscles loosen up, who cares if it's "mental"?

Massage is probably best reserved for relatively minor aches and pains, such as stiff muscles, rather than for serious athletic injuries. And as we mentioned, massage should definitely *not* be used for deep tissue contusions (bruises). Massage should always be performed by a well-trained person.

MANIPULATION

Some athletes swear by chiropractic and other forms of manipulation; most doctors simply swear when the subject comes up. We are not afraid of controversy, and we don't duck this one. Throughout this book, we have frequently sided with athletes and taken positions that may seem a bit unorthodox to conventional medical practitioners who have not studied exercise physiology. But in this area at least, we must side firmly with the medical establishment. There is no evidence that manipulations are helpful for athletic injuries or for other musculoskeletal problems. We are not talking about stretching exercises or range-of-motion exercises as performed by a physical therapist, or maneuvers performed by an orthopedic surgeon to reduce (realign) dislocations. Chiropractic manipulations are quite another matter; in our opinion, they are of no proven benefit and could be harmful.

TRACTION

Traction devices exert gentle stretching forces on injured tissues. Traction can help eliminate muscle spasms and can enforce rest and immobilization so that injuries will heal faster. But traction devices can also be misused and abused; schemes such as inversion boots are just that — schemes. So here, too, we caution you against doing it yourself: if you need traction, it should always be prescribed and supervised by a physician, physical therapist, or trainer.

ELECTRICAL STIMULATION

When you exercise, your muscles contract because the cells are stimulated by tiny electrical currents originating from nerves. Physical therapists can stimulate your nerves or muscles directly by applying low-voltage electric currents to your skin. Electrical stimulation of nerves can help relieve pain, and stimulation of muscles can help reduce the atrophy of muscles that are immobilized after injuries. But electrical stimulation will not further increase the power of healthy muscles.

Electrical stimulation should be used only in conjunction with other treatment and rehabilitation tech-

niques. A wide variety of devices are available to generate low-level electric currents, but these treatments should be administered only by qualified therapists or trainers.

TAPING AND WRAPPING

It is virtually impossible to attend an athletic event from junior high school on up without seeing at least one player wearing an elastic bandage, tape, or brace. Indeed, many locker rooms resound with the sound of ripping tape before a game, and are littered with a tangle of tape afterward. Can hundreds of athletes be wrong about the benefits of tape? Not in this case.

External support such as tape, elastic bandages, and various braces can be very useful for exercise-related injuries. Immediately after an injury, wrapping can be used for compression, which will help reduce inflammation and edema or swelling. In the first post-injury days, wraps or splints can be used to reduce mobility and enforce rest, so that healing will occur. And later in recovery, when a return to activity is appropriate, tape or wraps can provide external support for injured ligaments or tendons that are not yet back to full strength, and they can prevent excessive motion that might lead to reinjury. Finally, external supports remind the athlete that he has had an injury, often serving as a warning to avoid excessive force or motion.

Like all good things, external supports have potential negative aspects as well. If they are too tight, circulation can be impaired. If they are used excessively, they may limit the restoration of full mobility and strength to the injured muscles and ligaments. Finally, because these supports do give the athlete a sense of security, they may even induce a mild sort of psychological dependence on the device itself. All in all, if external support devices are chosen appropriately, applied carefully, and used in conjunction with an active rehabilitation program, their benefits far outweigh these potential drawbacks.

Tape is one of the most useful forms of external support. Tape has the advantage of being inexpensive and, more important, of being infinitely adaptable to an injured athlete's particular problem and anatomy. The major problem with tape is that it must be applied by a skilled therapist or trainer rather than by the athlete himself. Although some of the newer waterproof adhesive tapes can be left in place for as long as two or three days, taping is generally a short-term proposition because tape tends to stretch out in the course of exercise and because perspiration and moisture will take their toll in a relatively short period of time. So in general, tape is best used when the injured athlete is ready to return to exercise. In these circumstances, tape is applied shortly before exercise and should be removed either right after exercise, or after two or three days of use. And if you've ever had adhesive tape removed, you are keenly aware of another drawback of taping.

To minimize the pain of removing tape, your skin should be shaved before the tape is applied. Skin irritation is another side effect of taping, so some trainers and therapists will use an underwrap of gauze or similar material to protect the skin, even at the cost of some support. If tape is applied directly to skin, an adherent such as benzoin can be sprayed on first to increase stickiness while also providing some skin protection. Tape is best removed with a tape cutter to minimize the need for pulling and tearing. Figure 11–3 shows a typical pattern for taping a sprained ankle.

Elastic or "ace" bandages are the most widely used type of external support. They are much more convenient to use than tape; most athletes can learn to wrap their injuries correctly in just a few minutes. In addition to being easy to put on, elastics are easy and painless to take off, and can be reused many times. However, they generally provide less support than tape, and a skilled therapist can direct pressure much more precisely with tape than with elastic wraps. Elastic bandages are an excellent way to provide compression during the acute phases of an injury. They can be helpful later in rehabilitation for some degree of support and security, but if stability and external support are very important, tape is preferred.

Elastic bandages come in various widths, from two to six inches. Use narrower sizes for small joints such as your ankle; use wider bandages to wrap larger areas such as your thigh. Figure 11–4 illustrates an elastic thigh wrap that provides pressure over a strain.

Elastic bandages are also manufactured in sleevelike configurations to slip right over a knee or ankle. This type of ready-made support is the easiest of all to use. However, since "one size fits all," you will give up the control and precision that you can get if you wrap your own injury to suit your own special needs. Some of these elastic sleeve devices are marketed as "braces," but they are much less supportive than true braces.

BRACES

Braces are the gold standard of external support. Modern technology has greatly expanded the role of external support. New methods and new materials allow custom building of these devices so that the athlete can attain support without unduly sacrificing mobility. Braces can be custom-fitted and custom-designed to fill specific needs. Most of us will never need these elaborate affairs, but if you have a chronic or recurrent injury that has not responded to simpler therapy, you should consider a trip to an orthopedic brace shop. Some of these devices can be expensive, and many of them look awkward, but they can be worth the investment of time and money if you really need them. If you have any doubts, you can obtain a "consultation" from Dr. J.: just turn on your TV and watch him soar to the basket wearing his neoprene knee brace, which allows him superior mobility while still protecting him from chondromalacia ("jumper's knee").

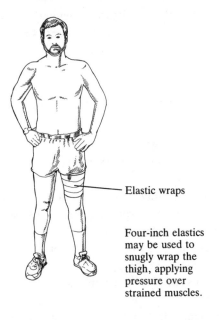

Elastic wraps

Four-inch elastics may be used to snugly wrap the thigh, applying pressure over strained muscles.

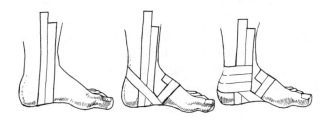

FIGURE 11–3: *How to Tape a Sprained Ankle*

FIGURE 11–4: *Elastic Wraps*

EXERCISE AND STRETCHING

Exercises for strength and flexibility are particularly important during the later rehabilitative phases following injury. Inactivity will cause an amazingly rapid decline in strength and flexibility. In some cases, diminished function can be documented as early as two or three days into a layoff, and if you add injury to inactivity, the loss of function will be even more pronounced. The goals of rehabilitation are to restore muscle mass, strength and endurance, joint flexibility, and coordination. No less important is the restoration of confidence, since many athletes become depressed and irritable after significant injuries and layoffs.

An exercise program should begin as early as possible. Even if the injured limb must be immobilized, a scheme should be devised that will exercise the rest of the body to maintain cardiovascular fitness and keep other major muscle groups strong. When it's time to mobilize the injured area, you will generally be taught isometric exercises first, so that muscles can rebuild strength without moving an injured joint through its full range of motion. Passive range-of-motion exercises may start at about this time; the therapist will gently move your joint without allowing your muscles to do any of the work. You will then progress to active range-of-motion exercises, and then to isotonic work, so that you will be using your muscles throughout their full range of motion. Eventually, you will probably be working with weights or exercise machines to build strength further. Your goal should extend beyond recovery to rebuilding yourself stronger than ever, so that you will avoid similar injuries in the future.

MEDICATIONS

Athletes use drugs for one of three reasons: to treat exercise-related injuries, to treat other medical problems, or to improve athletic performance. The first two reasons are certainly legitimate, but athletes using medications may require special precautions. Whereas the third reason is understandable, it is not acceptable; athletes using drugs to boost their abilities are courting disappointment (in the case of vitamins and nutritional supplements) or disaster (in the case of steroids or stimulants).

Most medications will not interfere with your ability to exercise safely, but if you require long-term medication, you should check with your doctor before you start your fitness program. If you incur an exercise-related injury, you may need medication as part of your treatment program. These medications fall into three broad categories: anti-inflammatory drugs, analgesics or painkillers, and muscle relaxants.

ANTI-INFLAMMATORY MEDICATIONS

There are a host of medications used to fight inflammation, and most of these drugs also fight pain. The net result is to reduce discomfort and speed healing, so that you can return to exercise and sports more rapidly.

Aspirin

Aspirin is the oldest anti-inflammatory drug and is still the benchmark by which other medications must be judged. For minor problems, such as mild tendinitis, as little as two tablets (600 milligrams) may do the trick. If you are recovering from tendinitis, for example, you may want to try several aspirin tablets within an hour or so of exercising. But if you have a more serious or chronic injury, you may require aspirin on a regular basis, using two or three tablets every four hours, up to a maximum of ten to sixteen tablets per day. Remember, however, that aspirin is not a cure-all; if you do not get relief, or if you still need regular doses after seven to ten days, you should consider other approaches and should consult a doctor.

Although aspirin is generally safe, there are potential side effects, including stomach irritation and bleeding. If you are prone to stomach upset, you can use buffered aspirin or aspirin combined with antacids; enteric-coated aspirin is best of all. But if plain old aspirin does not cause any side effects, we'd recommend that you use the least expensive generic aspirin preparation you can find, since the active ingredient is exactly the same in all aspirin formulations.

Newer Anti-inflammatories

A whole array of stronger anti-inflammatory drugs is now available with your doctor's prescription. Two old standbys are indomethacin (Indocin) and phenylbutazone (Butazolidin). These medications are more potent than aspirin, but can also have more side effects, including fluid retention and temporary mental changes as well as stomach irritation. Phenylbutazone can also interfere with blood cell formation, so we generally prefer indomethacin.

In the past few years, more than a half-dozen new

anti-inflammatory drugs have been marketed. Although these chemicals were first developed for arthritis, they are extremely useful for musculoskeletal problems resulting from exercise as well. This family of drugs is collectively referred to as the nonsteroidal anti-inflammatory drugs, or NSAID. All of these drugs fight inflammation and pain, and are very similar to aspirin itself. And like aspirin, their major side effects are stomach irritation. Another side effect, however, is that all of these drugs are much more expensive than good old aspirin. Why then use the newer drugs? A good question. In fact, if aspirin will do the job, we suggest that you stick with this time-honored, inexpensive preparation. But many people find the newer prescription anti-inflammatory drugs to be more potent than aspirin. In addition, they are much more convenient, since many of them can be taken only once or twice a day.

Figure 11–5 lists the chemical and brand names of the nonsteroidal anti-inflammatory drugs. Your doctor will start with the medication that he knows best, but you may have to resort to trial and error to find the medicine that's best for you. And remember that even these potent new drugs are not cure-alls. They should always be used as part of a comprehensive treatment and rehabilitation program, so that you will eventually be able to exercise vigorously without requiring medications of any sort.

If you have an injury that you can treat yourself and if you prefer a newer nonsteroidal anti-inflammatory drug to aspirin, you may not like calling or visiting your doctor for a prescription. Now you don't have to. After ten years of use as a prescription drug, ibuprofen is now available as an over-the-counter medication under the brand names Advil and Nuprin. The tablets that you can buy without a prescription are weaker than the prescription varieties (Motrin, Rufen), but you can get equivalent effects by simply taking two nonprescription tablets three or four times daily. You'll get all the anti-inflammatory and painkilling effects of ibuprofen — and all the potential side effects, too. Because you won't have the benefits of discussions and warnings from your doctor, read the label thoroughly, and be careful. Use the lowest dose that will work, discontinue the medication as soon as possible, and be alert for stomach irritation and other side effects.

CORTISONE

Cortisone and its derivatives are the most potent of all anti-inflammatory drugs, but they also have the most serious side effects. Because of these side effects, steroid pills are almost never given for athletic injuries; in our view, prescribing cortisone pills for tendinitis is trying to kill an ant with a sledgehammer.

Cortisone and related steroid hormones can also be injected directly into inflamed tissues. These are the "cortisone" shots given to competitive athletes so they can get on with an important game. Steroid injections

FIGURE 11–5: NONSTEROIDAL ANTI-INFLAMMATORY DRUGS

Chemical name	Brand names
Diflunisal	Dolobid
Fenoprofen	Nalfon
Ibuprofen	Motrin, Rufen (prescription)
	Advil, Nuprin (nonprescription)
Indomethacin	Indocin
Ketoprofin	Orudis
Meclofenamate	Meclomen
Mefenamic acid	Ponstel
Naproxen	Naprosyn, Anaprox
Oxyphenbutazone	Oxalid, Tandearil
Phenylbutazone	Butazolidin
Piroxicam	Feldene
Tolmetin	Tolectin
Sulindac	Clinoril
Suprofen	Suprol

can be very helpful for some cases of severe localized inflammation, such as bursitis. These medications can sometimes be combined with local anaesthetics such as Novocain to get rapid relief from pain and sustained relief from inflammation. In skilled hands, steroid shots can be very helpful, but there are potential problems, the greatest of which is thinning and weakening of tendons, which can even lead to tendon rupture; hence, steroids should never be injected directly into tendons. In fact, steroid shots should be reserved for situations in which safer forms of treatment, such as ice and aspirin, don't do the trick. And cortisone shots should be used sparingly; in general, we would recommend no more than two or possibly three injections spaced at least a month apart.

ANALGESICS

Analgesics are painkillers. Aspirin and the other non-steroidal anti-inflammatory drugs are analgesics, but not all analgesics are anti-inflammatories. The most common example of a painkiller that does not fight inflammation is acetaminophen, which is marketed as Tylenol, Datril, and many other brands. Acetaminophen causes less stomach irritation than aspirin and is just about as potent in reducing pain. However, acetaminophen does not fight inflammation, so if your stomach can tolerate aspirin we'd much prefer the dual-purpose effects of aspirin to the single-duty benefit of acetaminophen for treating musculoskeletal injuries.

A great many potent painkillers are also available by prescription; examples of prescription analgesics include codeine, oxycodan, propoxyphene and pentazocine. These medications are very effective in reducing pain, but all have potential side effects and may be habit forming. Your doctor should use these medications only after less-potent drugs fail; these drugs should be used for brief periods of time under close supervision. And, as a rule of thumb, if your pain is strong enough to require a prescription analgesic, your body has not recovered from your injury enough for you to resume athletics.

MUSCLE RELAXANTS

Muscle spasm is an important component of many exercise-induced problems. When muscles are injured or excessively stretched, they often go into spasm. In turn, muscle spasms cause stiffness and pain, and can provoke inflammation of joints and tendons. Heat,

stretching exercises, rest, and anti-inflammatory drugs are the best ways to treat muscle spasms. But in some cases additional medications may be required to overcome spasms. This is particularly true if strong muscles develop spasms, such as the muscles of your back or neck.

Muscle relaxants are prescription drugs, which require medical supervision. Examples include diazapam (Valium), methocarbamol (Robaxin), carisoprodol (Soma) and orphenadrine (Norflex). Each of these drugs can help reduce painful spasms and can therefore speed your recovery from injury. But because there are potential side effects, you should use these drugs sparingly and only under close medical supervision. And muscle relaxants should always be part of a comprehensive treatment program including anti-inflammatories or analgesics, heat, and rest or even traction.

UNAPPROVED DRUGS

Dimethyl sulfoxide, or DMSO, is now gaining underground popularity among many athletes to treat muscle and joint problems. DMSO is not approved by the U.S. government for any human use except for a rare type of bladder inflammation. However, DMSO is widely available for veterinary use in nonbreeding dogs and horses.

DMSO was discovered by a Russian chemist in 1866 as a by-product of paper manufacturing. Today this chemical is widely used as an industrial degreaser solvent. How did an industrial solvent obtain underground popularity as a "wonder drug" for arthritis, sprains, and strains? We are not sure how this came about, but we certainly discourage the practice. Although thousands of people have tried DMSO, there is no scientific evidence that it will help any musculoskeletal problem or athletic injury. In fact, careful scientific studies of tennis elbow and tendinitis have found that DMSO is ineffective. We also know that DMSO can cause cataracts in animals, and there is reason for concern about side effects in man. We can certainly sympathize with athletes who want to return to sports as soon as possible after an injury. Unfortunately there is no quick fix.

Androgens (male sex hormones) increase muscle bulk, and they have been used by many power athletes to increase muscle size and strength. The bodybuilders and weight lifters are right in that androgens can increase muscular bulk — but there is no good evidence that male hormones increase strength and actually improve performance. And even if strength were increased, the potential side effects are too high a price to pay; androgens can produce many harmful effects, ranging from acne to high blood pressure, heart disease, temporary sterility, breast enlargement, and liver disease. The scandal of the 1983 Pan-American games has brought the problem of androgen abuse out into the open, but it has been going on for years in Europe, America, and elsewhere. Hopefully this renewed publicity, together with improved drug-detection testing, will finally begin to control the entire problem of illicit drug use and abuse by competitive athletes.

Street drugs are, unfortunately, abused by a shockingly large number of professional athletes. Amphetamines (speed), cocaine, and narcotics have absolutely no place in exercise or sports. These illicit drugs will not improve athletic performance in any way and they are extreme health hazards, to say nothing of their profoundly destructive psychosocial effects. Avoid them.

Don't be tempted to try unapproved drugs. Instead, rely on the tried and tested combinations of physical therapy and anti-inflammatory medications. Be persistent but be patient — it is every bit as important to preserve your general good health as it is to recover from your athletic injury. When well-tested medications are used in combination with physical therapy, you'll be able to recover from your athletic injury, rehabilitate yourself, and continue to exercise for fitness, health, and enjoyment.

Androgens and illicit drugs can be disastrous for health and are obviously grounds for disqualifying athletes from competitive games. But even "innocent" medications, such as cold remedies, and prescriptive drugs, including some used for asthma, can be grounds for disqualification as well. These days it seems that referees need a degree in pharmacology to keep it straight.

12

Specific Medical Complications of Exercise and Sports

This chapter presents a glossary of common sports injuries, dealing both with your internal organs and with your musculoskeletal system. We will not attempt to be encyclopedic; although we'll try to cover the most common problems, you won't find every sports injury here. Nor will you find all the details about medical treatment; our goal is not to turn you into a doctor, but to explain how your body works, how you can recognize important sports-related problems, and how you can get started on a treatment program.

This chapter is designed primarily as a reference for the athlete who develops problems from sports, but it is not meant to stand alone. The best type of treatment is prevention, which is the focus of the earlier sections of this book. Here, we deal with the simpler problems that you can recognize and manage by yourself. But remember that our advice is necessarily general, and your problem could represent an exception to these rules. Above all, be sure to get competent professional advice for any problem that seems severe, prolonged, or unusual. There is nothing more precious than your body and your health.

When most people think of medical complications of exercise and sports, they quite naturally think of injuries to muscles, bones, and joints. But exercise involves much more than muscles and bones; vigorous exertion can stress virtually any organ system in your body, and as a result any of these systems can be injured.

EXERCISE AND YOUR INTERNAL ORGANS

HEART

The most highly publicized complications of exercise involve the heart. We believe that aerobic exercise is beneficial for your heart; exercise-induced cardiac problems are quite uncommon, but when they occur, they can be very serious. Whereas older athletes are most vulnerable to such tragic complications, heart problems can also occur in apparently healthy young athletes. There are several things you can do to minimize your risks. First, understand how exercise affects your heart, so that you are aware of both the benefits and risks (see Chapter 1). Next, review your health status to see if you have risk factors for cardiac disease; collaborate with your physician so that you can get the medical tests you need to be sure your heart is healthy (see Chapter 5). Finally, listen to your body: it is crucial for you to identify and report any warning symptoms that suggest heart problems during exercise.

The most typical warning signal is chest pain. In its classic form, heart pain comes on with exertion or emotion and is relieved by rest (or by medication such as nitroglycerine). The pain is often described as a heavy or dull pressure in the midchest, and it may radiate to the jaw, shoulder, or arm, usually on the left side. But heart pain can masquerade as indigestion, gall bladder attacks, or rib pain. And in some cases, there is no pain but only a mild discomfort or sensation of profound fatigue. The moral: If you have any suspicious symptoms, check with your doctor as quickly as possible, and don't exercise until you have medical clearance to do so.

A number of other symptoms could suggest heart problems, even in the absence of chest pain. These symptoms include a rapid or irregular heartbeat, unusual shortness of breath or fatigue, excessive perspiration, nausea, light-headedness, pallor, or wheezing. In the heat of competition it can be easy to dismiss these symptoms as a side stitch or as simple exhaustion. Don't minimize your symptoms — it's much safer to halt play and get help than to risk serious illness.

Most of these symptoms are caused by coronary artery disease, in which blockages prevent the heart from getting all the oxygen it needs during exercise. But you should know about uncommon heart problems such as infection or inflammation of the heart muscle, called "myocarditis." This is the result of viral infections and is worth thinking about because it may be partially preventable. If mice are forced to exercise during certain viral infection, they have had a high incidence of myocarditis. We don't know if these observations have any applicability to man, but it does seem prudent to restrict vigorous exercise during infections. It's very doubtful that exercise would be harmful during a typical siege of the sniffles. But if you have fever, muscle aches, and fatigue, which can suggest the spread of virus throughout your blood and system, it makes good sense to avoid strenuous exercise until you're better. For some of us, such restraint can be difficult. If you are addicted to exercise, you can use spells like this to do gentle stretching exercises, which will facilitate your return to training when the virus is gone.

What should you do if you feel ill while playing a sport? If you or your partner experience chest pain, undue shortness of breath, wheezing, excessive perspiration, unusual nausea, or general weakness, you should stop play immediately, rest quietly, and if the symptoms don't dissipate immediately, arrange prompt transportation to expert medical evaluation. Profound weakness or sudden collapse during exercise obviously mandates the same prompt medical attention. Remember that there are many causes of collapse, ranging from a severe allergic reaction (called anaphylaxis) to heat stroke, to disorders of the heart rhythm, to actual stoppage of the heart (cardiac arrest). If a heart stoppage occurs, you would not ordinarily be able to get an ambulance in time to save the victim unless you are prepared to administer cardiopulmonary resuscitation (CPR) while help is on the way. Because of this, we strongly suggest that everyone consider taking a CPR course sanctioned by the Red Cross. These courses are offered at many community centers, Y's, and adult education facilities. A few hours of instruction could pay big dividends; the life you save could be — your partner's.

If chest pain is the most common symptom of heart attacks, then denial is the second most common. One reason many people fail to report symptoms to their doctors is that they are afraid that they will be permanently prevented from exercising. This concern is not unfounded, but fortunately it is only half true. The diagnosis of heart disease does not mean that you will be unable to exercise, but it does mean that you'll require medical evaluation, time, and supervision to get you back on your feet. In fact, exercise is now an accepted form of rehabilitation and treatment for people with heart disease.

Doctors have come a long way in understanding the benefits of exercise after a heart attack. At one time patients were kept on strict bed rest for six weeks or more. The results were predictable: profound weakness, fatigue, and depression. Whereas these changes were initially attributed to heart damage, we now know that as little as one to three weeks of bed rest will produce a 20 to 25 percent decrease in cardiac work capacity, a 10 to 15 percent decrease in skeletal muscle mass and strength, and a substantial decrease in blood volume, which causes low blood pressure and thick blood with a propensity to clot formation. Early ambulation after a heart attack will prevent all these problems, and now most patients are out of bed within two to three days. In fact, the total length of hospitalization is now only ten to fourteen days after an uncomplicated heart attack.

By the time of discharge from the hospital, most patients recovering from heart attack can begin a program of gentle walking. At four to six weeks, patients can return to an appropriately equipped medical center for supervised exercise on a stationary bicycle. Needless to say, they require supervision and monitoring during this early exercise period. If all goes well, by ten to twelve weeks, more strenuous exercise training can begin. At the Massachusetts General Hospital, our cardiac rehabilitation program uses the stationary bicycle, walking, and jogging. All patients are medically evaluated and undergo stress testing to measure both oxygen uptake by the lungs and the heart's response to exercise. Each patient gets an individualized exercise prescription based on these evaluations. They then begin a three-month rehabilitation program, coming to the bike lab or track three times a week. Each session begins with a warm-up period of calisthenics and stretching and then includes thirty minutes of dynamic exercise. As the patients improve, the intensity of exercise is increased, so that by the end of three months many patients can jog three miles continuously. A cool-down period concludes each session. Progress is evaluated by measurements of weight, blood pressure, and repeat stress testing to evaluate work capacity and heart function. If all goes well, patients are graduated from the program at the end of three months. But graduation is really only the beginning, for these people can now continue on with unsupervised exercise.

The results have been spectacular. Most patients who've completed the program remain hooked on exercise. They have uniformly achieved a marked increase in work capacity, and many have better blood pressure and blood cholesterol levels despite the use of fewer medications. Our alumni frequently return to the track to exercise with new patients, and we have an annual reunion each March for a five-mile fun run. Although we don't encourage competitive racing, a number of our graduates have participated in road races up to and including the truly spectacular achievement of successful marathon completion.

If running is safe for these patients, exercise should be safe and beneficial for you. We have stressed potential problems in this section in order to give you a balanced account, with guidelines for your protection, but for the great majority of people, careful planning, appropriate medical screening, and a sound program should result in aerobic exercise free of cardiac difficulties.

LUNGS

Exercise does not cause lung damage. However, if air pollution is heavy, temporary lung difficulties can cause coughing, breathlessness, or poor athletic performance. Exercise at high altitudes can result in a severe breathlessness caused by a very serious accumulation of fluid in the lungs, called "pulmonary edema." Anyone engaging in climbing should be acquainted with the symptoms and prevention of mountain sickness.

Another lung problem, which is a rare complication of exercise, is the so-called spontaneous pneumothorax, in which a part of the lung collapses. Sudden shortness of breath and chest pain are the warning signs. Prompt medical attention is necessary, often including hospitalization and placement of tubes to reinflate the collapsed lung.

A much more common but much less serious lung complication of exercise is asthma. Not all people with asthma are susceptible to exercise-induced asthma. And some people can develop wheezing during exercise even though they don't have asthma under other circumstances. Exercise-induced asthma can produce coughing, wheezing, or shortness of breath during or shortly after exercise. In general, the severity of exercise-induced asthma is proportional to the intensity and duration of exercise. Environmental temperature is equally critical. Cold, dry air is the main culprit. Hence, exercise-induced asthma is most likely to occur during intense winter sports such as cross-country skiing or running, and is least likely to occur during warm-weather sports.

If you have exercise-induced asthma, your doctor can prescribe medications that may allow you to exercise even during the winter months. Although standard asthma medications may work, it is important to remember that drugs that stimulate the sympathetic nervous system are not accepted at international competition. Treatment with aminophylline derivatives can help prevent exercise-induced asthma, and these drugs are generally accepted for competitive sports. Another acceptable drug that can be very helpful is called Cromolyn, an inhalation drug. This medication is particularly desirable because it has few stimulatory side effects. Although Cromolyn is widely used for children, it is not commonly prescribed for adults. So if you have exercise-induced asthma, you may want to remind your doctor about this medication.

Even with medications, people with exercise-induced asthma should avoid extreme cold. A long warm-up period and a face mask for outdoor sports may help you adapt to cool weather. But the best defense of all is simply to exercise indoors when it is very cold. Swimming is a particularly desirable sport for people with asthma, because of both the warmer temperatures and the higher humidity.

Even ordinary, allergic-type asthma is no barrier to athletic competition — if the illness is under good medical control. Just ask Olympic sculler Ginny Gilder. She is one of seventy-five asthmatic athletes who entered the 1984 Olympic Games — and collectively won a total of forty-one medals.

EXERCISE AND YOUR BLOOD

Even though your bloodstream bathes all your organs, and your circulation is greatly speeded up during exercise, there are relatively few direct effects of sports on the blood system. For the sake of simplicity, think of your blood as four different elements: plasma, white blood cells, red blood cells, and platelets and other clotting elements.

Plasma is the watery fluid element of blood. When you exercise strenuously you generate lots of heat; in order to dissipate that heat you will sweat profusely. The result can be a fall in the volume of plasma in your circulation. In everyday terms, you will be dehydrated, which can cause many other problems. Protect yourself with adequate fluid replacement (see Chapters 4 and 7).

The white blood cells in your circulation are crucial to fight infection. After exercise, the number of white cells in your blood will rise. However, this effect is only transitory and does not seem to have any real importance. Although many runners and athletes claim that they have many fewer colds since they started exercising, there are no really good scientific studies to support this claim. All in all, exercise does not seem to have any important effects on the white blood cells, either helpful or harmful.

Your red blood cells can be affected by exercise. Some people who exercise regularly and strenuously can develop a so-called sports anemia or pseudoanemia. True anemia reflects an absolute decrease in the numbers of red cells in your body. However, in "sports anemia" the total red cell count is normal, but the *percentage* of red blood cells in your circulation is slightly lower. The reason is that regular exercise can stimulate an increase in your total blood volume, so that even if your red cell numbers are normal, the *percent* of red cells may be decreased. This is nothing that you will ever notice in terms of symptoms. But if you are a regular athlete and a routine checkup discloses mild "anemia," ask your doctor to consider the possibility of pseudoanemia or sports anemia before he puts you through a lot of tests and treatments.

Even less commonly, exercise can help contribute to a true anemia. In certain people the vigorous pounding of running or other sports can injure small blood vessels, which in turn damage the red blood cells in the circulation, so that they are destroyed early. Finally, athletes are sometimes cautioned to take extra iron supplements because iron is lost in sweat or in the intestinal tract. In fact, the amount of iron lost is extremely small; iron-deficiency anemia should not be a problem except in menstruating female athletes who eat low-iron diets.

The final components of your blood are your platelets and clotting proteins. Laboratory tests have shown that exercise makes platelets less sticky and can also activate the blood's mechanisms for dissolving clots. You will never feel any of these effects, and they are not known to cause any bleeding problems whatsoever. In fact, on theoretical grounds they may be helpful since these mechanisms may help prevent harmful blood clots from forming within your arteries.

In summary, the only way in which regular exercise can adversely affect your blood system is by producing a mild anemia, and in most cases this is nothing more than an artifact or pseudoanemia. So if you have any abnormalities of your blood system, don't simply attribute them to exercise; instead, get a thorough medical evaluation to exclude potentially serious illness.

EXERCISE-INDUCED ALLERGIES

Allergic reactions produce feelings of fatigue, flushed skin, and itching; in more advanced cases, allergies produce hives or even diffuse swelling. The most severe form of allergy is "anaphylaxis"; swelling of the lips and tongue, respiratory distress, wheezing, belly pain and nausea, fainting, and collapse are all signs of anaphylaxis.

Whereas most allergies are caused by exposures to foreign chemicals, exercise can produce all of these allergic reactions. Fortunately, exercise-induced allergy and anaphylaxis are really quite uncommon. These episodes tend to occur during strenuous exercise in warm weather, often in people who have allergies to foods or pollens.

Although the symptoms of exercise-induced anaphylaxis can be very alarming, the outlook is excellent. Most people will recover with rest in a cool place. Antihistamines or adrenaline can be used in more serious cases. In fact, most people who have had such episodes can return to exercise without subsequent problems. However, if you've had exercise-induced anaphylaxis, you should check with your doctor before returning to strenuous sports. You will probably be advised to avoid vigorous exertion in very warm weather, and to carry antihistamines, adrenaline, and a medical alert identification in case of emergency.

INTESTINAL COMPLICATIONS OF EXERCISE

Although many athletes experience stomach and bowel

complaints, serious disorders of the digestive tract are really quite rare. A feeling of heartburn and nausea can be troublesome, and occasional athletes may experience vomiting after very strenuous exertion. All of these complaints generally improve with just a few minutes of rest, but if you experience these symptoms, you can try milk, antacids, or dietary manipulations to try to prevent recurrences. The same is basically true for abdominal cramps and diarrhea (the "runner's trots"), which can be caused by the tension of competition or by the physical stress of intense exercise.

The best advice that we can give you is to eat lightly before exercising and to avoid high-fiber foods if you are troubled by cramps. In fact, you should have only liquids within two hours of any reasonably strenuous exercise. If you are subject to cramps or diarrhea, you should avoid substances that may stimulate intestinal motility, such as caffeine and fluids with a very high sugar or salt content.

Intestinal bleeding has been detected in up to 22 percent of marathon runners. In most cases, the bleeding is so mild that it can be detected only in sensitive chemical tests. Exercise-induced bleeding is not itself serious, but if you have bleeding, you should have a thorough medical evaluation to exclude potentially important problems.

EXERCISE AND YOUR KIDNEYS AND BLADDER

The effects of exercise on the urinary tract have been observed by doctors for more than a hundred years. In most cases these are very subtle abnormalities, which can be detected only with laboratory tests, but in some cases they can cause alarming symptoms, such as bloody urine. Even in these dramatic cases, however, the abnormalities are self-limited and should resolve without leaving any kidney damage.

Every time you exercise, your muscles need more blood. As a result, blood flow is diverted away from your internal organs to your muscles. Changes in blood flow to your kidneys won't produce pain or other symptoms, but can produce transient abnormalities of your kidney function. Sensitive blood tests are needed to measure these changes, and the functions virtually always return to normal without any harmful effects. As we have already stated, however, you can help protect your kidneys by drinking adequate volumes of fluid before, during, and after exercise, especially in warm weather.

Exercise can also produce abnormalities in your urine. In most cases it will take a laboratory analysis to detect this. But if your doctor detects small to moderate amounts of protein or some "hyaline-granular casts" during a urinalysis after you've exercised, you should discuss the possibility of exercise-induced abnormalities before undergoing a difficult series of kidney tests. The best test of all, in fact, would be simply to repeat your urinalysis before you exercise; if it's normal, you can be quite sure that the proteins or casts in your urine after exercise are related to exertion rather than to disease of the kidneys.

Red blood cells can also be detected in the urine of many athletes after they exercise strenuously, and can even produce grossly bloody urine. Although these effects were first described in football players and others playing contact sports, it is now clear that bloody urine can also result from many noncontact sports, including running, swimming, and rowing. In fact, up to 18 percent of marathon runners will have at least microscopic amounts of blood in their urine after racing. Some doctors feel that the blood comes from the kidneys, whereas others believe that it comes from the bladder. Although there is disagreement about the cause of the bleeding, there is a general consensus that the problem is benign and self-limited. Even so, if you notice blood in your urine after exercise, you should always report this to your doctor so he can check you over to be sure that you don't have a urinary tract infection or another kidney disorder unrelated to exercise.

EXERCISE AND THE REPRODUCTIVE ORGANS

Menstrual abnormalities are fairly common in highly trained female athletes. Girls who begin intensive training in swimming, running, or ballet before puberty can experience a delayed onset of the menstrual cycle. Older girls or women who begin training after they have started menstruating may notice that their periods became scanty and may even develop amenorrhea, or loss of menstrual periods. In some studies, up to 50 percent of female athletes have reported menstrual abnormalities, but in most cases these are minor complaints rather than complete absence of periods. The likelihood of menstrual abnormalities depends upon the intensity of exertion, so these problems are most likely to occur in highly trained competitive endurance athletes.

The exact causes of menstrual abnormalities are uncertain. Weight loss is one important element. Body fat is responsible for producing some of the body's estrogens, or female hormones. In adult women, 22 percent body fat is considered necessary to maintain normal menstrual function. Competitive long-distance runners may have as little as 7 percent body fat, and even recreational distance runners have less fat (about 15 percent) than do sedentary women (26 to 28 percent). Quite apart from the body fat issue, strenuous exercise may have direct effects on the pituitary gland (the so-called endocrine master gland) and on the levels of various sex hormones.

Exercise-induced menstrual abnormalities are not at all serious. It appears that menstrual function will return to normal with weight gain or decreased training. Long-term effects on reproductive function have not been noted.

However, there is some concern that decreased estrogen levels in women athletes can permit the loss of calcium from bone, resulting in fragile bones or osteoporosis. On the other hand, we know that exercise itself tends to *increase* the amount of calcium in bone. So all in all, the net effect of exercise on bone calcium levels in women athletes is uncertain and requires further study. At this point, theoretical considerations about estrogens and bone calcium are not compelling enough either to prescribe or to proscribe exercise.

Amid these concerns about the effects of exercise on female hormones is some good news from Dr. Rose Frisch and her colleagues at Harvard. Women who begin exercising during their college years are 50 percent less likely to get cancer of the breast or reproductive organs than are sedentary women. Whereas hormonal changes are probably responsible for this protection, normal reproductive function is preserved; the athletes had as many pregnancies as did the sedentary women. It may be premature to say that women can run away from cancer, but the evidence is encouraging.

Exercise is not known to have any consistent effects on male sex hormones or reproductive organs.

If exercise does not have lasting effects on reproductive function, can it still affect sexual behavior? There are widespread anecdotal reports that running and other endurance exercise promote sexual activity and prowess. Glowing testimonials, grateful letters, and magazine readership surveys notwithstanding, there is no scientific proof that regular exercise promotes sexual activity. A few available studies, however, hint that this may be the case; it's too early to say one way or another, but you may be interested in studying this question for yourself.

DIABETES AND EXERCISE

Exercise improves blood sugar metabolism by increasing the efficiency with which the hormone insulin binds to cells. In fact, exercise is one of the oldest treatments for diabetes, and people with mild to moderate diabetes may do very well with exercise, diet, and weight reduction instead of pills or insulin injections. But diabetics who take insulin require special precautions when they exercise because their blood sugar can decline to inappropriately low values. People with diabetes should always have a medical evaluation and supervision before they embark upon strenuous exercise programs. Often a simple decrease in insulin dosage will be all that is necessary, but people with diabetes should also be screened for coronary heart disease and should be instructed in meticulous foot care. Diabetics with active eye problems should avoid strenuous exercise. And anyone with diabetes who plays sports should wear a medical alert bracelet and carry sweets in case they should develop low blood sugar. But with these precautions and with good medical care, diabetics can compete at the highest levels; star athletes with diabetes have included baseball's Catfish Hunter, Ron Santo, and Bill Gullickson, football's Calvin Muhammad, and hockey's Bobby Clarke.

SKIN PROBLEMS RELATED TO EXERCISE AND SPORTS

You may not be accustomed to thinking of your skin as an organ, but in fact, it is one of the largest and most important organs in your body. Although you are undoubtedly aware of the cosmetic importance of your skin, you may not recognize the critical role your skin plays in preventing infection, controlling body temperature, and regulating fluid balance. Your skin is the interface between your internal organs and the outside world. As such, it is subject to disturbances originating either from within or from without; most sports-related skin problems begin with external problems, but if left untreated they can sometimes affect your internal health as well. All in all, even though these problems may be only "skin deep," they certainly merit careful attention.

BLISTERS

The most common causes of blisters are excessive friction, excessive pressure, and excessive moisture. Each of these factors irritates your skin; in response to this irritation, clear, serumlike fluid accumulates between the layers of your skin, causing the layers to separate. Small blisters are nothing more than a minor nuisance, but large blisters can be painful and can sometimes give rise to very serious infection.

Blisters tend to occur in areas of pressure or moisture. Foot blisters can be very disabling. To prevent them, you should always be sure that your shoes fit properly, and you should always break in new shoes gradually. Keep your feet dry with powder and with absorbent socks. In fact, if your feet sweat heavily, you may want to dry them, apply powder, and put on fresh socks during a pause in the action, such as between sets in a tennis match. But if your skin still tends to blister in pressure areas, you can prevent blisters by applying a small slippery plastic Band-Aid over the pressure point even before you put on your socks.

The same principles of prevention apply to other areas of the body where blisters may form, such as the racquet hand of tennis players and the hands of golfers and baseball players. Loosen your grip whenever possible, and be sure to keep your hands as dry as you can. Wearing golf gloves or batting gloves can be extremely helpful for some people.

If, despite these precautions, you still get blisters, you should know how to manage them. Small blisters should be left alone or covered with a thin Band-Aid, but if the blister is large and full of fluid, you'll feel better if the fluid is drained out. If you are faint of heart, you should see your doctor or podiatrist to have this done, but if you have a steady hand you can usually do it quite well yourself (see Figure 12–1). First, gently but thoroughly cleanse the blister with alcohol. Then flame a small needle until it is red hot, so that it's sterilized. After the needle cools, make a few puncture

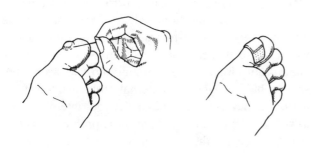

FIGURE 12–1: *How to Drain a Blister* (*see text for details*)

holes and gently squeeze out the fluid. Finally, wash once again with alcohol and cover the blister with a Band-Aid until it has healed.

CHAFING

Moisture and friction can also cause chafing, particularly in your armpit or groin. It's very hard to keep these areas truly dry during sports; to prevent chafing in these sensitive regions, apply a thin layer of Vaseline before you start exercising.

A similar problem in runners is so-called jogger's nipple. Prolonged friction of your running shirt can produce pain and even bleeding of the nipple in both men and women runners. Application of small elastic bandages before running will prevent this problem entirely.

DRY SKIN

Another common skin problem of athletes is dry, cracked skin, which can cause itching, pain, or both. The reason that athletes get dry skin is because they sweat and shower — both perspiration and water actually dry your skin by removing the natural oils that provide lubrication. The best way to handle this problem is by applying generous amounts of skin moisturizers immediately after you shower or bathe. Many effective lotions are available, but two of our favorites are Keri Lotion and Eucerin Cream.

PRICKLY HEAT

This is a common complication of summer sports. Prickly heat is a fine red rash, which produces itching and minor discomfort. The rash is caused by the blockage of sweat pores just at a time when they are working hardest. Although this is not a serious problem, it can be a lingering nuisance. Unfortunately, there is no magic remedy — keep your skin as dry as possible by removing excess sweat during sports, and use skin lubricants following your shower afterward.

ATHLETE'S FOOT AND OTHER FUNGAL INFECTIONS

Although we doctors may try to justify our education by making a diagnosis of *Tenia pedis,* your diagnosis of athlete's foot is every bit as correct. Whichever name you choose, you'll know this condition because of the itching and fissuring between your toes. A scaly rash can develop; in advanced cases your skin may become inflamed and can even develop sores and blisters.

Athlete's foot is caused by a fungus that is not transmitted from person to person, but that can indeed be picked up from environmental surfaces, including locker-room floors. Another fungal infection that plagues athletes is known in your doctor's office as *Tenia cruris*, and in the locker room as "jock itch" or "ringworm." Jock itch affects men more often than women, and because it is aggravated by moisture and friction, it is more common during the summer. Most often the upper thigh and groin are involved, with a deep red discoloration that becomes itchy and scaly. In some cases, you can see tiny little blisters at the margin of the rash, which are usually very sharply defined.

Although these superficial fungus infections are itchy, unsightly, and uncomfortable, they are not really serious. You should always do your best to prevent these problems by keeping your skin clean and dry, and by paying particular attention to the areas between your toes and in your groin and other body creases. If you get one of these infections despite these precautions, you can generally treat yourself quite effectively with a variety of over-the-counter medications. The most commonly used compounds are tolnafate (sold as Tinactin and Aftate) and undecylenic acid (sold as Desenex, Cruex, and other brands); both of these medications are available in powder or ointment form, and both are quite effective. In addition, at least six other medications are available from your doctor by prescription. In very severe cases (or if your nails themselves are heavily involved), your doctor may prescribe pills such as ketoconazole in addition to ointments and powders.

WHIRLPOOL DERMATITIS

A newly recognized skin problem for athletes is ironically enough caused not by sports, but by a commonly used treatment device — the whirlpool. If whirlpools are not adequately cleaned and chlorinated, their nice warm temperatures can provide excellent breeding grounds for certain bacteria. When this occurs, whirlpool users may develop an itchy red rash called whirlpool dermatitis. Although this is caused by a bacterium with a fearsome name (*Pseudomonas*), it is not a serious problem, and will generally go away by itself without antibiotic treatment. You may not need treatment, but your whirlpool will — it is more important to report this problem to the maintenance staff at your health club than to your doctor.

INSECT STINGS

Bee stings and other insect bites are certainly not unique to athletes, but any time you exercise outdoors in summertime, you are exposing yourself to the risk of stings. For most of us, a bee sting means nothing more than temporary pain, which is followed by swelling, redness, and itching at the sting site. An ice pack is the best first-aid treatment. Later on, cold compresses and antihistamine tablets can help relieve persistent discomfort.

But some people are highly allergic to insect venom, and a simple bee sting can cause terrible problems in these circumstances. Approximately two million Americans are in this highly allergic category, and at least forty die each year from severe allergic reactions (anaphylaxis). Up to half of these victims have no previous history of sting allergies, so even if you don't have an allergic history you should be aware of warning symptoms.

Symptoms of severe sting allergy include itching, swelling, or hives over areas of your body that are distant from the sting itself. More serious symptoms include weakness, faintness, wheezing, and trouble swallowing or breathing. Without treatment this can progress to severe respiratory distress, collapse, or shock. Fortunately, emergency injections of adrenaline and treatment with antihistamine medications can be life-saving.

If you are allergic to bee sting, you should wear a medical alert bracelet and always bring an emergency sting kit with you when you play sports. Be sure to instruct your partner in the use of these kits. Most important, be sure to see an allergist — modern techniques of desensitization can often protect you from these severe reactions *if* you begin a series of shots *before* the peak insect season, which is in late summer and early fall.

In addition, all of us can take simple steps to avoid insect stings. Don't wear bright-colored clothing or use perfumes that may attract insects. Cover all food and dispose of leftovers properly. Finally, insect repellents may also provide protection, but you will have to reapply them if you perspire heavily during summertime sports.

SUNBURN

From an aesthetic point of view, a suntan is considered attractive, and is often thought of as a desirable result of outdoor summertime sports. But in medical terms, a suntan is really a mild form of ultraviolet *injury*. If you are exposed gradually to the ultraviolet radiation in sunlight, the cells in your skin try to protect themselves by producing a pigment called melanin, which is responsible for the tan in suntan. But if you are fair skinned, and your sun exposure is abrupt, you will get a burn instead of a tan. A sunburn is just that, a first-degree burn of your skin similar to what you might get from a mild scalding. Your skin becomes red, warm, swollen, and tender.

Because intense ultraviolet exposure will damage and even kill cells in your skin, you should prevent sunburn by exposing yourself to sunlight only gradually at the beginning of the summer sport season. But you may even want to think twice about getting that nice, healthy-looking tan. Even mild sun exposure can, over a prolonged period of time, produce permanent damage to the skin. This can take the form of wrinkling, yellowing, or premature aging, and can even lead to skin cancer.

Does this mean indoor sports during summer? Indeed not. You can protect yourself very well with a few simple, commonsense measures. Remember that the sun's rays are strongest between 10 A.M. and 2 P.M., and that even cloudy days can be troublesome because an overcast sky will still transmit ultraviolet rays. Try to stay in the shade whenever possible, or bring your own shade in the form of a wide-brimmed hat or sun visor and light-colored clothing, which may help reflect the sun's rays. But we cannot recommend long pants and sleeves if you exercise vigorously in summer, because of the problems of heat retention. Fortunately, you can now protect your skin from ultraviolet damage with a variety of excellent sunscreen lotions.

The oldest types of sunscreen are physical agents such as zinc oxide paste. These work very well but are greasy and unsightly, so most people prefer to use newer compounds. A second group of sunscreens contain a chemical called para-aminobenzoic acid, or PABA. PABA lotions are very effective, but can cause some skin irritation and can stain light-colored clothing in some cases. Because of this, a final group of sunscreens has been developed that contains other ingredients such as cinnamates or benzophenones or padimate O.

You can choose whichever sunscreen is most pleasant to use. To compare sunscreens of different brands, look at the SPF (sun protective factor) rating. Higher numbers such as 10–15 provide the greatest protection and should be used by fair-skinned people who anticipate an intense exposure early in the season. On the other hand, if you have a darker complexion or if you wish to acquire a tan, you can use a sunscreen with a lower number, say 6–10. Whatever lotion you choose must be applied properly. It's best to apply the lotion at least one hour before you go out in the sun; because moisture will wash off the sunscreen, reapply the lotion after you sweat, swim, or shower.

If you are unfortunate enough to get a sunburn despite these precautions, stay out of the sun until you get better. Topical anaesthetic agents (the so-called *caines*) will help relieve pain, at least temporarily. However, you may develop an allergy to one of these chemicals, so we'd suggest trying cold compresses as the first resort. Skin moisturizers, zinc oxide, and even topical steroids can also be helpful. Aspirin tablets will also help relieve pain and inflammation, which can sometimes be severe enough to cause fever. Drink plenty of fluids, so you don't get dehydrated; if your burn is severe enough to cause blisters or weeping, see your doctor for help in preventing infection and other complications.

ENVIRONMENTAL ILLNESSES IN ATHLETES

Your exercise schedule should always take environmental conditions into account. By careful planning, you should be able to avoid most problems (see Chapter 7), but if symptoms of environmental illness occur during sports, you must be prepared to take prompt action to avoid serious damage.

HEAT ILLNESSES

There are three distinct patterns of heat illness in athletes. The mildest problem is *heat cramps*. These are painful involuntary spasms of the muscles that you are using most. Massage and stretching will generally alleviate the pain, and may even allow you to resume competition. Adequate hydration will go a long way toward preventing heat cramps.

A more serious problem is *heat exhaustion*. Whereas most athletes with heat cramps have normal body temperature, heat exhaustion is usually accompanied by a rise in body temperature to about 102 degrees. Other symptoms of heat exhaustion include fatigue, rapid breathing, headache, loss of concentration, light-headedness, and nausea. Profuse sweating is the rule, and as a result of this you may even feel paradoxically chilled at a time when your internal temperature is abnormally high. Despite all these symptoms, heat exhaustion will usually respond to simple first-aid measures if you take care of yourself properly. If you have warning symptoms of heat exhaustion, you must stop exercising immediately and rest quietly in a cool, dry place. A cold tub or shower or even ice packs would be extremely helpful. In addition, it's very, very important to drink large amounts of cool fluids so that your body will have enough fluid to bring your temperature down to normal.

The third type of heat injury is a true medical emergency. *Heat stroke* can occur as a result of strenuous exercise in the summer, but elderly or debilitated people can develop this problem even without the stress of exercise. For reasons that are not clear, one of the first symptoms of heat stroke is an inappropriate and abnormal cessation of sweating, so that the skin is flushed, dry, and very hot. Because sweating stops, body temperature rises rapidly, often to alarming levels of 106 degrees or higher. Confusion, grogginess, and then coma are major symptoms. Many serious abnormalities of blood chemistries occur, such as a rise in potassium levels and a severe acid load. Kidney failure, liver damage, and clotting abnormalities are common. In fact, without vigorous treatment heat stroke is a highly lethal disorder.

Heat stroke requires immediate expert treatment in a hospital emergency ward. If you suspect heat stroke in a fellow athlete, you should get medical help as soon as possible. Get the victim out of the sun and into as cool an environment as possible. Cold compresses or ice packs are extremely helpful. If the victim is conscious, he should drink cold fluids, but you should never try to force liquids into a groggy or stuporous victim.

COLD ILLNESSES

Frostbite begins with stinging or aching and then progresses to a numb feeling. The numbness can be very misleading, because you may mistakenly assume that the lack of a pain means that your body is safe. Quite the reverse is true — the lack of sensation is an important danger signal, even if there is no actual pain. Frostbite most often affects your fingers, toes, ears, or nose. These areas of your body will look white and waxy. Emergency treatment involves getting out of the cold as soon as possible, and rewarming your tissues in warm water of about 105 degrees. Because improper rewarming followed by refreezing increases tissue damage, rewarming should be delayed if necessary until

there is no risk of refreezing. During rewarming, your skin will become red and will be very painful. If the pain persists after rewarming, or if there is any discoloration of your skin, you should get immediate medical attention to be sure that there is no permanent tissue damage.

Exposure and *hypothermia* are even more serious problems. Hypothermia generally occurs during winter sports if injury, equipment failure, or exhaustion causes you to stop exercising before you can get warm. But even in temperate weather, immersion and wind chill can produce hypothermia.

The symptoms of hypothermia are gradual and insidious. Victims note extreme fatigue, mental confusion, and incoordination. They often have slurred speech, apathy, and impaired judgment, so they may not recognize that they are in danger in enough time to take corrective action. If hypothermia is allowed to progress without treatment, shivering occurs, and eventually the muscles become stiff and rigid. Shock will occur next, along with many metabolic changes; irregularities of the heartbeat are the most serious threat and can be lethal without prompt treatment.

Field management of hypothermia requires removing the victim to shelter as soon as possible. Warm, dry clothing is essential. In mild cases, the patient should drink warm fluids, and mild muscular activity may be encouraged. In more severe cases, rewarming with blankets and sleeping bags is critically important; external rewarming can be facilitated by wrapping the victim in the company of a healthy companion.

In mild cases of exposure these first-aid measures may suffice. But in more severe cases, and in true hypothermia, emergency evacuation to a hospital is mandatory.

ALTITUDE SICKNESS

High-altitude illness comes in several forms. The mildest is so-called *acute mountain sickness* or AMS. In its mildest form, AMS consists only of temporary headache, lack of concentration, nausea, and insomnia. But in more severe cases, vomiting, confusion, clumsiness, and even more serious problems can occur. Mild AMS is a self-limited problem that will generally subside with rest in several days. But other forms of altitude sickness can be much more severe. One of these severe syndromes is *high-altitude cerebral edema* or brain swelling. Here, headache and mild confusion rapidly progress to hallucinations and bizzare behavior or disorientation, drowsiness, stupor, and even coma. High-altitude cerebral edema is a true medical emergency, as is another form of altitude sickness that is called *pulmonary edema,* or fluid in the lungs. The symptoms of high-altitude pulmonary edema are breathlessness, cough, chest discomfort, and the production of frothy pink sputum. Both high-altitude cerebral edema and pulmonary edema can be fatal if not rapidly treated. Another form of mountain sickness, which is somewhat less severe, involves bleeding into the back of the eye, resulting in visual disturbance. Even though this complication is not likely to be fatal, it is serious and does deserve prompt medical attention.

We won't detail the medical treatment of mountain sickness, but we would like to stress the most important element in prevention: gradual ascent with plenty of time for acclimatization during each stage of your ascent. A medication called acetazolamide may help if it is taken preventively during ascent, but it is no substitute for gradual ascent and progressive acclimatization.

HEAD PROBLEMS

INJURIES

Head injuries are actually quite uncommon in athletes who are participating in lifesports or other noncontact sports. Quite the reverse is true in contact sports, in which head injuries can be devastating. Because this is a book about the use of exercise and sports for health and fitness, we are going to try to steer you away from contact sports, into activities that will give you the many benefits of endurance training without the hazards of trauma. But all of us should have at least a rudimentary knowledge of what to do about head injuries in ourselves or other athletes.

Here, too, prevention is the most important aspect of sports medicine. In the area of head injuries, prevention takes many forms, including avoiding contact sports and trauma, using proper equipment with good technique, playing by the rules, and tempering competitiveness with civility, whether you are swinging a tennis racquet or hockey stick, or jogging or biking along a busy roadway. But the prevention of head injuries also involves the use of specific protective devices. Serious bike riders, for example, should always wear protective helmets. Hockey injuries have decreased

dramatically since the advent of mandatory helmets, face masks, and mouth protectors. Safety glasses or goggles should always be worn for racquetball and squash, and we think they are an excellent idea for tennis as well.

If a head injury occurs despite this equipment, it must be taken seriously. If you receive a blow on the head and "see stars" or if you are dazed, you should stop play and rest quietly until your mind is totally clear. If you black out, even momentarily, if you are so badly stunned that you are temporarily confused, or if you sustain a loss of memory for the event that "rings your bell," you should assume you have had a concussion. Any player who has a concussion should check out of the game for the rest of the day and get a competent medical evaluation.

You should also know some important warning signs that can be clues to more serious problems: persistent headaches, nausea and vomiting, confusion, slurred speech, blurred vision, forgetfulness, uncoordination or an unsteady gait are all symptoms that mandate immediate medical evaluation. Sleepiness can also be a sign of serious problems, as can impairment of thought and judgment. Hence, the injured person is really not in a good position to monitor himself for signs of problems. Even if your condition seems quite good at first and your doctor tells you to go home, you should have somebody with you who can watch for these warning signs, so that you can be brought back to the hospital if necessary. Remember, too, that these warning signs can occur hours or even days after the injury itself.

As a spectator or player, you may sometimes be called on to aid an unconscious athlete. Unless you are medically trained or very sophisticated in first aid, your first response should be to get immediate help. If the victim is breathing easily, do not move him at all. Patients with head, spine, or back injuries should be moved *only* if this is necessary to clear their airway and establish good breathing. Otherwise, wait for medical help to arrive so that the head and spine can be stabilized before the patient is moved.

Obviously the unconscious athlete poses a potentially urgent problem. Here, too, our advice is relatively simple: get help. Your only first-aid responsibility should be to be sure that the ABC's are intact. First, be sure that the victim is positioned so the *airway* is open. Second, be sure that *breathing* is normal. Third, be sure that *circulation* is adequate by checking for a heartbeat or pulse.

HEADACHES

Headaches are very common problems both on and off the playing field. The most common causes of headaches during exercise are dehydration and overheating. Headaches, loss of concentration, and fatigue can sometimes be the only symptoms of dehydration or heat exhaustion, so remember to drink plenty of fluids before, during, and after your play, especially in warm weather. In the dog days of July and August, try to avoid exposure to direct sunlight and shift your exercise to early morning or late evening if at all possible. A visor can protect your eyes from glare; visors are preferable to hats because they allow your head to dissipate a surprisingly large amount of your body's heat. If you cover up with a hat, you may well increase the risks of overheating.

There are many other causes of headaches during exercise. Eyestrain can certainly be the culprit, particularly during sports that require visual concentration and hand-eye coordination. Glare can also strain your eyes and produce headaches, so you may want to try a pair of sunglasses if this seems to be your problem. Remember, however, to pick a pair of high-quality safety lenses if you are playing a sport such as tennis or baseball in which you run a risk of eye trauma.

Another cause of headaches is plain, ordinary tension. Tension headaches most commonly affect the back of the head and neck and come on at periods of stress or intense concentration. If you find yourself getting headaches from tension during sports, you should seriously rethink your competitive philosophy; exercise should be an outlet for pent-up energies and tensions, not a cause of stress.

Exercise itself can cause one variety of headache, the so-called benign exertional headache. Benign exertional headaches tend to come on with strenuous effort, particularly if it involves isometrics such as lifting heavy objects or pushing against a fixed resistance. These headaches can be quite severe and typically produce a pounding pain all over your head. The anti-inflammatory drug indomethacin (Indocin) seems particularly helpful for benign exertional headaches, although we do not know just how it works.

However, if you are prone to repeated or severe headaches during exercise, you cannot simply assume that you have one of these exercise-related problems. There are many, many other causes of headaches, including migraine and other vascular headaches, allergies, high blood pressure, infections, alcohol toxicity, sinusitis, mental problems, and even strokes or tumors. Fortunately, these serious cases of headaches are much less common than are the simple, ordinary headaches experienced by athlete and nonathlete alike. But if your headaches don't go away with rest, fluids, and aspirin or acetaminophen, or if they are unusually severe or recurrent, be sure to see a doctor for a thorough evaluation.

EYE INJURIES

The National Society to Prevent Blindness tells us that there are at least twenty-five thousand sports-related eye injuries in the United States each year that are severe enough to require emergency medical treatment. A great many of these problems can be prevented, chiefly by wearing appropriate eye gear. It is also important to think about your eyes *before* an injury occurs; your goal should be to keep your eye on the ball, so the ball won't get in your eye.

Your eye is surrounded by a group of strong bones called the orbit. The orbit provides protection for the eye, but unfortunately this protection is not complete. A strong blow can fracture these bones, producing a so-called blowout fracture, which will cause pain, swelling, and often double vision. Surgery is usually needed for blowout fracture, but on your way to the emergency ward, remember to keep an ice pack on the injured eye.

Whereas a strong blow with a blunt object is necessary to damage the strong bones of the orbit, even mild pressure can produce serious injuries if the object which hits you is small enough to strike your eye itself. The cornea is easily scratched; although corneal abrasions usually heal well with simple patching, infections can complicate healing and scars may result. The eye can sometimes be cut or lacerated, or internal bleeding into the eye (called "hyphema") may occur. Both of these problems usually require surgery. Finally, trauma can cause a retinal detachment, which also requires expert care on an urgent basis.

Eye injuries are too serious and too subtle for you to treat them yourself. In fact, even a general physician is usually not equipped to handle these problems, so you should be referred to an ophthalmologist. Perhaps one of the things that frustrates ophthalmologists most is that the great majority of sports injuries can be prevented. Courtesy, common sense, and concentration will go a long way toward protecting you from a stray ball, a stray racquet, or a stray finger. But appropriate protective gear is also extremely important. Wire or plastic cagelike devices can be used to protect your eyes during racquet sports or hockey. Even better are goggles or safety glasses made of impact-resistant materials such as polycarbonate plastic or CR39 plastic. People who wear glasses for visual correction should always use high-quality safety lenses and impact-resistant frames for sports. But even if you don't ordinarily wear glasses, you should seriously think about a pair of safety glasses or goggles for protection alone; this is mandatory for squash and racquetball and highly desirable for tennis. Even sports such as baseball and basketball can lead to eye injuries; lest you feel foolish or self-conscious about wearing goggles, remember that the towering center for the Los Angeles Lakers, Kareem Abdul-Jabbar, is not above wearing protective goggles when he plays ball.

EAR AND SINUS PROBLEMS

Swimmers and divers are the only athletes who are particularly vulnerable to ear and sinus problems. See page 209 for a discussion of these problems.

NOSE INJURIES

Nosebleeds are a common consequence of even mild trauma. Most often, the bleeding point is in the anterior or front part of the nose and will respond to simple first aid. You should rest quietly and comfortably in a sitting position while you apply pressure with an ice pack. If the bleeding doesn't stop, you'll need medical care, which may involve a nasal pack.

Because the nose is made up of rather fragile bones, fractures can also occur. If you are hit on the nose, apply ice as quickly as possible. If your nose seems misshapen or if your breathing is impaired, head for an emergency ward. The best time to reset a broken nose is within the first few hours after an injury, because after that, swelling may make proper alignment difficult or even impossible. On your way to the hospital, don't forget our wonder drug — ice.

MOUTH INJURIES

Like eye injuries, many mouth injuries can be prevented by wearing appropriate protective gear. When mouth injuries occur, they can be quite dramatic, but fortunately they are usually not terribly serious. Because your lips are very vascular, even a small cut can cause rather impressive bleeding. In most cases, ice and gentle pressure will stop the bleeding within a few minutes; even after the bleeding has stopped, you should reapply ice several times over the first few hours to help prevent swelling. However, if the bleeding persists or if the cut seems very deep, see a surgeon or oral surgeon for sutures.

Direct trauma can also loosen a tooth. If your tooth is in proper alignment and only slightly loose, you can handle the problem yourself simply by eating only soft solid foods and liquids for a few days until the tooth tightens up. But if the tooth is displaced or if you have a lot of pain, you should see your dentist. Your dentist can also do wonders with fractures of dental enamel; small fractures will respond simply to polishing, although larger fractures may need a crown.

On rare occasions you may have a tooth knocked out completely by a direct blow. If this happens to you, your first job is to find the tooth. Do not put it under your pillow as an offering for the tooth fairy. Instead, wash it off and try to replace it carefully into its natural position. If you can't get it back, put it in a glass of cool water. In either case, head for your dentist at once — it may be possible to save your tooth by attaching it to adjacent teeth to immobilize it while healing occurs, and then performing root canal treatments.

Although dentists are crucially important in dealing with these mouth injuries, we would like to caution you against expecting too much from your dentist. In the past few years there has been increasing interest in the field of sports dentistry or "oral orthopedics." It has produced tremendous advances in protective mouth guards, but in some cases it has also spawned unsubstantiated claims. A number of well-known athletes have taken to wearing mouth guards at night in the belief that they will relax the entire body and produce improved athletic performance. If you have jaw pain or headaches caused by grinding or clenching your teeth, this type of mouth guard will help. But unless you have this problem, don't expect your dentist to replace your coach.

MUSCULOSKELETAL PROBLEMS

NECK INJURIES

The neck is composed of many delicate structures packed

into a small space. The cervical, or upper, spine is composed of bony vertebrae separated by soft elastic disks. The spine is surrounded by strong muscles and ligaments, which provide stability, support, and also mobility. Finally, the major nerves and blood vessels for your shoulders, arms, and hands all pass through the neck, so neck injuries can sometimes produce pain or weakness in the arms.

Acute neck injuries are a major cause of concern. Injuries to the neck may produce nothing more than a muscle strain with pain and spasm, but because there is always the potential for spinal cord compression, significant neck injuries should be evaluated by a trained professional. The best advice is to avoid moving the injured athlete. This is particularly true if there is severe neck pain, and it is critically important if there is any numbness or weakness elsewhere in the body. Call for help, and let the first-aid team know the exact nature of the problem. Very careful immobilization will be required before the athlete can be transported to the hospital by stretcher and ambulance.

Fortunately, most neck problems are not this serious. The most common cause of neck pain in athletes and nonathletes alike is muscle spasm. Most often, a sudden unexpected motion produces excessive stretching in a muscle, which in turn responds with unduly strong contractions or spasms. Because the neck muscles are quite strong, the spasms are painful. Pain in turn leads to more spasm. Finally, the vigorous contractions can put pressure directly on nerves and blood vessels, resulting in impaired blood flow, tissue swelling, and nerve pressure, which further perpetuates the cycle of pain and spasm.

Neck spasms can be so severe that your neck can actually become stiff and locked or fixed in abnormal posture. Your doctor calls this spastic torticolis, your mother calls it a wry neck — either way, neck muscle spasms require prompt attention.

The first principle of treatment is rest — whenever a muscle is acutely stretched, inflamed, torn, or in spasm, it should be put to rest as much as possible until healing is under way. In the case of mild neck strains or spasms, this can be accomplished simply by staying away from sports for a couple of days. But in more severe cases it may be advisable to immobilize your neck as well. You can make a cervical collar by rolling a large bath towel into a tube, wrapping it loosely around your neck, and pinning it. Or you can get an official collar from your doctor or at a surgical supply house; foam collars are usually more comfortable than the rigid plastic types.

Whatever type you choose, be sure that it is well fitted so that it is comfortable and it holds your neck in a neutral position without forcing it backward.

If you need a collar, your goal should be to wean yourself away from it as soon as possible. Wear it early after the injury, but gradually reduce the number of hours you use it each day, so that you can do without it entirely within a week or ten days.

Even if the collar seems to help, it is very important to use other treatment methods simultaneously. Early after an injury, ice packs may help prevent swelling, pain, and inflammation in your injured neck muscles. After a day or two, however, heat is more helpful to relax muscles, and heat is especially useful during rehabilitation when you start to exercise your neck. Medications to fight pain and inflammation are also extremely helpful, and should be used as soon as possible after the injury; if aspirin doesn't do the trick, ask your doctor about the newer nonsteroidal anti-inflammatory drugs. If your spasms are unusually severe, you may need muscle relaxants as well.

Although you may be able to take care of mild to moderate neck problems by yourself, it is very important to see your doctor if pain persists despite treatment. In particular, if you have numbness or weakness in your shoulder, arm, or hand, you should get prompt medical attention to be sure that you don't have a pinched nerve. In most cases, your doctor will check for nerve compression and will order X rays of your neck. If there is evidence of a ruptured disk, nerve pressure, or neck arthritis, your doctor may prescribe traction or other treatments. Don't let this prospect frighten you — in most cases traction can be accomplished at home and is required only on a temporary basis.

Once the acute injury settles down, you should begin a rehabilitation program. At first you won't be able to exercise at all, but as your pain subsides you should begin gentle range of motion exercises (see Figure 12–2). These are best done in a warm shower because the wet heat will help relax tight muscles. For the first few days, the only exercise you should do is to rotate your head gently to the left and to the right; move your head slowly and exert gentle pressure toward each side, going only so far as you are comfortable. Hold your head in a position of maximum rotation for five to ten seconds and then return it to a neutral position. When your neck is better, you can start flexion and extension exercises simply by looking down toward your toes and then up toward the ceiling. Again, move slowly and don't go past the point of pain. Another helpful exercise

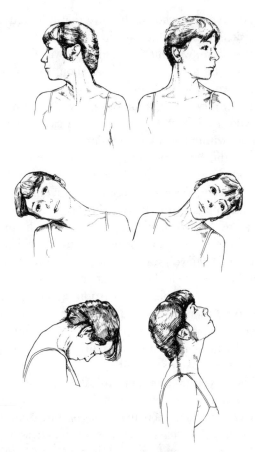

FIGURE 12–2: *Neck Exercises*

is to try to touch your ear to your shoulder by gently bending your neck laterally without shrugging your shoulder. A final simple maneuver is to shrug both shoulders upward toward your ears for a count of five, then relax and stretch your shoulders back as far as possible for another count of five.

When neck flexibility is restored and you are free of pain, you can start exercises to strengthen your neck. Begin with isometrics, which can be done easily by thrusting your head forward, backward, or to the side against the counterpressure of your clasped hands or a small towel held between your hands. Hold the contraction for seven seconds without moving your neck, rest for three seconds, and then repeat. Build up to a total of ten repetitions in each of the four directions. When your muscle strength is back, you can add isotonic exercises such as head and shoulder lifts or sit-ups with your hands clasped behind your neck (see Figures 6–14 and 6–74).

Whatever else you do, you will surely want to prevent further neck problems. The key is good posture. Your goal should be the so-called flat neck position, in which your chin is tucked in and your neck is held up and back. You should maintain this posture whether you are sitting or standing. Neck spasms can occur when you sleep, so it is important to retain good posture even in bed. If you sleep on your side, use only a small pillow under your neck to maintain a neutral position. If you sleep on your back, a three- or four-inch pillow should be placed under your neck rather than under your head. If you sleep on your stomach, try to get out of the habit because this position tends to force your neck into an unnatural posture, which can lead to spasms.

In addition to good posture, it is important to avoid excessive or abrupt motions of your head. In normal daily activities muscle spasms are most likely to result from excessive extension of the neck, as in looking upward. For example, you should not attempt to reach for heavy objects by lifting your hands over your head and looking upward; instead get a stool or stepladder high enough so that object is level with your eyes. In sports, too, try as much as possible to avoid sudden jerky motions of your neck, which can lead to spasms. Finally, be sure to warm up your neck muscles with gentle stretching exercises before you begin any strenuous activity.

At first it may be a nuisance to remind yourself constantly of these simple precautions. But after a while, they'll become second nature. Some thought and care on your part will certainly be worthwhile: if you use your head now, you won't have to get treatment for your head or neck later.

THE SHOULDER

In order for you to understand both the strengths and weaknesses of the shoulder, just imagine yourself passing a football, pitching a baseball, hitting a serve or overhand smash, or swimming the butterfly. Each of these motions requires an extraordinary degree of mobility of the shoulder joint, and each of them puts great stress on that joint. Although the shoulder is engineered for maximum mobility, this very freedom of motion means that it is also susceptible to overstress injuries.

The shoulder is a ball-and-socket joint. The ball is composed of the head of the humerus or arm bone, and the socket is composed of a smooth, depressed surface at the outer margin of the shoulder blade or scapula. Part of the scapula also comes around the top rear of the shoulder joint, where it joins with the collarbone (see Figure 12–3). The bony structures of the shoulder girdle are surrounded by numerous muscles, both big and small, which move the shoulder through its extraordinary range of motion. In addition, the shoulder is stabilized by a number of ligaments, and also by the capsule that surrounds the joint. Finally, the normal anatomy of the shoulder includes the bursae or fluid-filled sacs, which provide cushioning and lubrication for the shoulder as it moves through its range of motion.

If you think the shoulder is a complicated joint, you're quite right. With so many structures packed into such a small area, moving in so many directions with so much force, it's not surprising that shoulder pain can be quite difficult to figure out, even for your doctor. We'd like to introduce the main categories of shoulder pain so that you will be able to deal with at least milder shoulder problems on your own.

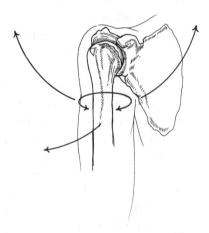

FIGURE 12–3: *The Shoulder*

Shoulder Separation

A fall on the tip of the shoulder causes this relatively common sports injury by tearing the ligaments of the joint. The result is a sprain, also known as a shoulder pointer or shoulder separation. Shoulder separations cause pain at the top of the shoulder, and may produce a snapping sound when you move your shoulder.

Mild shoulder separations can be treated with ice, anti-inflammatory drugs, and rest; you may need a sling for one or two weeks until the pain lessens, but you should move on to rehabilitation exercises as quickly as possible. Complete separations, however, should always be treated by orthopedic specialists, since surgery may be required.

Shoulder Dislocation

Whereas a shoulder separation involves only the small joint between the acromion and the clavicle, a true dislocation involves the main shoulder joint itself. In a shoulder dislocation, the head of the humerus pops out of its socket, causing severe pain and a marked reduction in mobility.

Although some athletes who have had recurrent dislocations can actually reduce ("relocate") the injury themselves, we believe that a skilled physician should always be the one to perform these treatments. The treatment, however, does not stop with replacing the ball in the socket; even after the joint is back together, you will need a period of six to eight weeks of immobilization in a sling, followed by a comprehensive rehabilitation program. These exercises are extremely important to rebuild your shoulder strength. Rehabilitation is important for two reasons: first, to restore strength and motion of the shoulder, and second, to prevent recurrent dislocations. Unfortunately, shoulder joints that have been dislocated two or more times are prone to repeated episodes, which can occur with any throwing motion. The more dislocations you have had, the easier it is to relocate the shoulder — but the more likely you are to have recurrent episodes. Ultimately, you may lose strength and mobility, and can even develop arthritis in the shoulder joint as a result of recurrent dislocations. Because of this, surgery may be indicated in some cases to restore the integrity of the joint and prevent dislocations.

Bursitis

Although there are many fluid-filled bursal sacs around the shoulder joint, the most common form of shoulder

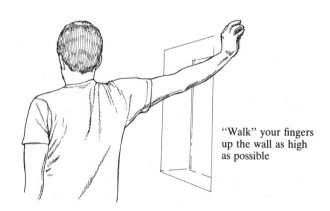

"Walk" your fingers up the wall as high as possible

FIGURE 12–4: *Wall-Climbing Exercise*

bursitis involves the sac at the tip of the shoulder just below the acromion. This problem can result from overuse, and will cause constant pain in the shoulder, which can even be severe enough to keep you up at night. You'll have tenderness at the tip of your shoulder, and motion of the shoulder joint will be painful.

Since this is another form of "itis," aspirin or other anti-inflammatory medications can be very helpful both to reduce inflammation and to diminish pain. Your natural inclination will be to avoid moving your shoulder if you have this type of bursitis. Whereas rest is very important for most inflammatory injuries, excessive rest can be very harmful to the shoulder. You should begin an early program to mobilize your shoulder, using pendulum and wall-climbing exercises (see Figure 12–4). If you don't get your shoulder moving early, it can become very stiff or "frozen." If anti-inflammatory pills and exercises don't do the trick, an injection of cortisone into the bursa can be very helpful.

Tendinitis

Tendinitis of the shoulder joint can be quite hard to distinguish from bursitis. One clue is that the pain of bursitis tends to be constant, whereas the pain of tendinitis may actually diminish as you loosen up your shoulder with use. In addition, X rays are normal in bursitis, but in some cases of chronic tendinitis X rays will show deposits of calcium along the tendon. The treatment for bursitis and tendinitis is basically the same. Early mobilization is important, even in the face of shoulder pain. A few minutes of pendulum and wall-climbing exercises can help avoid many hours of painful rehabilitation from a frozen shoulder.

The Painful Shoulder Syndrome

All of the conditions we've been discussing cause shoulder pain, but another very complex type of painful shoulder injury can occur in any athlete who performs repetitive motions involving forceful overhead movement of the arm. Examples include the service and overhead shots in tennis, passing a football or pitching a baseball, and the freestyle, butterfly, or backstroke in swimming. This type of injury goes under many names, including "swimmer's shoulder," the "impingement syndrome," and the "painful arch syndrome."

No matter what sport causes this injury, the problem lies in the same groups of muscles and tendons. Overhead movement of the shoulder calls into play a group of four muscles, which are collectively known as the rotator cuff. Repetitive use of these muscles can cause strains or inflammation in the muscles or the tendons that attach them to bone. If inflammation is the major injury, pain will be your major symptom. However, if fibers of the muscles or tendons are actually torn, you can also develop weakness and limited motion.

The pain of rotator cuff injuries is most marked at the outer or lateral part of the shoulder, just below the tip of the shoulder at the top end of your arm. The pain will be greatest when you attempt to elevate your shoulder between 45 and 120 degrees. You can also have tenderness of your shoulder, which may be so severe that you'll find it impossible to sleep on your side.

Needless to say, it's best to treat these rotator cuff problems as early as possible. Milder cases of inflammation usually respond nicely to cutting back on activities that involve overhead motions of the arm, along with using ice and anti-inflammatory medications. Rehabilitation exercises for flexibility and strength are extremely important. In more severe cases, you may have to avoid serving or throwing motions altogether until the pain has settled down. In such severe cases, steroid injections may be indicated. The most serious of these injuries, however, involve actual tearing of rotator cuff muscles or tendons. A special X ray called an arthrogram, in which dye is injected into the shoulder joint, may be necessary to establish the diagnosis of a rotator cuff tear. Mild tears may respond to a comprehensive rehabilitation program, but severe tears may require surgical repair. Rotator cuff tears have jeopardized or ended many athletic careers, particularly of baseball pitchers, so they should always be managed by an orthopedic surgeon with special expertise and experience in this area.

Reconditioning and Rehabilitation

Exercises for strength and flexibility are extremely important in the recovery from any shoulder injury. We have already discussed and illustrated pendulum and wall-climbing exercises, which constitute the earliest program to maintain flexibility immediately after an injury. You should move on to more comprehensive strength and flexibility exercises (see Chapter 2).

When you have rebuilt your shoulder with these exercises, you can return to play. However, it is extremely important that you resume competition in a graded, logical fashion so that you don't reinjure your shoulder. We can think of no better advice than Dr. Frank W. Jobe's program. Dr. Jobe is one of our leading authorities on the shoulder, and he has performed nearly miraculous surgical repairs of rotator cuff tears, which have allowed players to beat the odds and return to competitive sports. Dr. Jobe suggests a six-point regimen for a return to throwing:

1. Briefly massage and stretch your shoulder before throwing. A careful warm-up period is extremely important to limber up your shoulder before you even pick up a ball or racquet.
2. Perform throwing or serving motions without a ball or racquet.
3. Lob the ball easily, wearing your warm-up jacket. If your sport is tennis, perform shadow serves without actually hitting a ball. If your sport is swimming, move your arm through your stroke pattern before even getting into the water. Begin playing easily, whether this involves gently lobbing a ball, hitting a few soft serves, or swimming at a slow speed.
4. Gradually increase the intensity of your work until you have built up to full strength.
5. After you complete your play, put on a warm-up jacket or sweatshirt and perform a full set of stretching exercises to cool down gradually and stretch out your shoulder.
6. Finally, spend twenty or thirty minutes with an ice pack on your shoulder to prevent recurrent inflammation.

THE UPPER ARM

In the absence of trauma, arm injuries are relatively uncommon in athletes. One problem that can occur is inflammation of the biceps muscle or its tendon. This is particularly likely to occur at the upper end of the arm near the front of the shoulder joint. Sometimes chronic inflammation can result in a "snapping shoulder," a snapping sound produced when a thickened biceps tendon snaps out of its groove. The snapping shoulder does not require any treatment unless there is associated pain. Biceps inflammation or tendinitis does require treatment, but usually responds quite nicely to the PRICE program (see pages 251–252). An even less common problem involving the biceps is actual rupture of the long head of the muscle. This typically occurs at the time of a forceful contraction, and causes the abrupt onset of pain and tenderness, which resolves gradually over a few days. You'll know that this involves more than just inflammation, however, because you'll see a bulge in the front of your arm. A trip to your doctor

will be necessary to confirm the diagnosis and plan treatment. The only way to get rid of the bulge is to undergo surgical repair of the ruptured muscle. If you use your biceps maximally during sports, repair may be needed to restore full strength. However, some athletes can get along surprisingly well even without surgery.

THE ELBOW

The elbow is composed of three bones: the largest is the humerus or upper arm, which meets the smaller radius and the even smaller ulna of the forearm at the elbow joint (Figure 12–5). This arrangement allows two important motions at the elbow joint; bending and straightening is the major motion, but the forearm can also move in a rotary fashion. The elbow joint is a delicate apparatus because of its broad range of motion, its relatively weak bones, and its lack of padding with large muscles. In addition, important nerves and vessels lie close to the joint and also near to the skin surface, where they may be damaged by direct injuries.

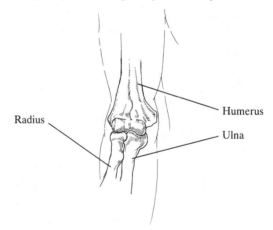

Radius   Humerus   Ulna

FIGURE 12–5: *The Elbow*

Most sports-related elbow injuries are due either to direct trauma or to repeated use of the joint, as in racquet sports, golf, or sports that require lots of throwing. Sprains and strains of the elbow usually result from contact sports, and are particularly troublesome if the elbow is bent back excessively, the so-called hyperextension injury. Strains and sprains should be treated in the usual fashion with ice, rest, compression, and elevation; tape is very useful to stabilize and immobilize the joint, and a sling can be helpful to protect the elbow further. However, if you sustain elbow trauma and experience severe pain and rapid swelling, particularly in the context of a hyperextension injury, you may have a dislocation. You should have this checked out by your doctor as quickly as possible, because a dislocated elbow can put pressure on nerves and blood vessels. Similarly, a fracture of any of the bones that make up the elbow joint also requires prompt and expert attention.

A direct blow to the elbow can also cause a condition called "olecranon bursitis." Although this name sounds fearsome, it is usually a fairly mild problem, which you may recognize readily by its common name of "beer drinker's elbow." This popular name derives from the fact that pressure on the elbow joint from any cause — including the surface of a bar — can lead to an accumulation of fluid in the bursa, or sac, behind the elbow joint. You'll notice a soft swelling behind the elbow, but your elbow itself should be able to move normally without pain. Ice and pressure are usually very helpful; an elastic bandage will ordinarily suffice, but you may need a sling for a day or two. If, however, the swollen bursa is also red and hot, your doctor will probably want to tap the fluid out to be sure you don't have an infection or gout. Drainage can sometimes be useful even for ordinary elbow bursitis, although the fluid usually reaccumulates unless steroid medications are injected into the sac. You can protect yourself against recurrences by wearing an elbow pad or a neoprene elbow sleeve during sports.

By far the most common and troublesome sports-related elbow problem is epicondylitis, also called tennis elbow, pitcher's elbow, and thrower's elbow. The same problem can even occur in nonathletes who overuse the forearm and elbow; we've seen dentists, carpenters, and hairdressers with "tennis elbow."

There are actually two distinct varieties of "the elbow." Classic tennis elbow involves the outer, or lateral, part of the elbow. This same ailment can result from throwing, whether a baseball or a javelin. Among tennis players, "the elbow" occurs most frequently in middle-aged, middle-quality players, and is the result of poor backhand technique combined with weakness or stiffness in the forearm muscles that extend (straighten) the wrist and fingers. In contrast, involvement of the medial, or inner, epicondyl occurs in some golfers and also in some tennis players; in this case, however, the tennis players at risk are highly skilled amateurs or pros who experience excessive stress caused by exaggerated spin serves, such as the American twist serve.

The major symptom of tennis elbow is pain. Movement and strength are usually fairly normal, but the pain can be so intense as to prevent playing. Although the reason for this pain is hotly debated, most experts believe that the problem is inflammation and swelling at the epicondyl, a small region where the tendons meet the bone at the elbow. In addition, small microscopic tears in the muscles or tendons may help explain the symptoms.

How can you tell if you have tennis elbow? X rays are normal, and there are no simple laboratory tests to make a diagnosis. But with the aid of a friend you can perform a simple test for tennis elbow (see Figure 12–6). Hold your arm at your side, bend your elbow to 90 degrees, and hold your fingers parallel to the ground. Have a friend push down on your hand while you try as hard as you can to resist his pressure by lifting your hand up. If you feel pain in the outer elbow, you probably do have tennis elbow. You can confirm this by making a fist and having your friend squeeze your outer elbow — pain and tenderness also suggest that you have "the elbow."

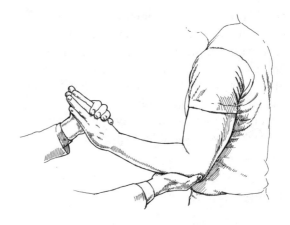

FIGURE 12–6: *Testing for Tennis Elbow*

To test for medial tennis elbow ("golfer's elbow"), hold your arm in the same position and have your friend press up against your palm while you exert downward force. Pain on the inside of your elbow — together with tenderness when your friend squeezes here — strongly suggests that you have the less-common medial variety of "the elbow."

Epicondylitis or tennis elbow affects up to 10 percent of tennis players at one time or another. If you are one of the unlucky victims, what can you do about it? Your first goal should be to reduce inflammation. If your pain comes on suddenly and is severe, you should elevate your elbow, apply ice, and apply pressure by wrapping a snug elastic bandage around your elbow. Rest is also very important early on; if pain is very intense, you may even want to use an arm sling or forearm splint to provide support. However, such complete immobilization can produce stiffness and weakness, so you should try to get your arm moving again as soon as the pain is diminished. This is another good example of how our principle of selective rest can be helpful — move your elbow and arm as much as possible, avoiding only those motions that produce pain. You can even return to play if you avoid strokes that cause pain, such as the backhand in the case of classic tennis elbow and the serve in the case of inner tennis elbow or golfer's elbow.

Rest and ice, however, may not be enough to ease your pain. In that case you should try anti-inflammatory medications such as aspirin or similar drugs. At first you may need to take these medications on a regular basis; as your rehabilitation progresses, you can taper the dosage, finally taking as little as two aspirins one hour before you play.

The most powerful anti-inflammatory drug is cortisone. Doctors can inject cortisone directly into the point of pain, and this treatment will reduce inflammation and ease discomfort. However, in the case of tennis elbow, we would advise steroid injections *only* if simpler measures fail, because the injections themselves can cause thinning and weakness of tendons. Even if steroid injections are your last resort, you should probably not take more than several shots. Finally, in some cases surgery may be suggested for extremely refractory cases of tennis elbow. Operations can be very helpful in extremely difficult cases, but we'd advocate at least six months of diligent conservative treatment before even contemplating surgery.

Once ice, rest, elastic bandages, and anti-inflammatory medications have done their work to reduce acute pain and inflammation, you can begin the second phase of your treatment program: active rehabilitation. You should exercise to improve your strength and flexibility (see Chapter 6). Wrist curls are particularly important (see Figures 6–49 and 6–50 and page 286). Although your elbow and forearm are the inflamed areas, your problem may stem from weakness, inflexibility, or muscle imbalance elsewhere in your upper body, which is forcing you to overuse your forearm to compensate. Even a weak grip can contribute to tennis elbow. Therefore, it is important to exercise your entire arm, shoulder, and trunk to take some of the load off your elbow. In fact, you should start with your other muscle groups first, adding elbow and forearm exercises only after the inflammation has subsided.

A few simple precautions will also help when you return to tennis. Always warm up thoroughly before you even hit a ball. In cool weather you should wear a long-sleeved jersey, and you should massage your elbow or even use a heating pad to warm it up before you play. At first hit only forehands. When you are ready to add backhands and service, do so gradually, hitting at half-speed at first. And after you play, be sure to apply an ice pack to your elbow. A whirlpool or ultrasound may also help reduce inflammation after play.

A little attention to your tennis equipment may also help (see pages 240–241).

A small device that may help is a forearm support. This is a wide band of adjustable, nonelastic fabric designed to be worn just below the elbow. The support should be snug but not so tight that it interferes with blood flow. If the support causes pain or swelling, it is too tight. Wear the support only while you are playing, and loosen it up briefly between games.

The most effective preventive medicine for tennis elbow sufferers, however, should be administered by a teaching pro. Good technique is the key to preventing tennis elbow. In the case of classic, or outer, tennis elbow, a good backhand is crucial. Never "lead with your elbow." Use your rehabilitation phase to relearn proper technique. In fact, you may even want to learn a two-handed backhand, since two-handed players rarely suffer from tennis elbow. If you have the less common inner, or medial, variety of tennis elbow, work on your service technique and stay away from fancy twist serves.

Epicondylitis can be a terribly frustrating problem for tennis players, pitchers, and golfers, but don't let your frustration get the best of you. With patience, persistence, and the treatment program outlined above, you should be able to return to full activities without pain.

THE FOREARM

The forearm is composed of two bones, the radius and the ulna (see Figure 12–7). The ulna is larger at the elbow end, and is a major component of the elbow joint, whereas the radius is larger at the wrist end, and is a major component of the wrist joint. These two bones are linked together by a network of ligaments, and are surrounded by muscles, which serve principally to bend and straighten the wrist and fingers. In addition, the bones of the forearm can undergo rotary movements around each other, which enable you to turn your hand over in a palm-up or palm-down fashion.

Overuse of your forearm muscles can produce acute

or chronic muscle strain. This is most common in the extensor muscles that run along the back of your forearm, and occurs particularly in gymnasts or other athletes who must keep these muscles contracted for prolonged periods of time. This ailment has been called "forearm splints" because it is in some ways analogous to shin splints in the leg. Treatment of forearm strains involves the same principles as other muscle strains, with early rest, ice, and compression, as well as anti-inflammatory drugs if necessary. You can help protect and rest your forearm with an elastic bandage, with tape, or a forearm splint. But even if you use one of these methods, be sure to avoid prolonged immobilization of your fingers so that they don't stiffen up. When pain subsides, you can proceed to rehabilitation. Begin simply by bending and straightening your wrist, and by turning your hand palm up and palm down. When all these motions can be accomplished comfortably, you can perform these exercises while holding a three-pound dumbbell.

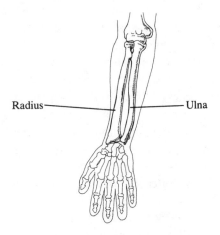

Radius ——   —— Ulna

FIGURE 12–7: *The Forearm*

When you are ready for sports, always remember to warm up thoroughly. Two aspirins before you play can be helpful, and you may want to wear tape or elastic wraps when you first return to competition. And as usual, remember to apply ice immediately after play.

THE WRIST

The wrist is composed of eight small bones, the carpal bones, which are bound together by strong ligaments (see Figure 12–8). The blood vessels and nerves that supply the hand pass over these bones and under some ligaments; as a result, wrist injuries that produce swelling can put pressure on these nerves and blood vessels.

Wrist sprains are very common in athletes. Although we call these sprains, in many cases they are actually strains, since tendons are involved more often than ligaments. In either case, acute wrist sprains and strains are most often caused by falls, particularly if you land on your open palm with your arm straight so that the wrist and hand are forced backward or "hyperextended." Chronic wrist sprains can occur from repeated overuse in sports that require a lot of wrist action, such as rowing and basketball. Finally, chronic irritation can produce inflammation of the wrist. Like other forms of inflammation, you'll recognize this problem by pain, redness, and swelling; there may also be crackling sounds when you bend and straighten your wrist.

All of these wrist problems are best managed early with the PRICE regimen (see pages 251–252). You can easily immobilize your wrist with an elastic wrap or a splint, and when you return to play you may want to continue using a wrap or tape for support.

A variety of exercises can help you rehabilitate and recondition your wrist when the acute pain and swelling have subsided. You can begin by simply moving your wrist in all directions — it can be very helpful to do this in a basin of warm water to help loosen up your wrist. Next, you can proceed to towel twisting, which is exactly what it sounds like. Roll a small bath towel into a tube, grip it in both hands, and twist it back and forth in both direction.

Another good exercise is wrist curls; first you can perform curls without any weight, but as you improve, hold a three- and then a five-pound dumbbell in your hand (see Figures 6–49 and 6–50). Do both front and back wrist curls to strengthen the muscles on both sides of your wrist. For front wrist curls, place your arm flat on a table, letting your hand extend over the edge with your palm facing up. For back wrist curls assume the same position, but with your palm facing down. Finally, you can build up your wrist by doing wrist rolls against resistance. You can do this by attaching a two- or three-pound weight to a long string, and suspending it from a cut-off broom handle. Let the weight dangle almost at floor level and hold your arms straight out in front of you at shoulder height with your palms down. Grasp the broom handle in your hands, and roll the handle until the string is wound entirely around it.

Although sprains and strains are by far the most common wrist injuries, you should always make sure that you don't have more serious problems. In particular, a fracture of one of the eight small bones of the wrist is easy to overlook; if you have severe or persistent wrist pain, you should always get X rays to exclude this possibility. Arthritis, gout, and infections can also involve the wrist. See your doctor if your problem seems unusual or severe.

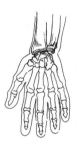

FIGURE 12–8: *The Wrist*

A common, mild wrist problem is the so-called ganglion. This is a painless swelling on the back of the wrist. Although ganglions are not caused by sports, they can sometimes become painful if you exercise your wrist a great deal. In most cases, a ganglion is merely a bulging and swelling of the smooth membranes that surround the tendons. These so-called synovial sacs are usually filled with fluid, and are soft and movable, but in some cases they can be quite firm. In most cases, you should treat a ganglion simply by ignoring it. The time-honored method of whacking your wrist with a heavy book to rupture the ganglion is doomed to failure, because the fluid will reaccumulate. Although your doctor can remove the fluid with a needle and syringe, it will also reaccumulate after this procedure. So, if the ganglion is a cosmetic problem or if it interferes with your wrist motion, surgery is the only way to assure a cure.

THE HAND

The hand is one of the most marvelous and complex parts of the human body. The hand is composed of five large metacarpal bones in the palm, and each finger has three small bones called phalynxes, except for the thumb, which has only two (see Figure 12–9). These bones meet in a series of complex joints, and motion is made possible by many small muscles, some of which originate in the forearm and some of which are entirely within the hand itself. A network of blood vessels provides nutrition to all these structures, and many small nerve branches provide delicate sensation and fine motor control.

Because the hand is such an intricate apparatus with many small structures packed into a compact space, we advise extreme care in dealing with hand injuries. Although you can take care of mild problems yourself, we believe that you should get expert evaluation for hand problems more readily than for any other athletic injuries except perhaps head and eye problems.

Direct trauma to the hand can produce contusions or fractures, and the muscles and ligaments of the hand can experience strains and sprains. You can manage these problems in the ordinary PRICE fashion (see pages 251–252); remember, however, that bleeding or infection in the hand can produce terribly serious problems because there is little room for swelling in these tightly packed structures. Get medical attention if you have any doubt about your hand.

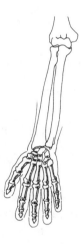

FIGURE 12–9: *The Hand*

Finger injuries are very common. Sprains are generally managed with ice, splinting, rest, and elevation. "Baseball finger" is an injury that can happen in any sport involving catching a ball. This problem occurs if you catch the ball on the tip of your finger so that your finger is abruptly bent inward. The result can be a so-called mallet finger or dropped finger — you won't be able to straighten out your fingertip because of a rupture of the tendon that extends the fingertip. You should treat this problem yourself as soon as it occurs with ice and a splint; your doctor should supervise definitive treatment, which usually involves application of a splint for as long as eight to ten weeks. You should always have X rays taken, because if a large fragment of bone is broken off, surgery will be required.

Dislocations of a finger are also fairly common, particularly in volleyball, basketball, or baseball, in which the fingertip can be "jammed" if struck head-on by the ball. Ice and splinting are the first-aid treatment you should know; your doctor will obtain X rays. Unless there is a major bone chip, splinting for three weeks or so should take care of the problem.

Many athletes take dislocated fingers rather casually and attempt to realign the injury themselves. If the dislocation occurs between the hand and the base of the finger (the so-called MCP joint), you should not under any circumstances attempt to reduce the dislocation yourself. Resist all temptation to pull on the finger; instead, put on an ice pack and head for your doctor for X rays and definitive care.

A less serious type of dislocation involves the middle joint of the finger. This has been called "coach's finger," because oftentimes a coach or fellow player will yank on the injured finger to realign it. In many players this simple maneuver will work, but we strongly advise X rays and expert medical care in all cases. Although some athletes will resume play immediately after this type of dislocation is realigned, we discourage this practice. Your hand is just too delicate and valuable to take any chances with it.

Rehabilitation is the final step in recovery from any hand injury. You can regain your hand strength with a variety of exercises. Begin simply by repeatedly gripping your fist, and also by spreading your fingers apart and then bringing them together. These exercises are best done at first in a basin of warm water. When your strength begins to return and your joints are flexible once again, you can squeeze on a small rubber ball or use a hand-grip strengthener to build your muscles up to normal.

A variety of sports can cause minor hand and finger problems. Bikers may develop so-called handlebar palsy, caused by excessive pressure on the outside of the hand if it rests heavily on the handlebar for miles on end. Handlebar palsy produces weakness of the fifth finger but does not impair sensation in the finger. If you bike seriously, you can prevent this problem simply by changing your hand position frequently while you are cycling, or by using a padded handlebar.

Even your fingernails can be injured, sometimes seriously enough to produce temporary incapacity. Subungual hematomas sound dreadful, but are really nothing more than a black and blue under the nail. Because there is so little room for swelling, however, this is usually very painful. You can get immediate relief from pain by drilling a small hole through your nail to relieve the pressure. Most of us would want to have this done

by a doctor — but your doctor will probably use nothing more sophisticated to perform this little operation than a heated wire, such as a straightened paper clip, or a small, short beveled needle. Your fingernail can also become infected at the nail base. This will produce pain, swelling, and redness, and there may be a small amount of pus drainage as well. You can usually handle this problem with warm soaks four times a day, but if the infection starts spreading up your finger, or if you have fever or chills, head for your doctor's office at once to get antibiotics. In some cases you may even need nail surgery.

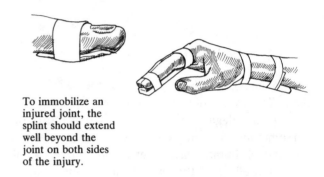

To immobilize an injured joint, the splint should extend well beyond the joint on both sides of the injury.

FIGURE 12–10: *Splinting Techniques*

THE BACK

You don't have to be a ski racer, road racer, or bike racer to qualify for back pain — you just have to belong to the human race. Low-back pain is one of the most common afflictions of modern man, affecting up to 80 percent of all Americans at one time or another. We are in the midst of an epidemic of backache. The costs of this epidemic are truly staggering, involving twenty million doctor visits and two hundred thousand operations each year — to say nothing of all the pain, suffering, and disability. Yet despite the fourteen-billion-dollar annual price tag for back pain in America, back pain is poorly understood, and is among the most controversial subjects in medicine today.

It has been argued that back pain is the inevitable price that humanity pays for a two-legged, upright posture. Indeed, as evolution has taken us from a four-legged gait to standing on our own two feet, we have increased the pressure and stress put on the back, especially the lower back. But back pain is not an inevitable consequence of evolution. Quite the contrary; in fact, back pain is a side effect of "social progress." In underdeveloped countries, back pain is much more common in the upper classes than in workers. Similarly, in industrialized societies the epidemic of back pain is a relatively new problem. Sedentary living, obesity, poor posture, poorly designed chairs and mattresses, an excessive dependence on the automobile, and psychological stress have all contributed to the rise of back pain in the modern world.

It is our belief that physical fitness and regular exercise can help prevent many cases of backache. But in all fairness, we must point out that exercise is not a cure-all. A quick perusal of the sports pages will demonstrate that athletes are not immune to back problems. In many cases, contact sports and trauma are responsible for back pain in competitive athletes, but even without trauma, back problems can occur. For example, in August 1983 Tracy Austin was forced to withdraw from the U.S. Open because of back pain, despite being seeded fourth. And in that same month, slugger Jim Rice of the Boston Red Sox required hospitalization and traction for back pain, even though he was in the thick of the American League home run championship derby (which he won). Austin and Rice are very different types of athletes playing very different sports, and they are but two examples of the way in which backache can strike even highly conditioned athletes. Even so, backaches are probably more common in sedentary executives than in athletes playing noncontact sports. If you understand your back and take care of it properly, you should be able to play sports without problems; moreover, a sound exercise program will strengthen your back and actually help prevent back problems in everyday life.

Understanding Your Back

The human back is a very complex set of structures (Figure 12–11; see also Chapter 2). Your "backbone"

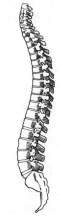

FIGURE 12–11: *The Back*

is, of course, not a bone at all, but a column of twenty-four individual bones, called vertebral bodies. The vertebral bodies are separated by intervertebral disks, which act as shock absorbers. Nerve roots run from the spinal cord out between the vertebral bodies to your muscles, where they are responsible for your strength, your sensation, and your reflexes. A series of strong ligaments help hold the vertebral bodies together to provide stability, and strong muscles run along the sides of the spinal column to provide additional support. Not to be forgotten are the abdominal muscles and the pelvic and hip muscles, which can be very important to help maintain the normal curvature of the back and support a share of the body's weight.

The Causes of Backache

Despite the frequency of this complaint, the exact causes of most cases of back pain remain controversial or obscure. Some authorities believe that the intervertebral disk is responsible for many cases of back pain, while other physicians invoke the sacroiliac joints or other forms of arthritis. But we believe that in up to 90 percent of cases the problem is mechanical: most cases of back pain, whether in athletes or in sedentary people, are due to strains and spasms of the back muscles and sprains and inflammation of the ligaments.

Once back pain is viewed in this context, you can see that the problem is really not unlike other musculoskeletal complaints in athletes. And indeed, the causes of back pain are really very similar to the causes of muscular injury in sports. One major predisposing cause is the lack of flexibility; tightness in the hamstrings, pelvis, or back itself can lead to abnormal mechanics and predispose to back pain. A similar cause is the lack of apropriate warm-up periods. Muscles that are cold tend to be stiff and tight, and are very vulnerable to strains or "pulls." Excessive stress is perhaps the most common precipitating cause of back pain. This can result from the recurrent overuse of muscles that are tight or tired, or from a single overstress caused by an ill-advised motion; for example, a single unfortunate twist during a tennis serve or golf swing can cause the problem.

Whatever the precipitating cause, back pain tends to be severe and persistent because a nasty cycle of events is set into motion. Muscles respond to pain and stress by contracting. The strong contractions or spasms are themselves painful, and they tend to perpetuate themselves because pain causes more spasms. In addition, muscle spasms decrease the blood supply to the muscle tissue itself, causing inflammation — a further cause of pain and hence spasm. Not surprisingly, nerve endings become irritated by the pressure and inflammation, producing more pain.

Back pain caused by this cycle of strain, spasm, inflammation, and pain can be very severe. My own experience in the dark days before I (HBS) got into shape is quite typical. I remember vividly the ill-advised weekend tennis game which caused my trouble. I pulled a muscle during a serve (a fault, no less) and had pain so severe that I actually fainted for the only time in my life. Severe pain kept me in bed for a week, and kept me uncomfortable for two weeks more. Happily, my back problems are a thing of the past now that I exercise regularly and stretch diligently. But the severity of my pain caused by "simple" spasms is quite typical of what can happen.

Even though simple muscular back pain can be extremely severe, it is important to be alert for warning signs of more serious problems. Nine times out of ten your pain will be due to strain, sprain, spasm, and inflammation, but you should be alert for more serious problems. Radiation of pain into your leg can be a sign of a herniated intervertebral disk that is pressing on the nerve root. Numbness or weakness in your leg strongly suggests disk disease, with nerve pressure, and is an indication for prompt medical attention. Similarly, bowel or bladder dysfunction suggests nerve pressure and requires medical attention. Even if these dramatic warning symptoms are absent, severe or persistent pain always merits a doctor's advice.

Pain that increases when you lie down or that fails to respond to usual treatment is another possible clue to serious problems. If fever, chills, or drenching sweats accompany back pain, you should get prompt medical attention, because serious infections can occasionally cause back pain. Back pain in children or adolescents or in the elderly always requires expert evaluation. Finally, the sacroiliac joint can also be the cause of low-back pain. This is actually quite a common problem, both in athletes and in sedentary people. Sprains of the joint are generally responsible for the nagging, low-back pain that develops.

Treating Your Aching Back

If the origins of backache can excite controversy, then the treatment of back pain can incite war.

As in most areas of medicine, heated controversy exists because of a lack of facts. Medical studies have failed to demonstrate the superiority of any one form of treatment over another. You should always be suspicious of any dogmatic claims for any one treatment program; there are just no quick cures or surefire treatments for most back problems.

Controversy notwithstanding, we'd like to give you a few guidelines for the treatment of your aching back. Remember that we are talking here about musculo-ligamentous pain and not about the less common but more serious varieties of backache that require individual medical treatment.

The first principle is rest. During the acute stages of back pain, any activity can produce more muscular stress and lead into the cycle of spasm, inflammation, and pain. The pressure on your back is actually greatest when you are sitting, so you'll be most comfortable resting on a flat, hard surface such as a very firm mattress, a mattress resting on a bedboard, or on the floor. The most restful position is flat on your back with two low pillows propped under your knees. The sooner you get off your feet, and the more you rest, the more rapidly your pain will resolve. Significant back pain is one situation in which we strongly advise you not to "play through it" — you can save yourself a lot of pain and grief by avoiding repeated stress.

Another important element in treatment is heat. Whereas most acute muscle injuries respond best to ice, back pain usually responds better to heat unless you catch it very early — in which case ice can help.

Aspirin remains the standard drug to fight pain and inflammation, but the newer anti-inflammatory agents can also be extremely helpful. All of the medications in this category have a dual effect because they will decrease both pain and inflammation. But if your pain is very severe, you may have to use additional prescription analgesics such as codeine and other potent pain-killers. As for drugs that fight muscle spasm, there are many muscle relaxants on the market; since these all require prescriptions, your doctor will have to decide which one is best for you.

Fortunately, in most cases prescription drugs are not necessary. Ordinary back pain will respond to rest, aspirin, and heat. But one additional element is also extremely important: patience. Even the most diligent treatment program takes time to work. Your goal, of course, is to return to sports and to build up your back so that it is stronger than ever. But don't try to rush it. A premature return to sports can often cause a new cycle of pain and spasm.

This treatment program is very straightforward, following the same guidelines used for muscle and ligament injury elsewhere in your body. Needless to say, many other forms of treatment are available for back pain. Traction can be useful, but we're not at all sure that it adds anything to strict bed rest. Similarly, massage can be of some help in relaxing tight muscles, but we remain very skeptical of more aggressive forms of spinal manipulation. Acupuncture is a total unknown from a scientific point of view, but if it seems to help you, we certainly have no objections. Finally, a device that can help some people is a lumbosacral corset, which can temporarily provide external support. When your back is less painful, however, you should begin a gradual exercise program to build up the strength of your own muscles, so that you will no longer need external support from a brace.

Rehabilitation and Prevention

If you've ever had back pain, you will be a great enthusiast about the prevention of recurrent episodes. The first step in prevention is weight control. Obesity puts extra stress on all of the structures of your back; no wonder that an old adage among orthopedists is "You can never be too thin for your back."

A very important way to prevent back problems is with good body mechanics. Your mother was right — posture is important (see Figure 12–12). Stand with your head up, chin in, and shoulders back. Try to keep your abdomen flattened in and your pelvis tilted slightly forward to prevent excessive curvature of your lower

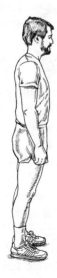

FIGURE 12–12: *Correct Posture*

spine. There is also a correct way to sit. Avoid thick, cushiony seats in favor of chairs with firm backs and seats. Don't slouch. Use a low footrest if you have to sit for prolonged periods. Posture is even important when you sleep: select an extra-firm mattress or place a half-inch plywood bedboard under your mattress. Sleep on your back or on your side but not on your stomach, which exaggerates the curvature of your lower back and can stress your muscles. Use only a thin pillow under your neck or, if you sleep on your back, put a pillow under your knees.

Lifting and bending must be done properly to avoid back problems. You should never bend over from your waist — instead, bend at your knees and hips, keeping your back relatively straight. If you are lifting a heavy object, keep it close to your body. And always get help with bulky or awkward items.

Whether in sports or in daily life, you should always stretch and warm up before you do anything strenuous. And try to move with smooth, gradual motions instead of sudden, jerky motions, which can provoke spasm. Similarly, you should always allow your back muscles to cool down gradually after exercise instead of allowing them to become chilled.

Exercises are extremely important to build flexibility and strength. Remember that you should *never* start an exercise program while your back is acutely painful. After the pain is better, however, you can start out with gentle exercises such as pelvic tilts and William's exercise (see Chapter 6). When you're free of pain and comfortable with these simple exercises, you can gradually begin a more vigorous program to build up your back. Your goals should be: (1) to build both flexibility and strength of your lower back; (2) to build abdominal muscle strength; and (3) to develop flexibility of your hip flexors and hamstrings (see Chapter 6 for all these exercises).

Remember that all of these exercises must be done gradually and carefully. If your back begins to ache in the course of your exercise program, ease off. Return to the first principles of treatment, including rest, heat, and aspirin, and then gradually restart an exercise program. You may even want to consult a physical therapist about your posture and gait, as well as about the exercises themselves. The YMCA's healthy back program can be a good place to start a regimen to prevent recurrent back problems.

When can you return to sports? When you are free of pain. Always remember to start off gradually, and always include diligent warm-up and cool-down periods. Above all, pick your sport according to your body's dictates; the best sports are those with rhythmic, predictable motions that you control. Swimming is particularly good for the back; the crawl and backstroke are especially desirable, but the butterfly can stress the back and should be avoided. Walking is excellent for people with ordinary muscular back problems; jogging is also safe, but it's particularly important to wear good shoes and to find a soft surface. If you have actual disk disease, however, the pounding involved with jogging and running can increase your problems and hence should be avoided. Biking can be a mixed blessing for backache sufferers; in general, if you bike in an upright posture, your back will be just fine; but if you bend forward in a racing posture, you can stress your back with unfortunate results. Finally, sports that involve twisting motions, such as tennis and golf, can trigger back spasms. Most people who have had back pain can eventually resume both of these sports, but you should always be sure that your back is in shape before you pick up your racquet or clubs.

THE ABDOMEN

The abdomen contains many of your vital organs: your stomach, intestines, liver, and spleen. In addition, your pancreas and kidneys lie at the rear of the abdomen. Any one of these organs can be damaged by blunt trauma in contact sports. These are potentially very serious injuries; happily, these accidents are very rare in non-contact sports.

A svelte profile is often equated with fitness; we're all for the "flat-belly" look, but more than vanity is involved in keeping your abdominal muscles strong. They are very important in helping you maintain good posture and, therefore, in taking some extra stress off your back.

Weak abdominal muscles are also subject to pulls or strains. Such strains are likely to occur with sudden reaching motions, such as a service or overhand in tennis. You'll know you have a pulled abdominal muscle because you'll get a steady pain over the injured muscle, both during and after exercise. In this respect, a pulled abdominal muscle is quite different from a side stitch: a side stitch is very painful during exercise, but usually quiets down promptly with rest; a pulled muscle will go on aching. The reason for this difference is that the side stitch is a transient cramp, whereas a strain of the abdominal muscles involves stretching or even tearing of muscle fibers.

If you think you have an abdominal muscle pull, test yourself at home — you may well be able to save yourself from a trip to the hospital. Lie on your back on a firm surface, and tense your abdomen by raising your head and legs simultaneously, or by raising your legs against resistance. If this test duplicates your pain, it is likely that you have a strained abdominal muscle rather than a potentially more serious internal problem.

The treatment of an abdominal muscle pull is similar to other muscle strains. Ice is helpful in acute injuries, but later on, or in chronic strains, heat can be very soothing. Similarly, you should rest at first and then move to active rehabilitation. Prevention and rehabilitation involve strengthening your abdominal muscles, which is best accomplished by doing bent-knee sit-ups, starting gradually at first until your strength improves (see Chapter 6).

THE PELVIS

The pelvis is a circle of strong bones and ligaments which has two functions: to transfer weight from the trunk to the legs, and to provide protection for the internal organs, including the female reproductive tract, the lower urinary tract, and the rectum.

Most sports-related pelvic injuries are caused by direct trauma; obviously, contact sports are implicated most often. Trauma can produce pelvic contusions (bruises) or even fractures. The most common variety of pelvic bruise is the so-called hip pointer, which is nothing more than a large hematoma or "black and blue." Despite its name, this injury does not actually involve the hip, but occurs higher up, at the crest of the ileum, or major pelvic bone. As a result, a hip pointer will produce pain, tenderness, swelling, and dark discoloration just below your waistline over the bony prominence (see Figure 12–13).

You should treat a hip pointer with ice and compression early on; when recovery is under way, use heat. As with all sports injuries, the best treatment is prevention — in this case by wearing padding during contact sports and, even better, avoiding trauma.

Although obvious trauma is the major cause of pelvic injury, you may develop small fractures of the pelvic bones even without any contact. These are the so-called stress fractures, which can occur from the trauma of repeated running, especially on hard surfaces. Most often, a stress fracture will produce pain at the front of your pelvis (the pubic symphysis), but sometimes it can happen at the back where the pelvis meets your "tailbone" (the sacroiliac joint). Pain is the symptom of a stress fracture, and the only treatment is rest and time. Obviously, wearing good footwear to cushion shock and running on soft surfaces whenever possible will help prevent these problems.

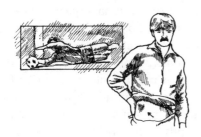

FIGURE 12–13: *A Hip Pointer*

Finally, remember that pelvic pain can sometimes reflect diseases of the internal pelvic organs. So if your symptoms persist, and particularly if pain is accompanied by fever, urinary tract or rectal symptoms, or disorders of the female reproductive organs, see your doctor to get a detailed evaluation.

THE HIP

The hip is a ball-and-socket joint. The socket is formed by the pelvic bones, and the ball is the head of the thigh bone, or femur. This arrangement allows great mobility of the hip joint. Stability is provided by strong ligaments and, especially, by the large strong muscle groups that surround the hip.

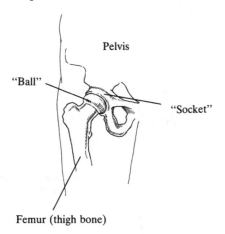

FIGURE 12–14: *The Hip*

Although discomfort in the hip region is quite common in athletes, in most cases this is caused by inflammation in the surrounding structures rather than by difficulties in the hip itself. Because of the great mobility of the hip, sprains of the ligaments are quite uncommon. However, the muscles and tendons that surround the hip can be strained, either by chronic overuse or by sudden, violent overstress. Hip muscle strain will show up as deep discomfort in your buttock or hip, particularly when you run; the pain will slowly diminish as you rest after play. As with other strain treatments, you should include the PRICE program (see pages 251–252) early on, with heat, anti-inflammatory drugs, and progressive exercises as you improve.

Bursitis is also quite common in the hip region, as there are no fewer than thirteen different bursal sacks around the hip. The most common type of hip bursitis produces localized pain and tenderness over the outer portion of the hip (see Figure 12–15). If you have this

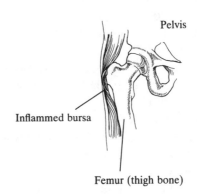

FIGURE 12–15: *Greater Trochanteric Bursitis*

type of bursitis, the chances are very good that you will be able to keep on going with your sports as long as you ice the bursa down after play and take aspirin or other anti-inflammatory drugs. If the pain persists, you may have to rest for a day or two, and work back up to a full schedule slowly. Heat can be helpful in chronic cases, and if your case is unusually severe, your doctor may be able to help a great deal with a steroid injection.

Another cause of pain over the outside of your hip is inflammation of the iliotibial band, the longest ligament in the body, connecting your pelvis to your shinbone. This strong ligament is very important for maintaining erect posture, but it can be inflamed through overuse, such as can occur with excessive running. Because the iliotibial band runs right over the outer hip bursa, bursitis and inflammation of the ligament can exist simultaneously. Not surprisingly, the treatment is quite similar: once again the PRICE program is the answer.

Because overuse is the most common cause of inflammation of the iliotibial band, it's important to be sure that you don't have an abnormal gait that is causing abnormal stress. One readily correctable cause of an abnormal gait is leg-length discrepancy. Careful measurements have shown that most people have at least very slight differences in the length of their legs. Our bodies can compensate for slight discrepancies without difficulty, but if the difference between your leg lengths approaches one-half inch or more, you may develop knee, hip, or back pain. Usually the longer leg absorbs the greater stress, and is therefore prone to injuries. These problems can be readily corrected with a simple shoe lift. Finally, even if your legs are the same length, you may be developing hip pain because of muscle imbalance or inflexibility. If this is the case, exercises for strength and flexibility can go a long way toward preventing recurrences of your problem; in particular, stretching exercises for the iliotibial band can be very effective (see Chapter 6).

A very minor hip problem, which may cause you needless concern, is the snapping hip. Sometimes the iliotibial band will produce a snapping sound and a clicking sensation as it moves across the greater trochanter. Unless you have pain or stiffness, just ignore the sound; it does not reflect a disease or injury, and no treatment is necessary.

Thus far we've been considering disorders of the structures that surround the hip rather than problems of the joint itself. Actual hip problems are less common in athletes, but unfortunately when they occur they can be much more serious. Direct trauma can cause bruises, dislocations, or fractures, which are major problems indeed, and generally require surgical repair and a prolonged recovery period. Inflammation of the lining of the hip joint, or "sinovitis," produces deep hip pain, which increases with motion or even standing, and tends to settle down with rest. Aspirin or other anti-inflammatory drugs can help, but true hip sinovitis generally calls for rest, or at least a switch to non-weight-bearing sports such as swimming. The same is true of arthritis of the hip joint. Osteoarthritis, or "degenerative joint disease" (DJD), is the most common form of joint disease in the United States, and often affects the hip. DJD is not caused by exercise or sports, but comes on with advancing age, so it can crop up in older athletes. If the arthritis is mild, sports can be continued, some-

times with the aid of anti-inflammatory drugs. But for patients with moderate or advanced DJD, we recommend a switch to swimming or other non-weight-bearing forms of exercise. This advance also applies to people who have undergone corrective surgery for hip arthritis.

Hip pain can also be referred from the back, sacroiliac joint, or even from internal organs such as the kidneys, intestines, or pelvic organs. Hernias, groin strains, and thigh problems can also cause pain in the hip region. Finally, in some people true hip disease doesn't cause hip pain, but is referred elsewhere, particularly to the thigh and knee. All in all, pain in this region can be quite tricky. Hence, if your hip problem doesn't settle down promptly with self-treatment, see your doctor. X rays are particularly important to evaluate potential disorders of the hip region.

THE GROIN

Groin "pulls" are among the most disabling of the non-traumatic sports injuries. Although the pain of a pulled groin muscle is usually mild to moderate, these injuries are disabling because they are very slow to heal. The reason is that it's very difficult to rest these muscles properly since they are used constantly in daily activities such as walking. In addition, elastic bandages and other types of support simply don't work in the groin region.

As in the case of all muscle "pulls," the actual problem is either a muscle strain caused by tearing of muscle fibers, or tendinitis involving inflammation of the fibrous tissues that attach the muscles of the inner thigh to the pelvic bone (see Figure 12–16). These muscles

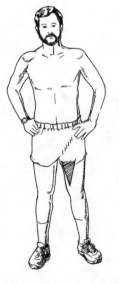

Shading indicates painful area caused by muscle sprain or tendinitis.

FIGURE 12–16: *A Groin Pull*

are prone to injury precisely because they are large and strong and often become tight and inflexible. The groin muscles can be injured by sudden starts and stops or by abrupt stretching motions, as in a fall or slip.

The early treatment of groin strains is the familiar PRICE regimen (see pages 251–252). Heat and anti-inflammatories such as aspirin will help later on. But in most cases, only the slow process of time will really heal these injuries. You will simply have to avoid any hard running until the pain has resolved almost completely. Then start gentle stretching exercises to get yourself back into shape before you resume vigorous exercise (see Chapter 6).

Another cause of groin discomfort is an inguinal hernia. Hernias are more common in men, but can occur in women as well. In addition to nagging discomfort, you will be able to see and feel a bulge in the groin region, which will increase if you cough or strain. The only curative treatment for hernias is surgical repair. Although some people may quite reasonably choose to defer surgery in favor of a truss or support, we strongly suggest that active athletes have their hernias repaired sooner rather than later. If you develop severe pain or discoloration, or if it becomes difficult to push the hernia back, you should see your doctor at once because urgent surgical treatment may be necessary.

A related question often asked by male athletes concerns the use of athletic supporters or jockstraps. Although most men do wear such supports, there is really very little medical evidence to suggest that they are helpful. In contact sports a protective cup is extremely important, but in all other cases it's simply a question of individual comfort and preference.

THE THIGH

The thigh is composed of the femur, a large bone surrounded by three strong muscle groups: the adductor muscles on the inside of your thigh, the large quadriceps muscles at the front of your thigh and at the back of your thigh, and the five large muscles collectively known as the hamstrings.

Strains or "pulls" of the quadriceps and, especially, of the hamstrings are among the most common injuries in athletes. These injuries are caused by a lack of warm-up, tightness, overuse, or muscle imbalance. Muscle imbalance is particularly important, because in many athletes the quadriceps are disproportionately stronger than the hamstrings. In normal circumstances, the quadriceps should be 50 percent stronger than the hamstrings; if your hamstrings are able to lift forty pounds, your quadriceps should be able to lift sixty. However, the quadriceps can become disproportionately strong as a result of sprinting, running up hills, cycling, and other sports. If this happens, the relatively weaker hamstrings (which are particularly important for distance runners) are prone to injury. You can test yourself to find out if your hamstrings are tight by lying on your back and trying to flex your leg at the hip, so that it is upright and perpendicular to the ground at a 90-degree angle. If you can't do this, you may have a hip or back problem — or you may just have tight hamstrings. For a good hamstring stretching exercise, see page 104; this exercise is also excellent for your warm-up routine before any sport that involves running. Treat thigh muscle pulls with the PRICE program (see pages 251–252), followed by heat, anti-inflammatories, and exercises for restoring strength (see Chapter 6).

Contact sports can also produce injuries to the thigh. The femur is a strong bone, so fractures require quite a severe blow. But deep muscle bruises can occur with even mild to moderate trauma; contusions of the thigh can be tricky because a surprisingly large amount of blood can be hidden in these muscles without producing any discoloration of the skin. You should be very careful to avoid massaging this type of injury, because massage can lead to even more bleeding. Instead, use ice and pressure to stop the bleeding early on. Later, heat and ultrasound treatments can help, but it may take four weeks or longer for a major thigh contusion to resolve fully. Elastic wraps can be very useful during the rehabilitation from both contusion and strains of the thigh.

THE KNEE

What do Joe Namath, Gayle Sayers, Earl Monroe, Dave Cowens, Mickey Mantle, Bobby Orr, Billy Jean King, Bernard King, and Harvey B. Simon have in common? All of these athletes have had knee injuries at one time or another in their careers (my own injuries have been quite mild, but I [HBS] can think of no other excuse for listing my name with great athletes). And the injuries which make headlines on the sports pages are only the tip of the iceburg; there are at least three hundred thousand athletic knee injuries in the United States each year. Although the knee can be injured during any form of exercise, some sports are more hazardous than others: skiing leads the list, with football, skating, track and field, soccer, and baseball rounding out the top six.

Why are knee injuries so prevalent in sports? The knee's anatomy accounts for its vulnerability. Although the knee is fundamentally a hinge joint, it's actually much more complex than simple bending and straightening motions would suggest. In fact, the knee joint also allows sliding and rotary motion. These motions permit the knee mobility that is essential for graceful athletic movements, but to permit these motions, the knee must be a fundamentally unstable joint, which is prone to injury.

The integrity of the knee does not depend on the alignment of the bones themselves, but on surrounding structures. On the outside of the knee, ligaments at the sides and rear provide stability. At the front is the kneecap, or patella, which gives protection. The inside of the knee joint is also stabilized by ligaments and by the two knee cartilages, which also act to absorb shock and to provide a smooth surface for the bones to glide on. Additionally, the thigh bone and shinbone are themselves covered by shiny cartilage, which allows gliding with low friction. The knee joint is lined by a fine joint membrane, which produces the fluid that lubricates and cushions the entire appratus. Finally, additional cushioning and lubrication are provided by the ten fluid-filled sacs, or bursae, in and around the knee.

Movement of the joint is controlled by the large thigh muscles, which also support and stabilize the knee. The fibrous tendons of these muscles pass across the knee, so that inflammation or tendinitis of these structures can produce knee pain, although they are not technically part of the joint apparatus itself.

Let's focus on minor knee problems that you may be able to manage yourself, then turn briefly to the major knee problems. Although we emphasize self-treatment of minor knee problems, we must stress that because the knee joint is so complicated, you should not delay in getting a medical evaluation if you have any doubt as to the cause or severity of your knee pain.

Overuse Injuries of the Knee

Almost all sports involve repetitive running, jumping, or bending of the knee. Because all of these motions stress the knee, overuse injuries can occur in any sport; not surprisingly, running, jumping, and basketball are the most common causes of this type of injury.

In addition to simple overuse, other factors may contribute to knee problems: muscle imbalance, inflexibility, poor biomechanics resulting in an abnormal gait, worn or poorly fitted athletic shoes, and excessive running or jumping on hard surfaces. You will recognize

this list because these are the common denominators of most nontraumatic sports injuries. And, in fact, the knee injuries that they can produce share the other common denominator of sports injuries: inflammation, or "itis."

Tendinitis

Any of the tendons that cross the knee can become inflamed, leading to knee pain. "Jumper's knee," for example, is particularly common in basketball players and involves inflammation of the patellar tendon below the kneecap; in severe cases, small tears may be present in this tendon as well. Long-distance runners commonly have more pain and inflammation on the outside of the knee joint due to inflammation of the iliotibial band. And breaststrokers who use the whip kick can get pain and tenderness of the inside portion of the knee; although "breaststroker's knee" is technically a sprain, it behaves very much like overuse tendinitis.

Bursitis

Any of the bursal sacs around the knee joint can become inflamed from overuse. As with other forms of athletic "itis," pain, swelling, and stiffness are common symptoms. The most dramatic example is prepatellar bursitis, better known as housemaid's knee. Because the front of the knee joint is quite lax, inflammation of this bursa can produce a dramatically large swelling in front of the knee. Even so, this is not a serious problem; like other forms of bursitis, it usually responds to ice, rest, and anti-inflammatory medications, with steroid injections in reserve for more refractory cases.

Synovitis

The knee joint lining can become inflamed as a result of overuse. This condition is also known as "water on the knee," and it's easy to see why. The synovial (joint) membrane normally produces fluid; in response to injury, it produces an abnormally large amount, which accumulates in the joint, producing swelling and stiffness. Synovitis usually responds very well to rest, ice, compression, and anti-inflammatory medications. But it's very important to be sure that the knee swelling is not the result of more serious internal derangements of the knee or other problems such as arthritis or infection. A careful examination can often help distinguish among these problems, but sometimes your doctor will have to order blood tests, X rays, and even tap some of the fluid out of your knee in order to be sure.

Chondromalacia

Chondromalacia is a good example of two common phenomena: (1) overuse can produce injuries, and (2) medical names are often a good deal more frightening than the actual injuries they describe.

In most cases, chondromalacia is a mild or moderate problem involving softening and inflammation of the cartilage lining the undersurface of the kneecap. Jumping, basketball, and running are the most common causes, but biking or any other sports that involve repeated bending of the knee can lead to this problem. Chondromalacia tends to be a bit more common in women because the kneecap is looser in its groove and is therefore subject to more irritation.

Chondromalacia produces knee pain, which is most pronounced when you are squatting or bending. These motions may also produce a creaking or popping sound as well as a crunching sensation. If you have chondromalacia, you will notice the pain when you walk upstairs and also when you get out of a deep chair after sitting quietly for a long time — the so-called movie sign. You can further suspect chondromalacia if your knee hurts when you press down on the kneecap while having your leg straightened out fully on the floor.

Treatment of Overuse Knee Injuries

All of these common knee problems respond to the PRICE regimen (see pages 251–252). Avoid the offending activity until the pain has settled down, and when you return to sports, do so gently. Wearing an elastic bandage or knee sleeve for compression may help, and it is very important to ice your knee down after activity. Aspirin or other anti-inflammatory drugs can be helpful, especially before you play, and careful stretching and warming-up exercises before sports are most important.

Exercises are also very important to help develop balanced strength of the muscles and tendons that surround the knee. Following athletic injuries you should always start with isometric exercises, which involve little motion, and then progress to range-of-motion exercises. Your doctor will outline your rehab program, and your physical therapist will provide the supervision which is so important.

Major Knee Injuries

Most knee pain in athletes is not terribly serious and can be treated exactly like overuse injuries of other parts of the body. But the knee joint is susceptible to certain major injuries, which do require specialized medical intervention. Many of these injuries occur in the course of contact sports. It's easy to see why football is the chief culprit here; all you have to do is watch a few tackles, from the backyard all the way up to the NFL, to be amazed that there aren't even more serious knee injuries among football players. Skiing is the other classic setting for major knee trauma. Anyone who's gone down even a few slopes has had the experience of the feet going one way while the body goes another — not surprisingly, if the knee is asked to bear the stress of these opposing forces, major injury can result. In addition to these rather florid situations, however, major knee problems can sometimes occur during virtually any sport. A case in point is Greer Stevens. Tennis is hardly a contact sport and, in fact, is generally quite easy on the knees. Stevens, however, snagged her shoe on an artificial court surface while she was pivoting, severely twisting her left knee. The result was major damage to her medial knee ligaments as well as to her cartilage. Greer Sevens required five hours of surgery and many weeks of physical therapy, but even so she was lucky: her knee regained nearly normal mobility and strength; in fact, she went on to win the Wimbledon mixed doubles championship the year after her injury. Nor do you have to be a tennis star to have this sort of problem. Any running or jumping sport can occasionally cause serious knee damage if a misstep or uneven surface causes you to stress your knee severely with a twisting type of motion.

Cartilage Tears

The two knee cartilages are very resistant to damage from simple overuse, but they can be badly injured by a rotary or twisting stress on the knee. This type of abnormal force can quite literally pinch the cartilage between the thigh bone and the shinbone and crush or tear it. The result is sudden pain and then swelling and stiffness, which occur over a period of hours. In the case of mild injuries, the swelling can subside with rest and time, and you may even get back to fairly normal activity with only minimal discomfort. However, the cartilages of your knee do not have their own blood supply, so they cannot regenerate or heal. As a result, moderate or major tears of the cartilage may result in permanent discomfort and even disability requiring surgical treatment.

Fortunately, surgery these days is much simpler than it used to be. The arthroscope is a wonderful instrument, which can be used to diagnose knee injuries with great precision, and which can also be used to repair torn knee cartilages and other selected problems. The arthroscope is a fiberoptic instrument about the diameter of a pencil, which can be inserted into the knee joint to allow direct inspection of the internal structures. Although this is a surgical procedure, it can generally be done on an outpatient basis, so you'll be home walking on the day of the operation and can usually resume nearly normal activity within weeks.

Although arthroscopy is a major advance, it is not indicated for all major knee problems. In some cases, simpler tests can be used to make a diagnosis; in other cases, such as major ligament tears, conventional surgical repair is still needed.

Knee Ligament Injuries

Like other ligaments in the body, the strong ligaments that provide stability for the knee joint can be sprained. Mild injuries can be managed with rest, ice, compression, and, after a period of time, a graded program of exercises to rebuild strength and mobility. In contrast, more severe sprains that involve significant tears in the ligaments require surgical repair and prolonged rehabilitation under careful supervision.

Dislocating Kneecap

Because the kneecap, or patella, rests in only a narrow groove, it can be dislocated relatively easily. In most cases, this produces only a popping sound and transient discomfort, which requires little attention. Exercises to strengthen the quadriceps muscles (see Chapter 6) can help prevent recurrent dislocations, and a knee wrap, sleeve, or neoprene brace will also help. If you have recurrent dislocations that are painful, or if the kneecap dislocates and locks in an abnormal position, surgery may be necessary. Happily, these cases are the exception rather than the rule.

Loose Bodies

Following various knee injuries, fragments of cartilage or even small chips of bone may come loose and float free in the joint. The original injury may have been long forgotten, but the loose body will serve as a reminder that all is not well. In some cases, the so-called joint mice cause nothing more than occasional grinding or clicking noises, which may be embarrassing but don't require any treatment. Sometimes loose bodies cause intermittent aching, stiffness, or swelling of the knee.

And if the joint mouse wedges into the joint apparatus itself, it can cause your knee to lock. No amount of exercise will get rid of these foreign bodies, nor are there any medications to chase away joint mice. Fortunately, most loose bodies within the knee can be removed relatively easily with an arthroscope, so that major surgery is not required.

Arthritis

Doctors are used to attributing most joint aches and pains to "arthritis," especially in middle-aged and older people. As you can see from the long list of knee problems we've been discussing, most cases of knee pain in athletes have other, specific causes. Exercise itself does not cause arthritis. But recurrent knee damage can eventually lead to degenerative joint disease or osteoarthritis, in which the smooth cartilage covering the thigh bone and shinbone is worn away. Less commonly, systemic diseases such as rheumatoid arthritis or infection can cause arthritis of the knee joint.

If knee arthritis is mild, you can continue to be quite active with the use of simple measures such as aspirin or other anti-inflammatory drugs and heat. However, you'd be well advised to concentrate on sports that do not involve weight-bearing, such as swimming. In occasional patients, knee arthritis can become progressively severe and even disabling. Although powerful medications and/or surgical treatment can help most of these patients, ski slopes and tennis courts will be out of the question for them. Remember, however, that virtually everyone can exercise in one form or another. If you happen to be one of the unlucky few who develop significant knee arthritis, check with your doctor, who will probably prescribe swimming as your form of exercise.

THE LOWER LEG

Leg pain is one of the most frequent complaints of injured athletes, particularly those who do a lot of running. The lower leg is composed of two bones, the tibia and fibula, surrounded by muscles. The muscles that extend your foot downward to raise you up on your toes and propel you forward are much larger and stronger than the muscles that bring your foot back up to its resting position after each stride. These large, strong muscles are the calf muscles, and the most powerful of these by far is the gastrocnemius, or "gastroc." The imbalance between the large, strong calf muscles and the much smaller, weaker shin muscles is a potential cause of overuse injuries. Another potential problem is that the lower leg muscles are divided into four rather snug compartments, each surrounded by dense, fibrous tissue. If the muscles become very large through training, or if injuries produce swelling, the tissues can be compressed, causing pain or even urgent problems.

Because the bones of the lower leg are not padded by bulky muscles, bruises and fractures can readily result from contact sports or falls. Fractures obviously need expert medical attention, whereas bruises or contusions will respond nicely to ice, elevation, rest, and time. Let's concentrate not on these traumatic problems, but on the more subtle causes of leg pain in athletes.

Calf Pain

The most common cause of calf pain is sprains of the gastrocs or calf muscles. When you begin running to get into shape for any sport, your calf muscles respond by becoming stronger and larger — and also tighter and stiffer. This combination of strength and tightness is an excellent recipe for injury. The final ingredient in this recipe is a lack of proper warm-up, because cold muscles are stiffer and all the more susceptible to injury.

The most common calf injury is muscle strain. This will usually cause a chronic burning or aching pain in the calf. If you have only a mild strain, you can continue playing sports by warming up thoroughly beforehand, and by applying ice immediately after play ceases. But if your pain is more severe, you should rest for at least a few days until the inflammation has subsided. Anti-inflammatory medications such as aspirin will also help. Finally, it is most important to embark upon a careful program of calf-stretching exercises (see Chapter 6).

Tennis leg is a variant of gastroc injury. Tennis leg tends to occur early in the season when players begin running on the courts without proper warm-up and flexibility drills. Sometimes a mild gastroc sprain precedes the muscle tear itself, so that players may remember a dull calf ache for several days prior to the abrupt onset of tennis leg. And the onset is dramatic indeed.

Tennis leg comes on with a sudden, sharp pain in the calf, particularly while serving or running. A popping or snapping sound may accompany the pain, which can be so severe that running is impossible and even walking without a support is difficult.

Tennis leg is caused by a tear or rupture of the inner portion of the gastroc muscle. So in a sense, it's nothing more than a rather severe and dramatic strain. Indeed, even though muscle fibers are torn, conservative treatment is generally successful. You may have to stay off your leg entirely for one or two days, and then walk with a cane or crutch for several days. Putting a heel lift in your shoe will also take strain off your calf and speed recovery.

Ice is very helpful, particularly if you can apply it immediately after the injury. You should ice your leg intermittently for the first forty-eight hours after the injury, and then shift to heat treatment for twenty minutes, three or four times per day. Then you are ready for gentle stretching exercises and, finally, for exercises to strengthen your calf (see Chapter 6).

Don't rush your rehabilitation — tennis leg can occur again. But with time, patience, and stretching and strengthening exercises, you should eventually be as good as new. And we hope you'll have learned your lesson and will stretch regularly and warm up carefully before you play.

The two smaller muscles of the calf, the plantaris and the soleus, can also be sprained or torn. Unless you are an orthopedist, it's rather hard to distinguish these injuries from strains of the calf muscle itself. Nor is the distinction particularly important, since the treatment regimen outlined above will be as helpful for the small muscles as it will for the gastroc itself.

Shin Pain

Pick a runner, any runner. Play word association. Say "shin." The response will invariably be "splints."

What are shin splints? For all their notoriety, there is no precise medical definition of shin splints. Athletes use the term to describe many variants of shin pain, which can be acute or chronic, and which can involve the inner or outer surface of the shin in its upper or lower portion.

In fact, there are many types of shin splints, each with a somewhat different cause. Overuse is certainly one of the most common causes. Any sport that involves substantial running entails repeated, heavy-duty use of the shin muscles. Muscle strain can result, producing chronic aching pain in the shin. If muscle inflammation (myositis) occurs as well, the muscles will swell. Remember that these muscles are surrounded by a tight compartment, and you'll understand why shin pain can be very severe at times. Overuse can also cause inflammation of the membrane that surrounds the shinbone, a process called periostitis. In addition, repeated running on a hard surface can lead to small stress fractures of the shinbone itself.

How can you distinguish among these causes of shin pain? Often you can't. Strain and myositis generally produce chronic aching, whereas the pain of a stress fracture tends to be sharper and more acute. The shin can be swollen and tender in any of these conditions, but stress fractures usually have the greatest tenderness and myositis has the most swelling. And in all these conditions, running will tend to increase the pain, often to an unbearable degree.

Even if you can't figure out the precise cause of your shin pain, you can start an effective treatment program. If it hurts you to run, don't. If you have a stress fracture, you may have to avoid running for as long as four to six weeks; if your problems are in the soft tissues, you will be able to resume activity much sooner. In either case, let pain be your guide. As the pain settles down, you can gradually begin running again, slowly building up to your normal level of activity. Ice is very helpful in the acute phases of shin pain, and elevation, compression bandages, and anti-inflammatory drugs will also be helpful.

However, prevention is every bit as important as treatment. Remember the many causes of these injuries: overuse, muscle imbalance, poor flexibility, poorly designed shoes, and running on hard surfaces. Each of these causes can be corrected by appropriate action on your part. Increase your mileage only gradually to avoid overuse injury. Remember that your calf muscles are much stronger than your shin muscles; exercises to strengthen the shin muscles and stretch the calf muscles will correct both imbalance and inflexibility. Choose well-designed, well-fitting athletic shoes, being particularly careful to have a flexible forefoot and a good heel lift with lots of cushioning. If your gait is abnormal, special orthotic devices in your shoes may help further.

Calf Cramps

For reasons that are not entirely clear, the calf muscles are particularly prone to cramps. Cramps are very brief muscle contractions, but because they are such strong spasms, they are extremely painful and will often stop you in your tracks. Calf cramps are caused by the same factors that can cause cramps in any muscle: overuse, fatigue, dehydration, cold temperatures, and lack of proper warm-up and flexibility.

When you get a cramp you should stop playing and gently stretch out the tight muscle until the pain is relieved. If available, ice will help. Then, gently resume play; if the cramps recur, however, you may have to call it a day.

As with other injuries, the best treatment is prevention. Stretching, warm-up, and good hydration are the key elements. Calf cramps can also come on spontaneously at night, both in athletes and nonathletes. Nighttime cramps are very effectively prevented by a prescription medication called quinine — the same chemical that is in tonic water. We have had some success preventing muscles cramps during sports by administering quinine before play, so if all else fails ask your doctor about this.

The Achilles Tendon

The Achilles tendon is well named: Achilles was the great Greek warrior who was noted both for his strength and for the vulnerability of his heel. In fact, the Achilles tendon shares these attributes of strength and vulnerability.

The Achilles tendon is a strong, fibrous band that attaches your gastrocs, or calf muscles, to your calcaneous, or heel, bone. Every time your calf muscles contract to raise your body up on your toes, your Achilles is subject to tremendous force. Even though the Achilles is one of the largest and strongest tendons in the body, it is still vulnerable to injury. For one thing, it is unique among tendons in that it lacks a protective sheath. In addition, if your calf muscles become overly strong or tight, the stress on your Achilles will increase, and since your Achilles is put to work every time you run or even walk upstairs, overuse can lead to problems.

The most common Achilles problem is tendinitis. Achilles tendinitis will produce pain and stiffness at the back of your heel (Figure 12–17). As with other forms of tendinitis, your symptoms may actually ease up after you warm up and begin exercise — only to return worse than ever when your game is over. In chronic tendinitis, you may even feel or hear a grating sensation when the tendon moves, because calcium can be deposited near its surface.

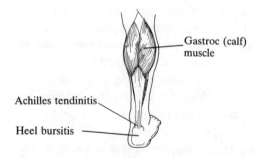

FIGURE 12–17: *Ankle and Heel Problems*

To treat Achilles tendinitis, use the PRICE program (see pages 251–252). In mild cases, you can get by with aspirin and warm-ups before you play, and ice massage afterward. But in more serious or chronic cases, you may have to avoid strenuous activity for a period of time; in severe cases, you may even have to stay away from stairs. A heel lift in your athletic shoes and also your street shoes can also be very helpful by taking some of the stress off your Achilles. Above all, to prevent recurrences be sure that you warm up and stretch your Achilles appropriately (see Chapter 6).

A more severe Achilles problem is partial or complete rupture of the tendon. Mild tearing of the fibers is nothing more than a first-degree strain, but when many fibers are torn you'll develop sharp, severe pain and you'll be unable to support yourself on your toes. If this happens, get medical attention at once. For partial tears, your doctor may choose conservative treatment with a cast, but in complete ruptures early surgery will probably be necessary.

THE ANKLE

Ankle problems are among the most common athletic injuries, but they are often misunderstood and hence mistreated. Since virtually all of us have turned an ankle at one time or another, we are likely to dismiss ankle pain as "just a sprain," thus omitting appropriate treatment. At the other extreme, we may erroneously accept the aphorism "Once sprained, always sprained," thereby tolerating chronic pain or weakness that could be corrected with proper therapy.

The ankle is a hinged joint that allows forward and backward motion every time you walk or run. The ligaments at the front and back of the ankle are relatively thin, but the ligaments on the outside and inside of the ankle are strong and thick to provide support. The ligaments on the inside of the ankle extend downward to the sole of your foot, where they provide support for the arch.

Although any of these ligaments can be sprained, either singly or in combination, the most common ankle injury is a sprain of the ligaments at the outside of your ankle. Mild or first-degree sprains will cause pain and slight swelling without loss of strength or mobility. More serious or second-degree sprains will produce more swelling, often with purplish discoloration caused by bleeding into the tissues. In addition, a second-degree sprain will involve some actual weakness of the ankle joint.

Most serious of all are third-degree sprains, which involve tearing of the ligament, either partially or completely. You should suspect a third-degree sprain if the injury causes you to fall or if it is accompanied by very severe pain, immediate swelling, or a popping sensation. If you suspect a third-degree ankle sprain, you should put on ice and a compression bandage and head for the emergency ward; you will require at least a cast and perhaps even surgery. If you neglect proper treatment, you may be left with chronic instability of your ankle, which will necessitate more extensive reconstructive surgery in the future.

Fortunately, most ankle sprains are mild enough so that you can treat them yourself. Here again the PRICE program (see pages 251–252) is the key. Later, rehabilitation is crucial to rebuilding strength so that chronic or recurrent ankle problems can be avoided. The first phase of rehabilitation is to restore flexibility and motion. At first, perform range-of-motion exercises in a basin of warm water; later, when your stiffness is diminished, you can move your ankle through its entire range without soaking it in water. Next, begin restoring strength. First you should do isometric exercises simply by pushing your foot from side to side against a chair leg or wall while you are seated comfortably. Then you can combine motion with exercises for strength by doing weight work. You can do this simply by filling a sock with sand so that it weighs one to three pounds. Drape the sock over your foot, and move your ankle in all directions. Increase the number of daily repetitions as you get stronger.

If your ankle sprain was severe, you will have started out on crutches, but by the time you are working with weights, you can resume walking. If your ankle is still tender, it's a good idea to start swimming or walking and running in water, because the buoyancy of water will support 90 percent of your body weight, leaving your ankle with only 10 percent of the load. You can then progress to normal walking and then to hopping exercises, first landing on both feet and later on the injured foot alone. Another good exercise is heel raising. Finally, you can start jogging, first in a straight line and then in large circles. Even when your ankle is normal, running can help it increase its strength further. If you run in circles or in a figure-eight pattern, you will increase the strength of all the ligaments of both ankles.

Thus far, we have said nothing about the most common treatment used for ankle sprains: tape or elastic bandages. Indeed, external support is very useful initially, because it permits earlier mobilization, and hence return to normal activities. But don't use tape or elastic bandages as a substitute for rehabilitation exercises. Instead, your goal should be to build up your ankle's own strength so that you can wean yourself from external support. Your ultimate goal should be to make your ankle stronger than ever.

The entire process of rehabilitation can take weeks or even months. Once you've gone through this painstaking procedure, you will undoubtedly want to continue exercising both ankles to maintain strength and flexibility, so that you will avoid recurrent problems. High-top basketball shoes, tape, or elastic bandages can also help prevent recurrences, but strong ligaments are your best defense. If you do twist your ankle again, be sure to treat it with proper respect; dismissing injury as "just a sprain" can lead to lots of pain.

THE FOOT

The athlete's foot is one of the most overstressed parts of the anatomy. Every time you run or jump, you land with a force many times greater than your body weight — and that force must ultimately be absorbed by your feet. In most cases, your foot will be equal to the task. The humble foot is really a very complex structure, composed of twenty-eight bones, which interface at many joints and are held together by numerous small ligaments. The arches of the midfoot and forefoot provide a springy, elastic structure to absorb shock. Even the sole of the foot is specially designed to absorb shock; the skin is quite thick and is bound tightly to an underlying fat pad, which provides additional cushioning.

Despite nature's marvelous engineering job, the foot is often injured in athletics. A brand-new discipline, sports podiatry, has made tremendous strides in correcting problems of the foot, and has also taught us that knee, hip, and even back pain can sometimes emanate from problems at ground level with the structure of the foot or with the biomechanics of the athlete's gait.

Whereas exercises can help with the Achilles and ankle, foot problems are rarely corrected by exercise alone. Instead, changes in equipment are almost always necessary to treat the injured foot. Sometimes a simple change in your shoe can correct foot injuries and, indeed, can prevent or treat problems elsewhere in your lower body. The shoe industry is certainly one of the most competitive and financially successful aspects of the exercise boom in America. But, in this case at least, the flashy designs and high-powered advertising do re-

flect a good product, since athletic shoes have improved enormously over the past fifteen years. Runners pound their feet the most and consequently suffer the most foot injuries. Happily, running shoes are the most advanced of all athletic footwear, but the principles of selecting shoes are basically the same for any sport (see page 190).

If shoe selection does not correct your foot problems, you may have to try a variety of felt pads, lifts, or moleskin protectors. We'll discuss some of these when we review common foot problems, but if you can't correct the problem yourself with these pads, your podiatrist may well prescribe an "orthotic" or foot support. The simplest and least-expensive orthotics are made of soft material such as felt. For even greater cushioning and shock absorbency, Sorbothane or Spenco can be used. Soft orthotics are generally best for temporary use, especially to provide cushioning and relief of pain. For long-term use, your podiatrist can make a cast of your foot, which is then used to custom-mold a semiflexible orthotic made of rubbery material. Semiflexible orthotics are ideal when you need good control of your foot motion to correct an abnormal gait. Rigid orthotics are also available, but these generally can't be worn during sports.

Although orthotics have been a great help to many athletes, they can also be oversold. Instead of investing in an expensive orthotic any time you have a twinge of pain anywhere from your waist down, you should always try to treat yourself first according to the PRICE regimen (see pages 251–252). But even if your problem persists, you should try an inexpensive, flexible orthotic before you invest as much as one hundred dollars in a permanent orthotic. As in most areas of sports medicine, you should be suspicious of exaggerated claims that costly orthotics will provide a "quick fix" for all injuries.

Heel Pain

Although the poet tells us that time heals all wounds, the athlete tells us that sports wounds all heels. There are many causes of heel pain. One common problem is bursitis — inflammation of the small fluid-filled bursal sac at the rear of the heel just below the Achilles tendon. Ice, protective padding, and sometimes anti-inflammatory medications should take care of this problem, but the best treatment of all involves a trip to the shoe store, stopping first at the garbage dump to get rid of the tight shoes that almost always cause the ailment. Padding and good shoes will also help prevent or correct heel bruises, which cause nagging pain with or without skin discoloration at the bottom of the heel.

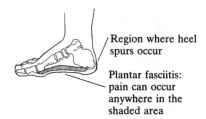

Region where heel spurs occur

Plantar fasciitis: pain can occur anywhere in the shaded area

FIGURE 12–18: *Foot Problems*

The bottom of the heel can also be the site of more severe and persistent pain. Sometimes X rays will show a bone spur, which is a bony outgrowth of the heel bone itself. But whether or not an actual spur is present, the basic problem here is plantar fasciitis, an inflammation of the thick fibrous tissues at the sole of the foot (see Figure 12–18). The key to treatment is a sponge rubber pad that raises the heel by one-quarter inch to provide cushioning and take some pressure off your heel by transferring your weight forward. If heel padding doesn't do the trick, it may be necessary to get a heel cup or to have your shoes modified by drilling a hole into the insole of the heel and then re-covering the hole with a foam pad. In more severe cases of plantar fasciitis, you'll need anti-inflammatory drugs, and you'll have to temporarily avoid any sport that involves running. And in uncommon cases, steroid injections or even surgery may be necessary. As usual, we would certainly advocate a long trial of conservative treatment before resorting to these more drastic remedies.

The Midfoot

Pain in the midfoot can be hard to diagnose because of the many small bones, ligaments, and nerves packed together in this region. The most common causes of pain in the midfoot are strains and sprains, which respond nicely to new shoes, arch supports, or orthotics. If the pain is severe, however, you may have a problem with one of your metatarsal bones. Each foot has five metatarsals, which are the long, slender bones extending from your heel forward to your toes. Running or even walking can lead to a "march fracture" or "stress fracture" of one of these bones. These are tiny hairline cracks, which can be so small that they may not show up on X rays, particularly early on. However, a special test called a bone scan can be used to detect early stress fractures. Because stress fractures never cause displacement of the bone, you will not need a cast to treat this sort of fracture. Instead, a few weeks of rest should do

the trick. You can even play sports on your "broken foot." Your body will tell you when it's safe to resume weight-bearing sports — when the pain is gone, you can return to your favorite sports, even if they involve running. But remember to wear good shoes and to run on the softest possible surface to avoid recurrent stress fractures.

You don't have to have a fracture to have pain in the metatarsal region. Excessive pounding can cause inflammation of one or more of the many tendons or bursal sacs in the midfoot. Even the nerves themselves can become injured because of excessive pressure. The most common example is the so-called Morton's neuralgia, or plantar neuroma. This typically occurs between the third and fourth metatarsals, producing pain that radiates backward toward the heel. Bursitis and tendinitis in the midfoot are generally aggravated by walking and running, but weight-bearing doesn't seem to increase the pain from a plantar neuroma; instead, lateral pressure duplicates the symptoms, so that athletes with this problem often find themselves leaving their shoes unlaced or even trying to exercise barefoot. Most of these problems will respond nicely to well-fitted shoes, arch supports, and felt metatarsal pads. Metatarsal bars can also be useful, but will probably be easier to wear in street shoes than in athletic shoes. In fact, if you have any sort of foot problem, it's important to wear excellent street shoes as well as athletic shoes. It hardly makes sense to spend a lot of time and money choosing fine athletic shoes, only to perpetuate your injury with a pair of worn or ill-fitting street shoes.

Toe Injuries

Toe injuries are so common that most sports claim them for themselves; nomenclature notwithstanding, "runner's toe," "tennis toe," and "basketball toe" are exactly the same injury. Any sport that involves running, particularly if there are abrupt starts and stops, can put excessive pressure on the toe. The result is bleeding under the nail, which produces pain and a bluish discoloration. Your doctor can provide immediate relief for this problem by boring a small hole through the toenail to drain out the blood and relieve the pressure. With a little practice you can even learn to do this yourself with a heated paper clip or small-gauge hypodermic needle. Sometimes the nail itself will fall off, but a new nail will grow in its place. The best treatment is, of course, prevention: choose a shoe with a large toe box so that you can avoid the "athlete's toe blues."

Ingrown toenails can affect athletes and nonathletes

alike. If you keep your nails well trimmed, you'll never have this problem; be sure to cut your toenails straight across instead of rounding out the side margins. If you develop inflammation and pain, you should treat yourself with warm soaks three or four times a day. Redness, swelling, and fever should prompt a trip to your doctor, who will probably prescribe antibiotics. Sometimes minor surgery on the toenail is even required.

Fractured or sprained toes cause pain and swelling following a stub-type injury. You won't need a cast for a broken toe, but you will need to limit weight-bearing sharply until the pain and swelling go down. It can be very helpful to tape the injured toe to its healthy neighbor for additional support.

Skin Problems

Many athletes develop problems with the skin of their feet. The two most common varieties are the infamous fungal infection called athlete's foot, and blisters (see pages 271–273). Corns and calluses can develop on your feet, usually in areas of excess pressure over bony prominences. Well-fitted shoes are the solution to this problem; small pads are also helpful to eliminate pressure and irritation. But if you have large calluses, you should see a podiatrist, who will carefully shave them down or use salicylic acid plasters as well as appropriate moleskin or felt pads.

We've ended this book of fitness with a litany of exercise-and sports-related injuries and illnesses. The last word about exercise, however, is not illness but *health*. With appropriate conditioning, proper progression, commonsense precautions, and, if needed, medical supervision, you can exercise vigorously without developing these problems. And regular exercise will be your key to fitness. Along with sound nutrition and stress control, exercise will help you attain and maintain total fitness. A long lifetime of health and fun will reward your efforts.

Appendix: Sources of Additional Information

AEROBICS AND CARDIOPULMONARY FITNESS

Cooper, Kenneth H. *The Aerobics Way*. New York: M. Evans and Co., 1977.

FLEXIBILITY AND STRETCHING

Anderson, Bob. *Stretching*. Palmer Lake, CO: Stretching Inc., 1985.

Hittleman, R. C. *Introduction to Yoga*. New York: Bantam, 1969.

STRENGTH

Sprague, Ken. *The Gold's Gym Book of Strength Training*. Los Angeles: Tarcher, 1979.

Todd, Jan and Terry. *Lift Your Way to Youthful Fitness*. Boston: Little, Brown, 1985.

For a directory of Nautilus Centers: Nautilus Sports Medical Industries, 305 East Ohio Ave., Lake Helen, FL 32744

For a guide of health clubs you can use when you travel: Travel Fit, 9089 Shell Rd., Cincinnati, OH 45236

PSYCHOLOGICAL FITNESS

Benson, Herbert. *The Relaxation Response*. New York: William Morrow and Co., 1975.

NUTRITION

Brody, Jane. *Jane Brody's Good Food Book*. New York: Norton, 1985.

———. *Jane Brody's Nutrition Book*, New York: Norton, 1981.

Krause, Barbara. *Calories and Carbohydrates*. 6th ed. New York: Signet Books, 1985.

Many useful booklets are available from the U.S. government. Write to Consumer Information Center, Box 100, Pueblo, CO 81022.

GENERAL HEALTH

The Harvard Medical School Health Letter (a monthly publication available from 79 Garden St., Cambridge, MA 02138).

WALKING AND RUNNING

The Athletics Congress, 200 South Capital Ave., Indianapolis, IN 46225

U.S. Orienteering Federation, P.O. Box 1039, Baldwin, MO 63110

Road Runners Club of America, 8111 Edgehill Dr., Huntsville, AL 35802

ROWING AND CANOEING

U.S. Rowing Association, 4 Boathouse Row, Philadelphia, PA 19130

American Canoe Association, P.O. Box 248, Lorton, VA 22079

SWIMMING

Councilman, James. *Competitive Swimming Manual for Coaches and Swimmers*. Bloomington, IN: Counsilman Co., 1977.

U.S. Swimming, 1750 E. Boulder St., Colorado Springs, CO 80909

U.S. Masters Swimming, Box 5039, Sun City, FL 33570

National Masters Swimming Program of the YMCA, 1765 Wallace St., York, PA 17402

BICYCLING

Bicycling magazine, Rodale Press, 33 E. Minor St., Emmaus, PA 18049

U.S. Cycling Federation, 1750 E. Boulder St., Colorado Springs, CO 80909

League of American Wheelmen, P.O. Box 988, Baltimore, MD 21203

International Bicycle Touring Society, 2115 Paseo Dorado, La Jolla, CA 92037

TENNIS

Levisohn, S.R., and Simon, H.B. *Tennis Medic*. St. Louis: C.V. Mosby, 1984.

U.S. Tennis Association, 729 Alexander Rd., Princeton, NJ 08540

Super Seniors Tennis, Box 5165, Charlottesville, VA 22905

SKIING

Woodward, Robert. *The Cross-Country Ski Technique*. Champaign, IL: Leisure Press, 1983.

U.S. Ski Association, Box 727, Brattleboro, VT 05301

SKATING

Petkevich, John M. *The Skater's Handbook*. New York: Scribner's, 1984.

BASKETBALL

Dunn, William H. *Strength Training and Conditioning for Basketball*. Chicago: Contemporary Books, 1984.

GENERAL

Amateur Athletic Union of the U.S., 3400 W. 86th St., Indianapolis, IN 46268

Woman's Sports Foundation, 195 Moulton St., San Francisco, CA 94123

YMCA of the U.S.A., 101 N. Wacker Dr., Chicago, IL 60606

About the Authors

Harvey B. Simon and Steven R. Levisohn are both graduates of Harvard Medical School. After postgraduate training, they joined the faculty of their alma mater, where Dr. Simon is Assistant Professor of Medicine and Dr. Levisohn is Instructor in Medicine. They both practice and teach medicine at Massachusetts General Hospital in Boston. Dr. Simon is a member of Harvard's Cardiovascular Health Center, which uses exercise, nutrition, and stress reduction to treat and prevent cardiovascular disease, and of the Massachusetts Governor's Committee on Physical Fitness and Sports. Dr. Levisohn is chairman and founder of Health Development Corporation, which designs fitness programs for industry. They are both members of the American College of Sports Medicine.

In addition to textbook chapters, articles, and lectures for medical audiences, Drs. Simon and Levisohn have written extensively on exercise and health for the public. They have addressed tennis players in their first book, *Tennis Medic,* and as Contributing Editors of *Tennis* magazine. Their articles have appeared also in many other national periodicals and newspapers.

Both authors practice what they preach. Dr. Simon is a dedicated swimmer and long-distance runner who has completed more than fifty marathons and ultra-marathons; he won the 1981 New England Athletic Congress Silver 50-mile Championship. Dr. Levisohn is also a veteran of many marathons and is an avid downhill and cross-country skier who plays tennis and cycles as well.

Index

Page numbers in italics indicate instructions for specific exercises